EAT THIS NOT THAT!

SUPERMARKET SURVIVAL GUIDE

Completely Updated and Expanded

BY DAVID ZINCZENKO
WITH MATT GOULDING

RODALE.

Portions of this book have previously appeared in *Men's Health.*

Rodale books may be purchased for business or promotional use or for special sales. For information,
please write to: Special Markets Department, Rodale Inc., 733 Third Avenue, New York, NY 10017

Printed in the United States of America

Rodale Inc. makes every effort to use acid-free ∞, recycled paper ♻

Book design by George Karabotsos

Cover photos by Jeff Harris / Cover prop styling by Richie Owings for Halley Resources

Photo direction by Tara Long

All interior photos by Mitch Mandel and Thomas MacDonald/Rodale Images

with the exception of page 104: © Christina Peters/StockFood (broccolini), Steven Mark Needham/FoodPix/Jupiter Images (corn),
© iStockphoto (carrots, pluot, and tomato), © Lew Robertson/StockFood (cauliflower), pages 122–123: © iStockphoto

Food styling on pages 59–77 by Diane Vezza

Illustrations on pages 10–11 by L-Dopa and pages 318–327 by mckibillo

Library of Congress Cataloging-in-Publication Data is on file with the publisher.
ISBN-13: 978–1–60961–241–2 paperback

Trade paperback and exclusive direct mail edition published simultaneously in November 2011.

Distributed to the trade by Macmillan

2   4   6   8   10   9   7   5   3   1   paperback

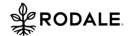

We inspire and enable people to improve their lives and the world around them.

www.rodalebooks.com

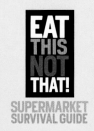

EAT
THIS
NOT
THAT!
SUPERMARKET
SURVIVAL GUIDE

Dedication

For the men and women
working in America's fields,
farms, and supermarkets.
Because of your hard work, we
have the choices that can keep
us lean, healthy, and happy.

ACKNOWLEDGMENTS

This book is the product of thousands of hours spent in the supermarket aisles, hundreds of conversations with nutritionists and industry experts, and the collective smarts, dedication, and raw talent of dozens of individuals. Our undying thanks to all of you who have inspired this project in any way. In particular:

To Maria Rodale and the Rodale family, whose dedication to improving the lives of their readers is apparent in every book and magazine they put their name on.

To George Karabotsos and his crew of immensely talented designers, including Courtney Eltringham, Mark Michaelson, Elizabeth Neal, and Laura White. You're the reason why each book looks better than the last.

To Clint Carter, the Rainman of the nutritional world. And to James Carlson and Hannah McWilliams. Your contributions are more valuable than you know.

To Tara Long, who knows how to bring even the most far-fetched ideas to life and shape them into something memorable. You're our ace in the hole.

To Debbie McHugh. It's impossible to believe we ever did these books without you.

To the Rodale book team: Steve Perrine, Chris Krogermeier, Erin Williams, Sara Cox, Mitch Mandel, Tom MacDonald, Troy Schnyder, Melissa Reiss, Nikki Weber, Jennifer Giandomenico, Wendy Gable, Keith Biery, Liz Krenos, Brooke Myers, Nancy Elgin, Sonya Maynard, and Sean Sabo. You continue to do whatever it takes to get these books done. As always, we appreciate your heroic efforts.

—Dave and Matt

Check out the other bestselling books in the *EAT THIS, NOT THAT!* and *COOK THIS, NOT THAT!* series:

Eat This, Not That!
for Kids!
(2008)

Eat This, Not That!
Restaurant
Survival Guide
(2009)

Cook This, Not That!
350-Calorie Meals
(2010)

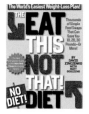

Eat This, Not That!
No-Diet Diet
(2011)

Eat This, Not That!
(2011)

CONTENTS

The American super is a wonder

There's a wonderful world where all you desire
And everything you've longed for is at your fingertips...

—BRUCE SPRINGSTEEN
"Queen of the Supermarket"

market

NO WONDER BRUCE SPRINGSTEEN SANG of "aisles and aisles of dreams" in his ode to checkout girls. In an interview with Britain's *The Observer Music Monthly*, he even declared, "They opened up this big, beautiful supermarket near where we lived....[A]nd I thought, this place is spectacular. This place is... it's fantasy land!"

But we can be as appreciative of its bounty as The Boss, and still be wary of the supermarket's dangers. As with every other sensory-rattling funhouse, in the grocery store, nothing is as it first appears. Friendly characters entertain our children while peddling junk that will blow up their waistlines and make them susceptible to diabetes. Words like "healthy" and "lite" are often meaningless phrases coated with fat and sugar.

Even the lowest-priced supermarket in your neighborhood is brimming with complete rip-offs—"health" foods that aren't healthy, "gourmet" foods that aren't gourmet, specialty items that just aren't that special. Yet the supermarket is a fact of everyone's life. The average American makes about 1.7 trips a week, and each one of those trips is a chance to gain weight, or to lose it. To save money, or to waste it. To set yourself and your family up for a lifetime of better health, or to deprive you all of the vital nutrients your bodies need to stay strong.

You make hundreds of health and financial decisions with each trip, yet there's not a lot of help to be found: The people stacking the boxes know where everything belongs, but they don't know what's actually in anything. Managers are seldom trained to do much more than settle coupon disputes, and at the checkout, you have the choice of a robot telling you to place items in bag, or a robotlike teenager swiping your family's food along a grimy scanner. Once you enter a supermarket, you're on your own.

And we're victims of that lack of helpful information: Only 27 percent of shoppers can correctly identify monounsaturated fat as a healthy fat, and nearly one in five people don't know whether trans fats are good or bad. (They're worse than bad. They're ugly.) No wonder two-thirds of the American population is overweight or obese. No one is telling us the truth about what's in the foods we're eating!

Well, that stops now. The *Eat This, Not That! Supermarket Survival Guide* is designed to make shopping faster, easier, cheaper, and, most important of all, healthier. And along the way, it's going to show you how to start losing weight fast— without dieting, without exercise. These pages are packed with thousands of simple grocery-store swaps that can save you 10, 20, 30 pounds or more—this year alone! Now, I know what you're thinking: Eating healthy is expensive. It doesn't have to be. You don't have to buy costly "health food" to get the weight-loss benefits of the *Eat This, Not That! Supermarket Survival Guide*. The simple swaps you'll find in this book will show you how choosing between two seemingly identical—and identically priced—products can save you hundreds of calories, and dozens of pounds, without impacting your wallet—or your taste buds.

Lose a pound every 9 days with swaps like this!

Consider this:

→ Who doesn't love Häagen-Dazs? But here's a secret: Not every pint of Häagen-Dazs loves you back.
Its Chocolate Peanut Butter ice cream weighs in at 360 calories per half cup. But just switch to the company's Dark Chocolate and save 200 calories with every 1-cup serving. Do that every night and you'll drop a pound every 18 days, and cut out one-third of your sugar intake at dessert!

→ Remember when I warned you about "health" foods that aren't?
You'd think Healthy Choice Complete Meal Sweet & Sour Chicken would be, you know, healthy. In fact, it's got more sugar than a Reese's-flavor Klondike bar. Opt for the Oven Roasted Chicken, however, and you'll save 150 calories per serving, and 10 grams of sugar.

→ How about a small frozen pizza? DiGiorno makes a Traditional Crust Supreme Pizza and a Flatbread Melts Chicken Parmesan. But the only "traditional" thing about the first item and its whopping 790 calories is the middle-aged spread you'll get—long before middle age. (You'll save 410 calories by picking the Parmesan—that kind of swap can save you a pound every 9 days!)

Drop 20 pounds in 1 year with this simple swap!

Now, a lot of us equate eating healthy with spending hours poring over nutrition labels. And most of us have neither the time nor the patience for that: According to "Shopping for Health," a Food Marketing Institute study that was partially funded by Rodale, the proportion of shoppers who read nutrition labels as of 2010 was just 64 percent. (That number is down 7 percent from 2007. Busy, anyone?) And nutrition labels can be confusing: A 2008 USDA study found that only 49 percent of people actually changed their buying decision based on what they saw on a nutrition facts label.

Well, that's where the *Eat This, Not That! Supermarket Survival Guide* comes in. Now, I still want you to read nutrition labels when you can, because the more you educate yourself, the greater your ability to protect yourself and your family. But even if you don't, you'll still be able to make smart swaps and save pounds on almost every purchase. (And if you don't have your copy of the *Eat This, Not That! Supermarket Survival Guide* with you, make sure you download the *Eat This, Not That!* app for your phone!)

Ready to start changing your life?

Why Your Weight Is Not Your Fault

Ever go to a parent-teacher night at an elementary school and try to squeeze into your fourth-grader's desk chair? Embarrassing, right? Our adult bodies are simply wider, heavier, and differently proportioned than our children's are.

Well, if we could build a time machine and travel back—not to Cro-magnon days, but to our grandparents' day—we'd find much the same thing. The chairs would be smaller. So would the clothing. And guess what else would be smaller?

The meals and snacks.

Consider, for example, the humble bag of potato chips, washed down with a soda. Since the days when Fonzie was ruling the drive-ins and diners of America, the average salty-snack portion has increased by 93 calories, and soft-drink portions have increased by 49 calories, according to an analysis of combined data from the Nationwide Food Consumption Survey 1977 and the Continuing Survey of Food Intakes by Individuals 1989 and 1996, which created a sample of more than 63,000 people. So if you were to indulge in a bag of chips and a soda once a day, you'd be eating 142 more calories every day than Fonzie would have. And that's just in one snack! (No wonder it was so easy for the Fonz to be cool.) It takes 3,500 calories to create a pound of fat on your body. By eating the same snack every day that people from our grandparents' era (with its much lower rates of obesity) did, we automatically ingest enough calories to add a pound of flab to our frames every 25 days—that's 14 pounds of fat a year!

But it's not just our snack foods that are loaded with more calories. The supersizing

"There were days I'd go to bed looking one way, and I'd wake up thinner."

BEFORE:
245
pounds

"In the South, we tend to avoid talking about obesity or weight loss—it's kind of a sore subject," says **Tim Wadsworth**, a youth pastor in South Carolina. He weighed 180 pounds when he entered college in 2005, but every year at school added 10 to 15 pounds to his frame. The weight only got worse after marrying his high school sweetheart. "I looked in the mirror one day and said, 'What have I done to myself? I need to clean this up.'"

SMALL STEPS TO SMALLER PANTS

Tim's journey started with a pedometer. He clipped it on his pants and forced himself to walk 12,000 steps a day. If he fell short, he'd make an extra effort to get out and jog. After a month he was feeling better, but he was still overweight. That's when he decided to change his diet. First he cut sugars and refined grains, and then, to help with restaurant and supermarket decisions, he picked up the *Eat This, Not That!* book that he'd purchased for his wife a year prior. "I said, 'If I'm going to do this, I'm going to really step my game up,'" he says. Shortly after, the pounds started falling off. "There were days when I would go to bed looking one way, and I'd wake up thinner," he says. "I would look in the mirror and go, 'Oh wow!'" Suddenly his clothes were too big, and his friends started ribbing him that he needed to eat more cheeseburgers. His waist shrank from a 44 to a 32, but more importantly, Tim says he took getting fit as a personal calling from God, allowing him to become the healthy role model he wanted to be for the kids in his youth group.

THE SKINNY MINISTER

Dropping nearly 100 pounds helped Tim feel more confident when speaking in front of students, but what he found most surprising was the newfound boost of energy. While he used to need 8 or 9 hours of sleep a night, he now needs only 6, and although he used to feel tired and lethargic after a day of preaching ("We called it a holy hangover," he jokes), he now bounces back quickly. Recently Tim began working at a new church, and to the members there, he's always been skinny Tim. "Then I show them pictures of me from a year ago," he says. "They literally can't believe it."

VITALS:
Tim Wadsworth, 26
Greenville, SC

HEIGHT: 5'11"

TOTAL WEIGHT LOST: 92 lbs

TIME IT TOOK TO LOSE THE WEIGHT: 1 year

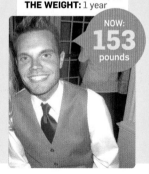

NOW:
153
pounds

of the American diet has infused all of our foods, and nowhere is that more apparent than at the supermarket. For example, in 1971, the average American male consumed 2,450 calories a day; the average woman, 1,542. But by the year 2008, American men were averaging about 2,504 daily calories (up 2 percent), while women were eating 1,771 calories (a whopping 15 percent increase, or 229 more calories every day!).

As a result, since the 1970s, the obesity rate in this country has more than doubled, with two-thirds of our population now overweight or obese. The health condition most directly tied to obesity—diabetes—now eats up one in every five dollars Americans spend on health care, and a recent study at Harvard found that obesity has become similar in magnitude to tobacco as the number one avoidable cause of cancer deaths. And the future looks even bleaker for our children: No matter what your weight may have been growing up, because of the way we're packaging and selling foods at restaurants and supermarkets, your child faces three times the risk of obesity that you did.

WHO BLEW UP THE FOOD?

A lot of people want to blame the obesity epidemic on too much TV, too little exercise, and too much gluttony. But that's blaming the victim, in my opinion. Why should the men and women of America have to give up a pizza and a pint of ice cream while arguing over *Monday Night Football* versus *Dancing With the Stars?* Indulgences like that make life worth living. And really—did they not have cheeseburgers and fries (and television) back in the 1970s?

Indeed, I'd argue that Americans are working harder than ever to keep themselves in shape. Every year, we spend an estimated $42 billion on diet books, $20.3 billion on health club memberships, and $5.2 billion on diet foods and weight-loss programs.

But unless you understand how food marketers have altered the reality of our weekly trips to the supermarket, it's impossible to truly see where the battle lines fall in the fight against fat. See, the food industry spends $30 billion a year on advertising—70 percent of it pitching convenience foods, candy, sodas, and desserts. And while they're busy using dancing leprechauns and talking teddy bears to sell you on how the new shrink-wrapped food of the month is going to make you the most popular mom or dad on the block, they're obscuring the real story. And the real story is this: The food we consume today is different from the food that Americans ate 30 years ago. And the reasons for that are as simple as they are sneaky.

We've added extra calories to traditional foods.

In the early 1970s, food manufacturers, looking for a cheaper ingredient to replace sugar, came up with a substance called high-fructose corn syrup. Today, HFCS is in an unbelievable array of foods—everything from breakfast cereals to bread, from ketchup to pasta sauce, from juice boxes to iced teas. So Grandma's pasta sauce now comes in a jar, and it's loaded with stuff just perfect for adding meat to your bones—and flab to your belly.

We've been trained to supersize it. It seems like Economics 101:

If you can get a lot more food for just a few cents more, then it makes all the sense in the world to upgrade to the "value meal." And since this trick has worked so well for fast-food marketers, your average product in the supermarket has become Hulkified as well. The problem is the way we look at food—we should be looking at cutting down on our calories, not adding to them.

We've laced our food with time bombs.

A generation ago it was hard for food manufacturers to create baked goods that would last on store shelves. Most baked goods require oils, and oil leaks at room temperature. But since the 1960s, manufacturers have been baking with—and restaurateurs have been frying with—something called trans fats. Trans fats are cheap and effective: They make potato chips crispier and cookies tastier, and they let fry cooks make pound after pound of fries without smoking up their kitchens. The downside: Trans fats increase your bad cholesterol, lower your good cholesterol, and greatly increase your risk of heart disease.

Our fruits and vegetables aren't as healthy as they once were.

Researchers doing a study that was published in the *Journal of the American College of Nutrition* tested 43 different garden crops for nutritional content and discovered that 6 out of 13 nutrients showed major declines between 1950 and 1999: protein, calcium, phosphorus, iron, riboflavin, and ascorbic acid. Researchers say it's probably due to farmers' efforts to achieve higher yields because plants that grow faster can be picked earlier. As a result, the plants aren't able to make or take in nutrients at the same rate.

We're drinking more calories than ever.

A study from the University of North Carolina found that, in 2002, we consumed 464 calories a day from beverages, nearly twice as many as in 1965. This increase amounts to an extra 23 pounds a year that we're forced to work off—or carry around with us. Many of the calories come from the HFCS in our drinks—especially, when it comes to kids, in "fruit" drinks that are often nothing more than water, food coloring, and sweetener. In fact, anything you have for your kids to drink in your fridge right now—unless it's water, milk, or a diet soda—probably has HFCS in it. Go ahead—read the labels.

We don't even know what's in our food.
More and more, marketers are adding new types of preservatives, fats, sugars, and other "new" food substances to our daily meals. Indeed, there are now more than 4,000 ingredients on the FDA's list of allowable food additives, and any one of them could end up on your plate. (And here's a terrifying fact: Only 373 of those 4,000 additives is "generally recognized as safe" by the FDA.) But often, they go unexplained (what is xanthan gum anyway?) or, in the case of restaurant food, unmentioned. Unless we're eating it right off the tree, it's hard to know what, exactly, is in that fruity dish.

All of these disturbing trends in our food supply are a lot to chew on—but chew on them we do, often because we feel we have no choice. Yet I believe there is a better way. I believe we can enjoy all the bounty of the supermarket—and heck, some pretty good TV shows, too—and not gain weight or lose control of our bodies and our health. I believe that taking control of our food, our weight, and our lives doesn't have to be difficult. I believe that if we have the knowledge and insight we need, we can and will make the right choices.

That's why I've written the *Eat This Not That! Supermarket Survival Guide.*

GNARLY FACT OF LIFE
A recent study from the University of Arizona claims that grocery-cart handles are dirtier than supermarket bathrooms, and half of them carry the *Escherichia coli* bacterium. Prepare ye Wet Wipes, germaphobes!

What You Can Gain from This Guide

If the information above is troubling—if it makes you concerned, even angry, about the ways foods are grown, packaged, and sold to you and your family—then let me be clear: The supermarket is filled—filled!—with great-tasting, healthy, satisfying options.

Finding them, and understanding what makes one food healthier and better for your waistline than the product sitting right next to it on the shelf, takes a lot of thought and research. Fortunately, we've done all the homework for you. All you need to do is reap the rewards. Here are just some of the ways this guide will make your life better.

YOU'LL SAVE TIME AND STRESS.

Deciding who should get your vote for president used to be a hard decision. Nowadays, it feels easy—choice A, or choice B? Compare that to the decision we make every time we sit down to watch TV—channel 1, or 2, or 10...or 134...or 705? Or the complex decision you have to make every time you try to decide on a new cell phone plan, or a book to read, or a brand of toothpaste to buy. But that's nothing compared to the challenge we all face every time we step into the supermarket: There are somewhere between 30,000 and 45,000 different food and beverage products on sale at your local grocery store. It's no wonder shopping trips seem to take forever! With the *Eat This, Not That! Supermarket Survival Guide,* you'll have the answers to complicated nutritional questions at your fingertips, so shopping becomes a snap!

YOU'LL LOSE WEIGHT AND LOOK BETTER.

The shopping advice in the *Eat This, Not That! Supermarket Survival Guide* is designed to specifically target belly fat—by filling you up with smart, healthy choices that rev up your resting metabolism and help keep you burning fat all day, every day—even while you sleep!

YOU'LL RESHAPE YOUR BODY.

Most "diet" plans force you to cut, cut, cut calories, until you're practically starving. And what do you get? Sure, you lose fat, but you lose muscle as well. And muscle is crucial to keeping your metabolism revving and giving you the lean, firm shape you crave. That's why I'm proud to say that the *Eat This, Not That! Supermarket Survival Guide* is not a diet book. It's not going to teach you to eat less, or to starve yourself, or to deny your cravings. Instead, it's going to teach you to feed your cravings with smart food choices that also will improve your body shape at the same time!

YOU'LL SAVE MONEY.

Each week, the average grocery shopper in the United States makes two separate trips to the supermarket and spends an average of $114.40 per trip (for families with children). At just under $230 a week for groceries, its no wonder we're all feeling financially pinched. But one of the advantages of the *Eat This, Not That! Supermarket Survival Guide* is that you'll learn how to get as much nutrition as possible in the foods you buy. As a result, you'll be wasting fewer dollars on empty calories, and instead be bringing home foods that keep your family fuller longer.

YOU'LL EARN MORE MONEY.

There's an old saying: Look the part, and you'll get the part. Well, more and more research is showing that people who are leaner and fitter are viewed as being more competent and successful than those who are overweight. And when people view you as competent, they are more likely to pay you what you deserve. Don't believe me? Consider this: A New York University study found that people packing an extra 40 pounds make 20 percent less than their slimmer colleagues.

YOU'LL GAIN GREATER HEALTH.

As I said above, the number one goal of this book is to cut out empty calories and add in nutrition—bringing you more nutritional bang for your buck with every bite. And by carving away belly flab, you'll cut your risk of heart disease, type 2 diabetes, stroke, and even cancer.

"A lot of diets say, 'You can't have this,' but nobody says, 'But you can have this instead.'"

BEFORE:
335 pounds

Katie Roemele grew up an hour outside of Pittsburgh, and her mom worked long hours in the city. That forced the Roemele family to eat late; Katie's biggest meal was typically just before bed. It was a routine with repercussions. By the time she reached third grade, she was overweight. "I never really identified myself by my weight or my size," says Katie. Not until early in 2011 anyway. Katie was singing with her chorus group when a cameraman snapped a photo. Looking at herself among the other girls, she was struck by her own size. "I don't see me in that picture at all," she says. "I don't see my personality. I'm the youngest person on that chorus by a good number of years, and I was one of the most unattractive." She vowed to find a solution.

VITALS:
Katie Roemele, 29
Pittsburgh, PA

HEIGHT: 5'8"

TOTAL WEIGHT LOST:
50 lbs (and counting!)

TIME IT TOOK TO LOSE THE WEIGHT: 4 months

NOW:
285 pounds

A FRESH TUNE

Katie found *Eat This, Not That!* through Twitter, and one of the first tweets she noticed inspired her to keep a food journal. "I don't even think I was consciously aware of the grazing I was doing," she says. She was shocked to discover that some of the foods she thought were healthy were, in fact, loaded with calories. She discovered that her favorite salad at Applebee's had 1,800 calories, so she began planning meals ahead of time. She also switched to smaller dinner plates and started eating breakfast every day. The changes are working. Within a couple of weeks of discovering *Eat This, Not That!*, her pants started fitting more loosely, and the girls she sings with took notice. "They'd say, 'You look so skinny! How much have you lost now?'"

THE COMPETITIVE EDGE

Four months in and already down 50 pounds and three pants sizes, Katie has no intention of letting up. Her goal is to get down to 150 pounds; at the pace she's going now, she'll be there by summer 2012. Every Sunday morning she weighs herself and e-mails the outcome to one of her friends, who responds with a message of motivation. It's a little trick to remind herself to keep cutting calories. "A lot of the diets out there say, 'You can't have this,' but nobody says, 'But you can have this instead,'" she says.

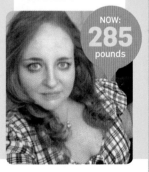

Fat's Dominos

OVERWEIGHT PEOPLE ARE:	50 percent more likely to develop heart disease (obese: up to 100 percent)	Up to 360 percent more likely to develop type 2 diabetes (obese: up to 1,020 percent)	16 percent more likely to die of a first heart attack (obese: 49 percent)
Roughly 50 percent more likely to have a total cholesterol level of more than 250 (obese: up to 122 percent)	14 percent less attractive to the opposite sex (obese: 43 percent)	Likely to spend 37 percent more a year at the pharmacy (obese: 105 percent)	Likely to stay 19 percent longer in the hospital (obese: 49 percent)
20 percent more likely to have asthma (obese: 50 percent)	Up to 31 percent more likely to die of any cause (obese: 62 percent)	19 percent more likely to die in a car crash (obese: 37 percent)	120 percent more likely to develop stomach cancer (obese: 330 percent)
Up to 90 percent more likely to develop gallstones (obese: up to 150 percent)	590 percent more likely to develop esophageal cancer (obese: 1,520 percent)	35 percent more likely to develop kidney cancer (obese: 70 percent)	14 percent more likely to have osteoarthritis (obese: 34 percent)

"*Eat This, Not That* reshaped my thought process about food completely."

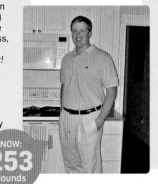

BEFORE:
323
pounds

David Coleman is a tall guy with a big frame. In high school he was an athlete, but even a daily training schedule didn't drop him below 250 pounds. When David left high school for college, he left athletics behind, and that's when he started gaining weight. "I was putting on pounds without even thinking about it," he says. In college he started lifting weights and eating more salads, but his body continued to grow. He was overweight and he knew it, but the gravity of the situation didn't hit him until he graduated.

A SIMPLE SOLUTION FOR A BIG PROBLEM

Shortly after that, David went to visit his parents, and he noticed a copy of *Eat This, Not That!* sitting on their bookshelf. As he flipped through the pages, his weight started to make sense. "I was shocked," he says. "The foods I thought were healthy were actually the worst foods for me." David decided to try some of the swaps in the book, and almost instantly he noticed that he was losing weight. "*Eat This, Not That!* makes those first swaps so simple," he says. He purchased the *Eat This, Not That! Supermarket Survival Guide* and *Cook This, Not That!*, and his weight continued to drop.

BACK IN THE GAME

Over the past year and a half, David has trimmed 8 inches off his waistline, and he now feels like a recharged man. So much so that he decided to put his body back to work—he ran his first 5-K in November. "At my highest weight, I couldn't run half a mile without stopping," he says. "Now I have a lot more energy."

And his high school buddies? They noticed too. "At my high school reunion, no one could believe that I was back to my high school weight," he says. David continues to make swaps from the *Eat This, Not That!* books, and he and his girlfriend prepare recipes from *Cook This, Not That!* (The Chicken Cordon Bleu is his favorite.) To repay his parents for the accidental gift of weight loss, he bought them their own copy of *Cook This, Not That!*

Ask David if losing weight has any drawbacks, and he can think of only one: constantly shopping for smaller clothes. "I've gone through way too many new wardrobes!"

VITALS:
David Coleman, 24
Richmond, VA
HEIGHT: 6'3"
TOTAL WEIGHT LOST: 70 lbs
TIME IT TOOK TO LOSE THE WEIGHT: 18 months

NOW:
253
pounds

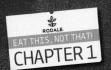

ANATOMY OF A SUPERMARKET

**EAT
THIS
NOT
THAT!**
SUPERMARKET
SURVIVAL GUIDE

Your supermarket shares much in common with your county fair

ANATOMY OF A SUPERMARKET

Roll your cart down the aisle and you'll be assaulted by bright lights, enticing smells, and row upon row of shameless hucksterism ("9 vitamins and minerals! Everyone's a winner!"). That's fine when the stakes are low, but going home with a 5-foot-tall Kung Fu Panda is far less important than going home with a trunk filled with food that will slim down that grizzly bear of a belly.

The truth is, the grocery store is your first stop in building a healthy lifestyle for you and your family. But it's also a business. Supermarkets are designed to make you spend as much money as possible, often on high-margin products loaded with cheap ingredients and non-nutritive calories. Major food conglomerates are far more concerned with their bottom lines than your waistline, and as a result, their foods are filled out with cheap, nutritionally sparse ingredients like refined white flour, hydrogenated oils, and hundreds of additives, preservatives, and sweeteners derived from staple crops like corn and soy.

The key to any good offense is a solid defense. You may be a well-meaning shopper, but without a thoroughly planned attack, an innocent weekly grocery run can turn into an all-out assault on your health and your finances. Thankfully, mastering the supermarket is far easier than outsmarting a carny. Smart shoppers share a set of characteristics, and by pawing through the research and spending countless hours in supermarkets, we've finally managed to crack the code. Adopt these 7 Habits of Highly Effective Shoppers and you'll be well on your way to being a master of the modern-day market.

3

1 Make Cash King

A 2010 study published in the *Journal of Consumer Research* tracked the grocery-shopping habits of 1,000 households over 6 months and found that shoppers who paid with cash bought fewer processed foods and more nutritious items than those who opted to use credit. The credit users not only bought more junk, they also spent an average of 59 to 78 percent more on their grocery bills. The explanation:

Credit and debit cards are more abstract forms of payment, so you don't use them as carefully as you do cash. The $4 price tag on a box of cheese crackers doesn't mean much when you don't have to think about the money that's about to leave your wallet, and as such, credit-card users are far more likely to make impulsive decisions in the aisles. Plan to drop by the ATM before your next supermarket trip.

2 Snack Before Spending

It's a no-brainer that an empty belly leads to increased food cravings, but hunger may also affect your decision-making skills more generally. In a 2010 study, researchers at University College London discovered that hungry participants made riskier gambling decisions than those who were satiated, leading the investigators to argue that the hormones your body releases when you're hungry influence your ability to think rationally. That means you're more likely to risk your health on bonbons than you are to invest in bananas, and once you get home, you're forced to live with the repercussions of that decision. The bottom line: An empty stomach is the enemy of rational shopping. Plan your market trips to fall right after meals, or fortify yourself by eating a handful of fiber-rich nuts just before shopping.

Enable your grocery GPS 3

Before you get in your car to drive somewhere you've never been, what do you do? You write down directions. Okay, you probably tap the address into an iPhone or an onboard GPS, but the objective is the same: You're trying to make all the right turns that will lead you to your destination. Similarly, if your destination is a healthy body and an affordable grocery tab, you need directions. The supermarket is a highly complex thoroughfare, and every turn brings you closer to or further from the body you want. Creating a grocery list helps you stay focused on what you want to buy, leaving you less susceptible to marketing tactics and impulse purchases.

Shop on Wednesdays 4

Most people leave their grocery shopping for Saturday or Sunday mornings, when the supermarket looks more like a ravaged battlefield than a center of commerce. Consider making midweek evening runs, instead. According to *Progressive Grocer,* only 11 percent of Americans shop on Wednesdays, and on any given day, only 4 percent shop after 9:00 p.m. So if you're shopping at, say, 9:00 p.m. on a Wednesday, you're able to get in and out quickly, which means you'll spend less time fighting impulse items in both the aisles and at the checkout line. As a bonus, you'll free up your Saturday morning for something more enjoyable, like cooking a healthy breakfast.

Take your cart for a stroll 5

Pushing a shopping cart instead of carrying a basket may help you make smarter supermarket choices. A study published in the *Journal of Marketing Research* found that, all other things being equal, the strain of carrying a basket made shoppers more likely to reach for quick-grab impulse items—like the crackers and chips concentrated at eye level in the aisle. If you're lugging around a heavy basket, you're not taking the time to read labels and reach for more nutritious foods.

5

6 Bring your reading glasses

With the exception of alcohol, every packaged food and beverage in the supermarket has an ingredients statement. By law, the more of an ingredient a product contains according to weight, the higher it appears on that list, so effective shoppers learn to ignore front-of-label claims and read ingredients statements instead. Claims like "made with whole grain" and "reduced fat" can fool you into thinking you're making healthy choices, but if your "reduced fat" food lists sugar as the first—or second or third—ingredient, then it's not doing you any favors. A good general rule for label scanning: The fewer the ingredients, and the easier those ingredients are to pronounce, the better.

7 Live on the edge

For practical and economic reasons, most supermarkets in America live by the same organizational principles. Long-lasting boxed and bagged foods end up in the center aisles, while perishable, single-ingredient foods like fruits, vegetables, lean meats, and dairy live along the outer walls. And that's where you should live, too. Every time you enter the supermarket, make a full lap around the outer wall before making strategic inner-aisle strikes for things like oatmeal and whole-grain crackers. The more time you spend working the perimeter, the healthier you'll be. To better understand the subtle ways supermarket organization can trick you into spending cash on empty calories, turn to page 10 for Anatomy of a Supermarket.

Are Healthy Food Stores Making You Fat?

One supermarket trend we really like: It's easier than ever to buy better-tasting food— that's also better for you. Case in point: the wide selection of all-natural, organic products and high-quality specialty items at Whole Foods Market, Trader Joe's, and the Fresh Market. We say kudos to them. And to the patrons who seek them out. But beware: These 21st-century "health food" stores can actually trick you into eating less healthfully. How? By making bad-for-you food even more appealing. Your best defense: knowledge. That's why we uncovered the secret ways these supermarkets supersize your stomach.

1 THEY DRIVE YOUR SENSES SENSELESS.

Those delicious in-store product samples that you find in every specialty supermarket? They not only whet your appetite for the product, but also encourage you to buy more food overall, according to a study from Arizona State University. In fact, the research indicates that even the smell of cooking food might contribute to this effect. The stores are well aware of this. In fact, the Fresh Market invites you to "help yourself to a sample of freshly brewed coffee" and brags that "fragrant smells fill the atmosphere."

2 THEY DRIVE CALORIE COUNTS UNDERGROUND.

When you buy a package of cookies the complete nutrition information is listed. But when you buy cookies made at an in-store bakery, you won't find calorie counts. That goes for all the bakery items, from the "gourmet muffins" at the Fresh Market, to the "bakery fresh chocolate chip cookies" at Trader Joe's, to the "gluten-free vanilla cupcakes" at Whole Foods. For perspective, just one of those Whole Foods cupcakes packs 480 calories. (The calorie count is listed online, but not in the store.) Knowing those numbers is critical: University of Mississippi researchers found that unhappy people —who are more likely to overindulge in comfort foods—ate 69 percent fewer calories when they checked the calorie content before digging in.

3 THEY MAKE THE JUNK LOOK GOURMET.

Ever notice that more-expensive products tend to come in fancier packages? Researchers at the University of Michigan recently found that food purveyors may actually use fancy fonts and labels to help justify higher prices. The scientists theorize that attractive fonts and labels give people the perception that they are getting more value for the higher cost. Think about it: Would you like a piece of cake—or a piece of *Cake?*

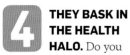

THEY BASK IN THE HEALTH HALO. Do you consider products from specialty supermarkets to be healthier than those from other grocery stores? If the answer is yes, you could be doing your waistline a disservice. When people guess the number of calories in a sandwich coming from a "healthy" restaurant, they estimate that it has, on average, 35 percent fewer calories than they do when it comes from an "unhealthy" restaurant, according to a study in the *Journal of Consumer Research.* Remember that the next time you reach for that package of Whole Foods' Organic Fruit & Nut Granola. One cup of this "healthy" product contains almost 500 calories.

THEY BULK YOU UP "IN BULK." On the Fresh Market Web site, the store claims to have the largest bulk snack selection "in town." But be careful what you buy in this bulk section: It may cause you to look like you fit in there. Why? By filling your own bag with a big scoop, you'll likely underestimate how much you've served yourself. Case in point: A Cornell University study found that nutritionists who were asked to serve themselves ice cream with large bowls and spoons dished out about 57 percent more than those given smaller bowls and spoons. Buy basic staples like spices, grains, and legumes in bulk, but make sure your snacks always come with serving sizes and calorie counts.

THEY BUFFET YOUR BELLY WITH BUFFETS. If you're watching your weight, don't step near the Whole Foods buffet. Cornell University researchers found heavier diners tend to overindulge in buffet settings. (Surprise!) Our real beef: While Whole Foods lists selections' ingredients on the buffet's ID labels, it doesn't provide nutrition information for any of them. And yes, one of the items is macaroni and cheese—or "pasta and cheese" as the chain calls it.

Anatomy of a Supermarket

There's a careful science to the way supermarkets are organized, and it isn't to make sure you have the most pleasant experience possible. Shelves are stocked and aisles arranged for one strategic end: to ensure you, valued consumer, spend as much money as possible before wheeling your cart back out those sliding doors. If you plan to make it out of the supermarket jungle alive, you'll need a map, a compass, and plenty of bug spray. Over the next four pages, we equip you with everything you need to escape unscathed.

GROCERY STORES
ARE BIGGER
THAN EVER.

The Food Market Institute says stores expanded from 35,000 to 47,000 square feet in the past 15 years. And with 38,000 items filling the aisles of the average market, it's never been easier to spend money on food that will sabotage your health and budgetary goals.

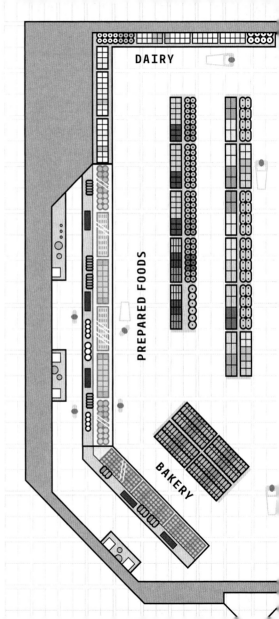

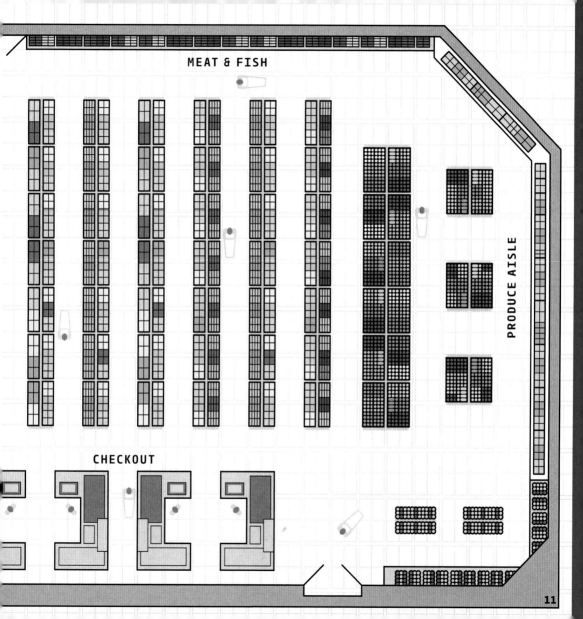

MEAT & FISH

PRODUCE AISLE

CHECKOUT

11

AVOID THE VEGAS EFFECT

Supermarkets are designed like casinos: clockless and nearly windowless expanses flooded with artificial light and Muzak, places where time stands still. Casinos force guests to navigate a maze of alluring gambling opportunities before they reach essential destinations: restaurants, bathrooms, exit doors. Same goes for the supermarket: The most essential staple foods—produce, bread, milk, and eggs—are placed in the back and along the perimeter of the supermarket to ensure that customers travel the length of the store—and thus are exposed to multiple junk-food temptations along the way.

SKIMP ON THE SNACKS

The densest collection of those temptations is found in the snack aisle, which on average packs in a waist-widening 446 calories per 100 grams of food. Cereals come in a close second, costing you 344 calories per 100 grams.

PREPARE YOURSELF FOR STEEP PRICES

The prepared-foods section of grocery stores has grown in recent years as consumers demand more quick, low-cost alternatives to restaurant meals. A 2010 survey found that 64 percent of people had purchased a ready-to-eat meal from a supermarket in the previous month, and experts estimated that the sector would grow to $14 billion by the end of 2011. Unfortunately, markups can be steep and nutrition is scarcely a concern for supermarkets looking to maximize profits. Your best bet on a busy night? A rotisserie chicken—healthy, versatile, and usually about $6 a bird.

CHECK YOURSELF OUT

Impulse purchases drop by 32.1 percent for women—and 16.7 percent for men—when they use the self-checkout aisle, according to a study by IHL Consulting Group. Eighty percent of candy and 61 percent of salty-snack purchases are impulse buys.

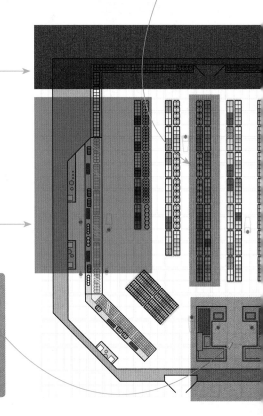

WORK THE PERIMETER

The produce section accounts for only 10 percent of a supermarket's sales, whereas the nutrient-depleted middle aisles make up 26 percent of sales. The most successful (i.e., healthiest) shoppers invert that ratio, spending the lion's share of their dollars in the produce and refrigerator sections and a small percentage in the murky middle aisles.

BUY YOUR LETTUCE LAST

Consumers tend to shop in a counterclockwise pattern, according to a study from the Wharton School, so grocers place the produce section at the front of the store. Why? Because research shows that shoppers who peruse the produce aisle first spend more time and money in the store.

GET TO KNOW THE BIG O

Organic foods and beverages have been one of the fastest-expanding sectors of the supermarket, with sales growing from $1 billion in 1990 to $26.7 billion in 2010. Organic foods can cost between 20 and 100 percent more than their conventional counterparts. To maximize your purchasing power in the organic-produce aisle, see page 101.

Anatomy of an Aisle

It's not just the overall layout of a supermarket that affects purchasing; no, every last square inch of real estate has been carefully considered by the engineers of profit. The biggest factor in the way your supermarket shelves are stocked? How much a manufacturer is willing to pay to have its products placed in prime positions. Called slotting, this pay-for-placement practice has come to dominate the arrangement of the modern supermarket, and consciously or not, it has tremendous impact on the products Americans stock their pantries with. Here's how to beat the system.

LOOK BEYOND WHAT THE FOOD INDUSTRY WANTS YOU TO SEE.

The top eight grocery chains now account for 50 percent of all supermarket sales, and with this increased clout, they're demanding that manufacturers pay higher and higher slotting fees for premium shelf space. By some estimates, manufacturers shell out $100 billion a year in shelf fees, representing more than half of the supermarket industry's profits.

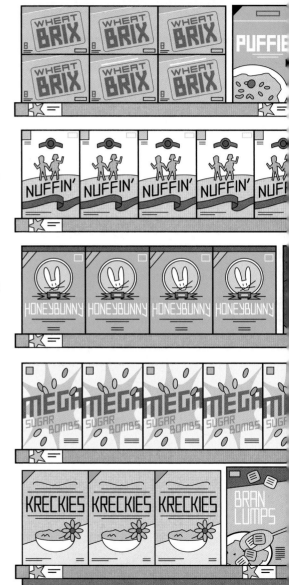

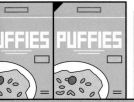
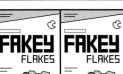

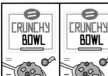

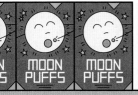
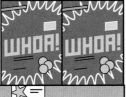
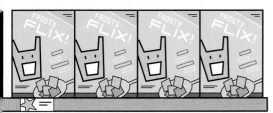
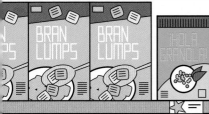

SHOP FOR CEREAL ALONE

The cereal industry spends more money each year—$229 million—advertising to children than any other packaged food category, according to the Federal Trade Commission. That also means they can afford to place sweet cereals on the lower shelves to catch the eyes of sugar-starved kids, who can then pester their parents for that colorful box of refined carbs.

LOOK HIGH, AND LOW

For a new product, the standard price of admission can run to up to $25,000 per item for a regional cluster of stores. Some have estimated the cost of rolling out a small product line in supermarkets nationwide at $16.8 million. At those prices, only the biggest manufacturers—the Krafts and General Millses and Frito-Lays of the food world—can pay to play, further solidifying their places as brand leaders. Always start by scanning the top and bottom shelves. If you do, we guarantee that you'll find crackers with more fiber, fruit snacks with less sugar, and canned goods with less sodium than those on the costly middle shelves.

SCAN FOR UNKNOWN BRANDS

As with the music and movies, sometimes the best stuff is the most obscure. Not only can bigger manufacturers afford better real estate, but they often pay to keep smaller manufacturers off the shelf or in disadvantageous locations. In California, independent bakers filed a lawsuit accusing Sara Lee of paying supermarkets to relegate local bagelmakers to only the top and bottom shelves. Sadly, these lesser-known brands are often healthier and more affordable than their big-name counterparts.

America's Worst Supermarket Foods

The average supermarket is now a minefield of more than 38,000 items. Quite a few can help strengthen your body, but even more can turn it to mush—and none more so than the 20 dietary detonators that follow. Know them and you can emerge from the aisles with the foods both you and your body will love.

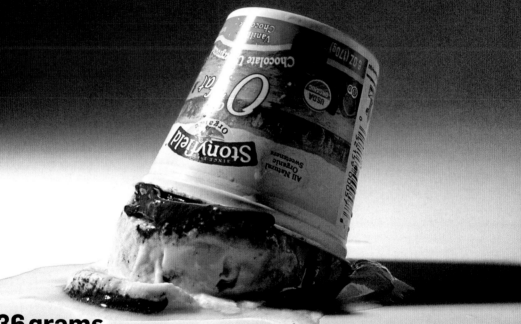

36 grams of sugar
Stonyfield calls it yogurt; we call it ice cream.

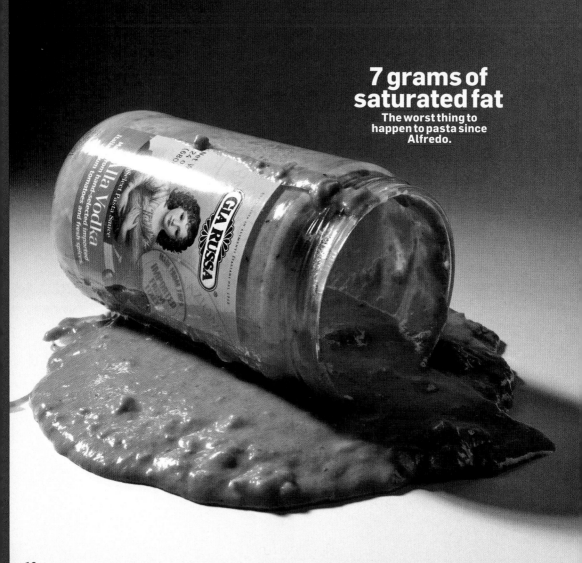

7 grams of
saturated fat
The worst thing to
happen to pasta since
Alfredo.

WORST CONDIMENT

20 Kraft Tartar Sauce Natural Lemon & Herb Flavor

(28 g, 2 Tbsp)
150 calories
16 g fat (2.5 g saturated)
180 mg sodium

In the real world, lemons and herbs are both essentially zero-calorie flavor boosters. But in the bizarro world of supermarket products, they constitute a 250 percent calorie tax on a normal bottle of tartar sauce—and every single extra calorie comes from cheap soybean oil. In fact, just 2 tablespoons of this Kraft-made kryptonite contain about 50 calories more than a full serving of tilapia. If your fish needs a friend, try cocktail sauce, salsa, or even Kraft's regular tartar.
Fat Equivalent: 10 strips of Oscar Mayer Center Cut Bacon

Eat This Instead!
Kraft Tartar Sauce
(30 g, 2 Tbsp)
60 calories
5 g fat (1 g saturated)
200 mg sodium

WORST COOKIE

19 Oreo Double Stuf Cakesters
(37 g, 1 snack cake)
170 calories
9 g fat (2 g saturated)
17 g sugars

The first four ingredients—sugar, palm oil, enriched flour, and high-fructose corn syrup—are each to be avoided individually, so in concert, they create one catastrophic cookie. Consume one of these a day and after a year, you'll have packed on 17 pounds of fat. Then you'll be shopping for double-stuff pants.
Calorie Equivalent: 80 Jujubes candy pieces

Eat This Instead!
Kashi TLC Oatmeal Dark Chocolate Soft Baked Cookies
(30 g, 1 cookie)
130 calories
5 g fat (1.5 g saturated)
4 g fiber
8 g sugars

WORST MARINARA SAUCE

18 Gia Russa Select Pasta Sauce Alla Vodka
(113 g, ½ cup)
200 calories
18 g fat (7 g saturated)
520 mg sodium

Don't blame the vodka for corrupting this tomato-based sauce. The real culprits here are heavy whipping cream, butter, and cheese—a fat-filled trio that pads this sauce with more caloric density than most ice creams. And let's be honest: You're going to eat more than one 1/2-cup serving. Make it 1 cup sauce with a couple cups of pasta and you've just hit 800 calories—and that's before factoring in the garlic roll and the glass of wine to wash it down with.
Saturated Fat Equivalent: 14 McDonald's Chicken McNuggets

Eat This Instead!
Amy's Light in Sodium Organic Family Marinara
(125 g, ½ cup)
80 calories
4.5 g fat (0.5 g saturated)
290 mg sodium

WORST WRAP

17 Mission Wraps Garden Spinach Herb
(70 g, 1 tortilla)
210 calories
4.5 g fat (2 g saturated)
510 mg sodium

A basic tortilla takes about four ingredients to construct—flour, water, oil, salt—but Mission uses no fewer than 30 ingredients to construct these wraps, and spinach falls under the "2% or less" portion of the ingredients statement. So what is this wrap made of? A lot of enriched flour and vegetable shortening, neither of which makes for a healthy wrap.
Calorie Equivalent: 4 Pizza Hut Traditional Buffalo Wings

Eat This Instead!
Flatout Flatbread Light Garden Spinach
(53 g, 1 flatbread)
90 calories
2.5 g fat (0 g saturated)
9 g fiber

▌16 Stonyfield Organic Whole Milk Chocolate Underground

(6 oz, 1 container)
220 calories
5 g fat (3 g saturated)
36 g sugars

What's your favorite candy-bar indulgence? Butterfinger? Reese's? Snickers? This yogurt has more sugar than all of them. The 9 teaspoons of sweetness in each container is enough to hijack your blood sugar and push your body into fat-storage mode. You'd be better off eating a modest scoop of ice cream.
Sugar Equivalent: 2 scoops of Breyers Original Rocky Road Ice Cream

Eat This Instead!
Yoplait Delights Parfait Chocolate Éclair
(4 oz, 113 g, 1 container)
100 calories
1.5 g fat (1 g saturated)
13 g sugars

WORST DRINK

▌15 SoBe Pina Colada

(20 fl oz, 1 bottle)
310 calories
1 g fat (0.5 g saturated)
77 g sugars

A 20-ounce Coke has less sugar, yet watchdog groups would have Coca-Cola in court if the company tried to plaster any health claims on its bottle.

So how does SoBe get away with touting the hibiscus and zinc in this drink? Simple: Without carbonation, SoBe's product is not a traditional "soft drink," so it's not on the radar of most health critics. This drink has nearly as much sugar as half a dozen Breyers Smooth & Dreamy Triple Chocolate Chip ice cream bars, and no mineral or herb can protect you from that.
Sugar Equivalent: 2 cans of Coca-Cola

Drink This Instead!
AriZona Arnold Palmer Zero Half & Half Iced Tea Lemonade
(24 oz, 1 can)
0 calories
0 g fat
<1 g sugars

WORST ICE CREAM

▌14 Häagen Dazs Chocolate Peanut Butter

(½ cup)
360 calories
24 g fat (11 g saturated)
24 g sugars

Do you know what the standard ½-cup serving of ice cream looks like? It's about the size of a hacky sack. So choosing poorly in the frozen section has caloric consequences beyond what the label suggests. Häagen Dazs is a perfect example of poor choices—the company is consistently among the worst on the shelf, and this carton packs

more than half your day's saturated fat into each scoop.
Saturated Fat Equivalent: 3 small orders of Burger King french fries

Eat This Instead!
Edy's Slow Churned Peanut Butter Cup
(⅓ cup)
130 calories
5 g fat (2.5 g saturated)
13 g sugars

WORST CANNED GOOD

▌13 Dennison's Original Chili con Carne with Beans

(256 g, 1 cup)
360 calories
14 g fat (6 g saturated)
1,030 mg sodium

Eat both servings in this can and you've just spooned down 38 percent more than the maximum amount of sodium most people should consume in a day. And thanks to the use of gristly beef cuts, you've also taken in more than half your day's saturated fat and 720 calories.
Sodium Equivalent: 112 Rold Gold Pretzel Sticks

Eat This Instead!
Campbell's Chunky Chili Roadhouse Beef & Bean
(1 cup)
230 calories
5 g fat (2 g saturated)
870 mg sodium

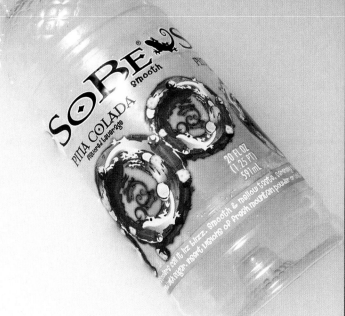

77 grams of sugar

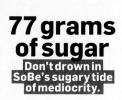

Don't drown in SoBe's sugary tide of mediocrity.

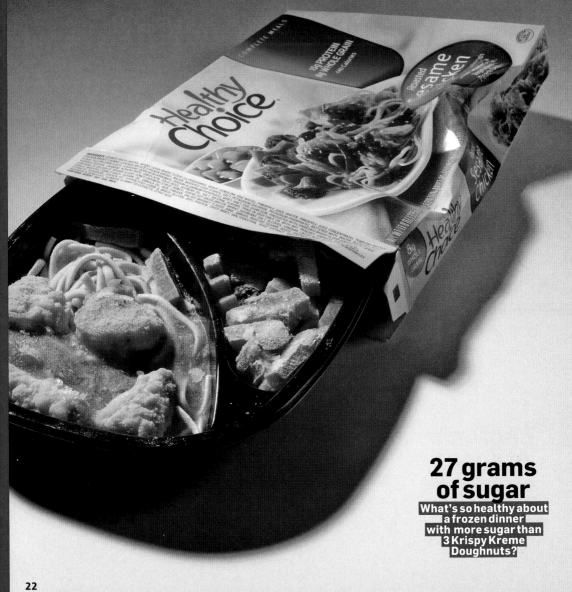

27 grams of sugar

What's so healthy about a frozen dinner with more sugar than 3 Krispy Kreme Doughnuts?

22

WORST CEREAL

12 Quaker Natural Granola Oats & Honey & Raisins

(102 g, 1 cup)
420 calories
10 g fat (1 g saturated)
26 g sugars

Granola must have a heck of a PR guy. After all, someone managed to convince an entire nation of eaters that clumps of oats and raisins glued together with sugar is somehow healthy. Five years as America's Worst Cereal, we hope, cuts through the spin.
Calorie Equivalent: 3 servings of Cookie Crisp cereal

Eat This Instead!

Kashi GoLean Crunch!

(53 g, 1 cup)
190 calories
3 g fat (0 g saturated)
13 g sugars

WORST "HEALTHY" FROZEN ENTRÉE

11 Healthy Choice Roasted Sesame Chicken

(335 g, 1 meal)
440 calories
9 g fat (1.5 g saturated)
470 mg sodium
27 g sugars

Reality check: The name says roasted chicken, but read the fine print and you see the meat is coated in flour and then cooked in vegetable oil. Sounds an awful lot like fried chicken, doesn't it? Then Healthy Choice soaks the pasta in pineapple juice and coats the fruit side dish in a sweetened syrup to deliver a candy bar's worth of sugar. Healthy? Hardly.
Sugar Equivalent: 3 Krispy Kreme Traditional Cake Doughnuts

Eat This Instead!

Kashi Southwest Style Chicken

(283 g, 1 entrée)
240 calories
5 g fat (1 g saturated)
680 mg sodium
3 g sugars

WORST PACKAGED SIDE

10 Pasta Roni Fettuccine Alfredo

(1 cup prepared with 2% milk and margarine)
450 calories
24 g fat
(7 g saturated, 3.5 g trans)
1,050 mg sodium

Alfredo is bad enough as it is, but Pasta Roni's version compounds the nutritional negligence with partially hydrogenated oil, monosodium glutamate, and a smattering of artificial colors. Each serving of this side dish has a meal's worth of calories, two-thirds of your day's sodium allotment, and 2 days' worth of trans fats. Safe yourself by boiling your own pasta and tossing it with olive oil and freshly grated Parmesan.
Sodium Equivalent: 97 Cheez-Its

Eat This Instead!

Pasta Roni Butter & Herb Italiano

(1 cup prepared)
300 g fat
11 g fat (3 g saturated)
780 mg sodium

WORST FROZEN TREAT

9 Mrs. Fields Ice Cream Cookie Sandwich

(129 g, 1 sandwich)
450 calories
19 g fat (11 g saturated)
41 g sugars

The classic ice cream sandwich of yesteryear represented an ideal balance of decadence and restraint, a compact package of vanilla and chocolatey goodness for less than 200 calories. Unfortunately, food manufacturers have ushered into the freezer section a new era for these treats, one defined by gargantuan portions and sky-high sugar counts. Sandwiched between Mrs. Fields' two giant cookie bookends are nearly a quarter of your day's calories and more than half of your day's saturated fat limit.
Fat Equivalent: 19 tablespoons of Extra Creamy Cool Whip

Eat This Instead!

Breyers Smooth & Dreamy Chocolate Chip Cookie Dough Ice Cream Sandwiches

(62 g, 1 sandwich)
160 calories
4 g fat (2 g saturated)
15 g sugars

Marie Callender's Southern Pecan Pie

(113 g, ⅛ pie)
450 calories
23 g fat (4 g saturated, 3 g trans)
44 g sugars

With three separate uses of partially hydrogenated oil and shortening, Marie Callender creates a slice of pie with more trans fats than you should eat in 36 hours and as much sugar as 97 M&M's. Regardless of brand, remember these two pie rules: Pecan pie is almost always the worst choice, and pumpkin nearly without fail is your best.
Fat Equivalent:
71 Chili Cheese Fritos

Eat This Instead!
Sara Lee Oven Fresh Pumpkin Pie

(131 g)
260 calories
10 g fat (4 g saturated)
20 g sugars

WORST KIDS' MEAL

Lunchables with Juice Nachos, Cheese Dip + Salsa

490 calories
21 g fat (4.5 g saturated)
890 mg sodium
25 g sugars

For all the heat school lunch programs have been taking lately, it's hard to imagine cafeteria slop being any worse than what's inside this box. The ingredients list reads like a college organic chemistry final, littered as it is with bizarre preservatives, fillers, sweeteners, and partially hydrogenated oil. The hardest part is deciding which part of the Lunchable is the worst: the sugary Capri Sun, the Nestlé Crunch bar, or the neon-orange cheese goo. Isn't it worth an extra few minutes to make sure your children go off to school with the best possible food in their bags?
Calorie Equivalent: 6 Applegate Farms Natural Beef Hot Dogs

Eat This Instead!
Lunchables with Fruit Ham + American Cracker Stackers

290 calories
9 g fat (3 g saturated)
530 mg sodium
22 g sugars

WORST INDIVIDUAL SNACK

Hostess Pudding Pie Chocolate

(128 g, 1 pie)
520 calories
24 g fat (12 g saturated)
40 g sugars

Skip past the enriched flour and water on the ingredients list and here's what you get: shortening, corn syrup, high-fructose corn syrup, sugar, modified corn starch, butter, chocolate liqueur, and on and on. Any one of these ingredients alone might prompt you to raise an eyebrow, but taken together they should invoke a gag reflex and a sprint for a new snack fix.
Calorie Equivalent: 5 Good Humor Cookie & Cream Bars

Eat This Instead!
Little Debbie Pecan Spinwheels

(30 g, 1 wheel)
100 calories
3.5 g fat (1 g saturated)
7 g sugars

WORST BREAKFAST

Jimmy Dean Breakfast Bowls Pancakes & Sausage Links

(244 g, 1 bowl)
710 calories
34 g fat (12 g saturated)
1,000 mg sodium
35 g sugars

Fat and sodium are the usual villains in Southern-style breakfasts, and both are in full force in JD's Pancakes & Sausage Links bowl. But here's the kicker: It also contains more syrupy sugar than a liquefied Snickers bar. You'd be better off eating two McDonald's Sausage Burritos soaked in syrup than you would be heating this container up.
Calorie Equivalent: 13 Little Debbie Powdered Mini Donuts

Eat This Instead!
Jimmy Dean D-Lights Turkey Sausage Muffin

(145 g, 1 sandwich)
260 calories
8 g fat (3.5 g saturated)
760 mg sodium
3 g sugars

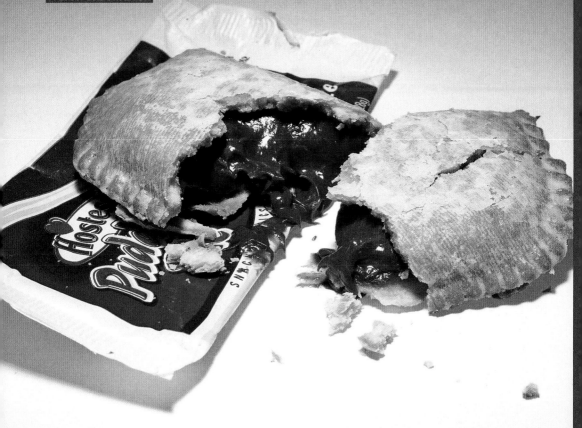

520 calories

Worst. Snack. Ever.

WORST STIR-FRY/SKILLET

Stouffer's Sautés for Two Steak Gorgonzola

(340 g, ½ package)
730 calories
26 g fat (14 g saturated)
950 mg sodium

Perfect for when you're dining with a mortal enemy. But if your table partner is someone you care about, spare him or her the nutritional assault. In total, this bag contains 1,460 calories and nearly one and a half times the saturated fat you should eat in an entire day. The reason: prime rib (among the fattiest cuts of beef) and four different cheeses.
Saturated Fat Equivalent: 5 Taco Bell Fresco Bean Burritos

Eat This Instead!

Bertolli Tuscan-Style Braised Beef with Gold Potatoes

(340 g, ½ bag)
310 calories
11 g fat (2.5 g saturated)
920 mg sodium

WORST FROZEN PIZZA

DiGiorno Traditional Crust Supreme Pizza

(262 g, 1 pizza)
790 calories
37 g fat
(13 g saturated, 3.5 g trans)
1,410 mg sodium

DiGiorno's line of Traditional Crust individual pizzas tops this category year after year, and for good reason. It has far more calories, sodium, and fat

(including dangerous trans fats) than any other pie in the freezer. Not even the company's newer stuffed crust individual pizzas are worse. The company's slogan may be "It's not delivery. It's DiGiorno," but you're definitely better off ordering Domino's than you are tussling with this pie.
Sodium Equivalent: 1 pound of oil-roasted peanuts

Eat This Instead!

DiGiorno 200 Calorie Portions Pepperoni Pizza

(170 g, 1 pizza)
400 calories
18 g fat (8 g saturated)
1,040 mg sodium

WORST FROZEN ENTRÉE

Hungry-Man Select Classic Fried Chicken

(406 g, 1 package)
1,030 calories
62 g fat (14 g saturated)
1,610 mg sodium

It should come as no surprise that Hungry-Man continues to find its way down to the bottom of our Worst Foods lists. But what is surprising is that these atrocious numbers don't tell the whole story of just how bad this brand can be. Sure, the calories, fat, and sodium are outrageous, but what concerns us most is that Hungry-Man fails to list trans fats on its nutrition label, despite federal regulations requiring it. And the thing is, every component of this plate—aside from the corn—contains a dose of par-

tially hydrogenated oil, the source of trans fats.
Calorie Equivalent: 8.5 KFC Original Recipe Drumsticks

Eat This Instead!

Stouffer's Homestyle Classics Fried Chicken

(251 g, 1 package)
360 calories
18 g fat (4.5 g saturated)
880 mg sodium

WORST PACKAGED FOOD

Marie Callender's Cheesy Chicken Pot Pie

(568 g, 1 pie)
1,140 calories
72 g fat (28 g saturated)
1,760 mg sodium

Don't fall for the nutritional sleight of hand: The company lists a serving as ½ pie, but few people are going to split what is essentially a single-person dish. Equally egregious is what's inside. Chicken fat is one of the first ingredients, followed by a bevy of oils, cream, cheese, and finally a string of unpronounceable chemicals that you might confuse with hazardous wastes. And the thing is, you wouldn't be far off.
Calorie Equivalent: Nine 12-ounce bottles of Guinness Draught

Eat This Instead!

Banquet Chicken Pot Pie

(198 g, 1 pie)
370 calories
21 g fat (8 g saturated)
1,040 mg sodium

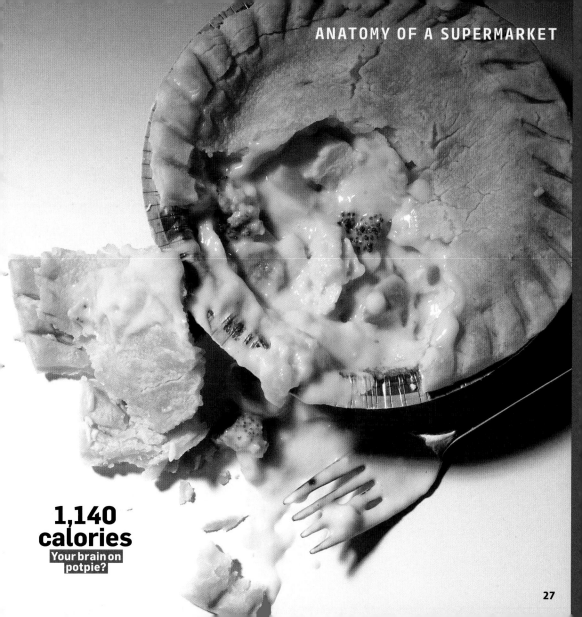

1,140 calories
Your brain on potpie?

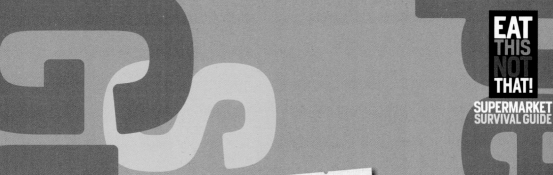

EAT
THIS
NOT
THAT!
SUPERMARKET
SURVIVAL GUIDE

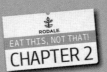

RODALE
EAT THIS, NOT THAT!
CHAPTER 2

YOUR SAVE-MONEY SHOPPING GUIDE

It's never easy

to talk about money.

At least every few weeks I make a special trip to see my niece and nephew, who live about an hour away. And inevitably, as night falls, they ask me why I have to leave, and why I have to go to work the next day. They're just 4 and 6, so they don't quite understand the intricacies of career management. So, I explain it to them in a way they can understand: "I have to go to work so I can make some money so I can buy some food."

But what started as a simple way to talk to kids has become, for many of us, something more serious. Over the past several years, the amount of work we all have to do in order to "buy some food" has been growing out of control. The USDA estimated that overall food prices would rise as much as 4.5 percent in 2011 alone. And the costs of some of the most important components of our daily meals are rocketing up at even faster rates: Beef was expected to rise by 9 percent in 2011, and dairy by up to 6 percent. (What are they feeding those cows, caviar?) Cooking oil is expected to go up as much as 7.5 percent as well. Nowadays, it feels like we're all walking around holding signs that say Will Work for Food.

And that's why mastering the supermarket has never been more important. In fact, I want you to look at this book not as a shopping and spending guide, but as an investing guide. After all, when you purchase groceries, you're not giving up a valuable resource. You're simply trading one resource (money) for another (nutrition). The more wisely you shop for food, the better your investment will pay.

Consider this: Nearly 45 percent of our food dollars are spent on restaurants, perhaps the worst investment imaginable. You fork over $15, $30, $45, or more for a family of four, and you get one meal, with maybe a doggie bag or two—and boom, that's it. Now you've got to go back to work to make more money to buy more food.

Spend that 45 bucks on groceries, however, and you could feed your family for days—if you do it wisely. The key is to think about investing in high-quality foods, not junk. Sure, the junk is cheaper, but it won't fill you up or satisfy your hunger.

With the right shopping strategy, you'll not only melt away the pounds, but you'll save thousands of dollars every year.

It will just make you fatter—and you'll still need to go spend more money on the nutrients your body needs. It's like that baby in the E*Trade commercials might say: Do your homework, run some analytics. But to invest wisely, you don't need to understand profit-and-loss statements or average cost-flow assumptions. You just

need to know the good food from the bad.

In fact, a Harvard study found that over the course of 4 years, the people who gained the most weight were the ones who bought the most potato chips (very little nutrition), sugar-sweetened drinks (zero nutrition), and red meats (nutritious, but expensive). On the other hand, those who lost weight bought the most vegetables, whole grains, fruits, nuts, and yogurt—all of which are packed with nutrition. Investing in more vitamins and minerals, more fiber, more protein, will pay dividends for your health while actually costing you less in the long run. Invest in sugar, fat, and empty calories, however, and you'll just have to work longer and harder, because you bought the nutritional equivalent of swampland in Florida.

Picking the smart food investments instead of the dumb ones is what this book is all about. But in this chapter, I want to give you a few smart tricks on not just what to shop for, but also how to shop for it—little secrets that will save you time and money while you cruise the aisles.

AVOID QUICKIES.
A study supported by the Marketing Science Institute found that shoppers who made "quick trips" to the store purchased an average of 54 percent more merchandise than they had planned to. Instead, be thoughtful in your planning—keep a

magnetic notepad on your fridge and make notes throughout the week about what you need. (Avoiding extra trips will cut down on your gasoline costs as well.)

BULK UP.

Discount clubs are great cost-saving alternatives, even if you have to pay a fee to join. It doesn't make sense to buy everything in bulk, of course—nobody needs a 2-gallon drum of capers. Focus on items you use a lot of and that won't spoil, like paper products and frozen foods. Some shopping clubs also offer discounted gas. Cha-ching!

WATCH YOUR WEIGHT.

Okay, so one box of crackers costs $4 and the other $4.50. But before you assume the $4 one is cheaper, take a closer look at the net weight. You'll often find that the more expensive box contains more food—and therefore is really cheaper. Checking the net weight is also a great way of making sure you're not paying for a lot of packaging, only to get home and discover that most of what's inside the box is air.

STAY LOCAL.

A 2004 Tulane University study found that having easy access to supermarket shopping was associated with increased household use of fruits (84 grams per adult equivalent per day). Map out the supermarkets both close to home and close to work, and while you're at it, look up the farmer's markets in the area at localharvest.org, an online database containing nearly every outdoor market nationwide.

EAT BEFORE YOU SHOP.

This is critical! A 2008 study published in the *Journal of Consumer Research* found that consumers, even when on a tight budget, are more likely to spend more if their appetites are stimulated before making a purchase. The study tested the reactions of women shoppers to a hidden chocolate chip cookie–scented candle in the room. Nearly 70 percent who got a whiff of the cookie scent said they would buy a new sweater even though they were on a tight budget, compared with only 17 percent of those who weren't exposed to the cookie smell. You just know the guys who run the bake shop at the supermarket have read this study too!

STOP THE RETAIL THERAPY.

Sadness increases the amount of money that shoppers are willing to spend, according to a 2008 study in the journal *Psychological Science*. Study participants who watched a sad video clip were willing to pay four times as much for a product than those who watched a neutral clip about nature were.

The (True) Cost of a Calorie

You have two options: Either you give us $5 for a hamburger, or you give us $7 for a hamburger, fries, and soda. Which is the better deal? The second scenario costs more, but you also get more food. Well you get more calories, anyway. Say your $5 fast-food burger packs in 500 calories. That's a penny per calorie. Add a medium order of fries and a medium soda, and for only a couple extra clams, you've doubled the number of calories in your order. Jackpot! Right?

Not so quick. What thin people understand is that calories are an inadequate measure of nutrition. Calories alone neither make you healthy nor provide sustained energy, and in many cases they do the exact opposite. Confusion about this point allows food processors to flood our aisles with the cheap ingredients and chemicals that can wreak havoc on our metabolisms and hormones. Instead of making us fit and energetic, cheap calories make us flabby and lethargic, and as such, we pay twice: First at the register, and again at the doctor's office. According to a study from the *American Journal of Clinical Nutrition,* lower-income families who put their food dollars toward low-cost, low-nutrient food have the highest rates of obesity, and in 2008 alone, obesity accounted for a staggering $147 billion in medical bills.

Here we've calculated the cost of 100 calories for 24 common foods. What you'll notice is that the cheaper the product, the more likely it is to contain excessive sugars, sodium, and other harmful ingredients. There are some exceptions, but the lesson here is simple: You want to put your food dollars toward nutrients, not just calories.

YOUR SAVE-MONEY SHOPPING GUIDE

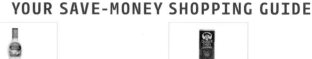

Maruchan Ramen Noodle Soup Chicken

WHAT ELSE YOU GET

99 calories of refined carbohydrates and soybean oil

18% of your daily sodium

Wonder Classic White Bread

WHAT ELSE YOU GET

98 calories of nutritionally shallow enriched flour and high-fructose corn syrup

24 grams of fiber-free carbohydrates

3 grams of sugar from high fructose corn syrup

Hidden Valley Ranch

WHAT ELSE YOU GET

14 grams of fat from soybean oil and buttermilk

An undisclosed amount of MSG, a flavor-enhancing amino acid known to cause head-aches in suscep-tible people

Blue Bunny Vanilla Ice Cream

WHAT ELSE YOU GET

1 tablespoon of sugar

11% of your daily calcium recommendation

Quaker Quick-1 Oats

WHAT ELSE YOU GET

3 grams of fiber, much of which comes from cholesterol-lowering beta-glucan

18 grams of quality, energy-sustain-ing carbohy-drates

10% of your manganese, which facilitates your body's use of numerous trace elements

$0.00 — $0.05 — $0.09 — $0.12 $0.13 $0.14 $0.15 — $0.17 — $0.20

Jif Creamy Peanut Butter

WHAT ELSE YOU GET

13 grams of heart-healthy fat

A dose of added sugars and oils

Ritz Crackers

WHAT ELSE YOU GET

6 grams of fat from soybean and partially hydrogenated oils

A hidden shot of high-fructose corn syrup

Oreo Cookies

WHAT ELSE YOU GET

2 teaspoons of sugar

7% of your day's fat

2% Milk

WHAT ELSE YOU GET

25% of your daily tryptophan, an amino acid required to produce mood-boosting serotonin

6 grams of complete protein

Bananas

WHAT ELSE YOU GET

1/3 of your day's vitamin B_6

467 mg of blood-pressure-reducing potassium

(Prices listed are for 100 calories of food)

35

Kraft Macaroni and Cheese (prepared with 2% milk and margarine)

Double your daily limit of deadly trans fats

Yellow #5 and yellow #6, food colorings that have been linked to behavioral problems in children

Coca-Cola

39 grams of sugar from high-fructose corn syrup

Phosphoric acid, a compound that erodes enamel and promotes tooth decay

Lucky Charms

10 grams of sugar, almost exclusively from marshmallows

4 different artificial colorings

Sirloin

6% of your heme iron, the kind readily absorbed by the body

10% zinc, a mineral that helps protect arterial walls

4 grams of oleic fatty acids, the heart-healthy lipids found in olive oil

$0.21 **$0.27** **$0.29** **$0.31** **$0.35** **$0.45** **$0.50** **$0.84**

Ruffles

6 grams of fat

100 mg of sodium

Almonds

2.5 grams fiber

9 grams of heart-healthy monounsaturated fat

More than a quarter day's worth of skin-protecting vitamin E

Eggs (Cage-Free, non-organic)

180 mg of choline, which your body needs to break down fat for energy

9 grams of highest-quality muscle-building protein

StarKist Chunk Light Tuna in Water

20 grams of pure protein

120% of your day's selenium, which can help prevent colon cancer

Organic Apples

5 g fiber

Quercetin, an antioxidant that regulates blood sugar by inhibiting the enzymes that break down carbohydrates

Organic Carrots

1,600% of your daily Vitamin A

50% of your day's vitamin K

Cauliflower

A surprising 25% of your day's omega-3 fatty acids

3 times your daily requirement for vitamin C

The lesson is simple: Put your food dollars toward nutrients, not calories.

 $0.89   **$1.06**   **$1.14**   **$1.76**   **$2.05**   **$5.14**

Atlantic Salmon

43% of your day's omega-3 fatty acids

Bioactive peptides in the protein that may help protect joint cartilage

13 grams of protein

Romaine Lettuce

40% of your day's allotment of 8 key vitamins and minerals

8 grams of fiber

Blueberries

8,400 micromoles of antioxidants, ranking it as one of the top cancer-fighting whole foods

4 grams of fiber

Worst Supermarket Rip-Offs

Walking into your average supermarket is a lot like being a contestant on *Jeopardy!* If you think hard, choose wisely, and give all the right answers, you can go home with a carload of cash and prizes. But make a few mistakes and you'll leave with an empty wallet—not to mention a lot of empty calories. In fact, even the lowest-priced supermarket in your neighborhood is brimming with complete rip-offs—"health" foods that aren't healthy, "gourmet" foods that aren't gourmet, specialty items that just aren't that special. Here are just some of the foods you're overpaying for.

Organic Onions and Avocados

The Environmental Working Group, an organization that studies pesticide contamination, ranks onions and avocados among the most-pesticide-free vegetables and fruits, respectively—even when grown conventionally.

In fact, as a general rule, anything you have to peel before you eat it (such as a banana or garlic, for example) is relatively low in pesticides. If you want to eat organic, splurge on produce with permeable or edible skin, such as peaches, lettuce, and apples.

Bottled Spices

What all those TV chefs say is true: You should try to refresh your spice cabinet as often as possible—at least once a year. Over time, spices' essential oils fade, and with them goes the flavor you're looking (and paying) for. So what's a savvy cook to do, pay $6 for a bottle of star anise you're only going to use twice a year? Absolutely not. Instead, shop at stores like Whole Foods and ethnic markets where you can buy all your spices from bulk containers that allow you to choose the amount. Fifteen grams of cardamom or cumin or coriander will cost you about a quarter of what a normal supermarket charges for a small bottle and will last you the better part of a year. Plus, high turnover ensures you're getting potent spices—not something that's been sitting on a shelf since Reagan left office.

Swordfish

A pound of swordfish can cost more than $20. Why? Supply and demand: Because it's scarce, it's viewed as a luxury. But you should consider its high cost a blessing: It probably has saved your family from slow, steady infusions of poison. Due to its abnormally high levels of mercury, the Environmental Defense Fund recommends that children and women who could potentially become pregnant cut swordfish from their diets entirely. A better seafood option: mahi mahi. It's a meaty, flavorful fish like swordfish, but it's nearly contaminant free, has about 30 percent fewer calories, and costs about half as much.

Gluten-Free Baked Goods

Gluten-free foods generally cost two to three times more than their gluten-containing counterparts, and unless you're among the less than 1 percent of people with celiac disease, there's no point in coughing up the extra dough. Gluten-free pastries and breads don't necessarily have fewer calories or more nutrients than regular products. A 2006 study published in the *American Journal of Gastroenterology* followed a group of gluten-free dieters with celiac disease for 2 years and discovered that 81 percent of them actually gained weight.

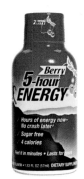

5-Hour Energy

There's a lot of hype about this bottle, but the only ingredient that provides any significant energy is caffeine, of which there are 135 grams in each bottle. That's less than you'd find in a 14-ounce cup of coffee (a Dunkin' Donuts 14-ounce medium has about 164 grams of caffeine). Cost for a cup of coffee: A buck or two. Cost for 5-Hour Energy: $3 to $4.

Tenderloin Steak

This is consistently one of the most expensive cuts of beef, but all you're buying is a little bit of tenderness. In fact, tenderloin isn't a particularly flavorful steak. So why does it cost so much? Because there aren't many tenderloin steaks on a cow, and because demand from diners looking for beef that cuts like butter tends to be high. Switch to skirt or flank steak instead. They're both lean cuts that pack far more rich, deep, beefy flavor. Marinate for at least 4 hours in a 50-50 solution of balsamic vinegar and soy and you'll have a steak you can cut with a spoon. Most importantly, it will cost you about half of what you would pay for that tenderloin. Remember this next time you're at the steakhouse, too.

Anything with a Cartoon on the Box

You know there's trouble when a food needs a mascot. A grinning cartoon character on the front of a box is a surefire sign of two things: 1) The box is filled mostly with cheap carbohydrates, and 2) most of the money you spend on it will end up in the pockets of marketers. See the Post Golden Crisp box here? The mascot on the front is known as Sugar Bear, which explains why more than half the calories come from sugar. This box is like a billboard for obesity.

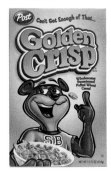

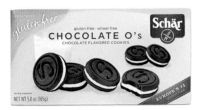

5 Diet Foods Not Worth a Dime

1

Quaker Instant Oatmeal Raisins & Spice
(1 packet)

150 calories
2 g fat
(0 g saturated)
14 g sugars

Somebody at the FDA must have been sleeping the day Quaker was approved to carry the oversized heart-health logo on its box. Sure, it's low in saturated fat and cholesterol, but it has more sugar than a bowl of Lucky Charms. Your best bet is to stick with Quaker's Old Fashioned oats and sweeten it yourself with fruit, but if you're set on the single-serving packets, go with the Lower Sugar variety. It packs in the fiber with a fraction of the sugar.

2

Yoplait Original 99% Fat Free Strawberry
(170 g, 1 container)

170 calories
1.5 g fat
(1 g saturated)
26 g sugars

Of all dubious label claims, "99% fat free" may be the most misleading; its presence on a package all but guarantees a profusion of added sugars. Just look at Yoplait's ingredients list to see the true picture. After milk, sugar is the first ingredient. Scroll down and you'll find high-fructose corn syrup, too. All told, you have more sugar here than a pack of Twix candy bars. We'll take a bit of fat over a load of sugar anyday.

3

Breyers Carb Smart Almond Bar
(1 bar)

180 calories
15 g fat
(10 g saturated)
5 g sugars

The fact that this bar has only 5 grams of sugar is commendable, but the fact that it contains half your day's saturated fat limit is not. It's a classic bait-and-switch: market a product as being low in one macronutrient (low carb!), then clobbering it with another while consumers have their guard down. Instead, look for a treat like Klondike that puts caps on both sugar and fat; cutting back on both will always be your best weight-loss strategy.

4
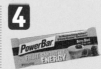

PowerBar Fruit Energize Berry Blast
(1 bar)

210 calories
3.5 g fat
(0.5 g saturated)
24 g sugars

Not only does it contain virtually zero fiber, but also the first ingredient is evaporated cane juice, otherwise known as sugar. Unfortunately, this is just but one of a long line of lackluster offerings from PowerBar. Switch to Kashi's GoLean Crunchy! and you'll earn a touch more protein and a ton more fiber. Plus, you'll drop your sugar load by almost half.

5

Arnold Whole Grains Health Nut
(2 slices)

240 calories
4 g fat
(0 g saturated)
4 g fiber

Don't blow your calories on the bread; save them for the delicious, nutrient-dense stuff you're going to stuff inside. Arnold's Whole Grains Health Nut earns the Worst Bread distinction by being high in calories and carrying a load of refined flour. Make your sandwiches on Nature's Own Double Fiber Wheat instead and you'll eliminate 140 calories and more than double your fiber intake.

Eat This Instead!
Quaker Lower Sugar Apples & Cinnamon

(1 packet)

110 calories
1.5 g fat
(0 g saturated)
6 g sugar

Eat This Instead!
Fage Total 2% Strawberry

(150 g, 1 container)

140 calories
2.5 g fat
(1.5 g saturated)
16 g sugars

Eat This Instead!
Klondike No Sugar Added Ice Cream Sandwiches

(1 sandwich)

100 calories
2 g fat
(1 g saturated)
3 g sugars

Eat This Instead!
Kashi GoLean Crunchy! Chocolate Caramel

(1 bar)

150 calories
3 g fat
(2 g saturated)
14 g sugars

Eat This Instead!
Nature's Own Double Fiber Wheat

(2 slices)

100 calories
1 g fat
(0 g saturated)
10 g fiber

The World's Healthiest $50 Shopping Cart

It's a common indictment against healthy foods: They cost too much. It's too expensive to eat healthy. In fact, a 2007 report out of the University of Washington found that healthy foods cost 10 times as much as junk foods. But here's the problem:

The study factored cost in terms of "calories." But your body doesn't want calories—it wants nutrients. In actual numbers, the study found that you'd pay $3.52 for 2,000 calories of nutritionally bankrupt boxed foods, but $36.32 for 2,000 calories of wholesome grub. That makes the bad stuff sound like a bargain, but remember: The $3.52 foods will make you fat and put you at greater risk for heart disease, diabetes, cancer, and other diseases. That won't seem like such a bargain when you see your health care bill.

Another flaw of the study: The shoppers weren't instructed to bargain shop for their healthy foods. Had they known what foods to buy—those that deliver fat nutritional packages with the leanest possible price tags—they would have fared far better. And that's what we've done here—prepared a $50 cart that will load your diet with days' worth of protein-, fiber-, and antioxidant-charged meals. In other words, a true bargain.

Avocado
($1.50)

Per 1/4 avocado:
80 calories
7.5 g fat
(1 g saturated)
3.5 g fiber

More than 50 percent of this fruit's fat comes from oleic acid, the kind found in olive oil, which has been shown to increase our absorption of fat-soluble nutrients like vitamins A and E. Dice with mango, onions, and cilantro for a quick salsa for grilled fish and chicken, or use it in place of mayo on your sandwich.

Lindt Excellence 85% Cocoa Bar
($2.69)

Per 40 g:
230 calories
18 g fat
(11 g saturated)
6 g fiber

When it comes to serious indulgence, you could do a lot worse. Dark chocolate contains resveratrol, the cancer-fighting compound in red wine. That's not to overlook the surprising 6 grams of fiber per serving. Eat a few pieces plain for dessert or use this bar as a substitute for milk chocolate in baking.

Fage Total 2%
(7 oz, $1.69)

150 calories
4 g fat
(3 g saturated)
8 g sugars
20 g protein

There is as much protein in this yogurt as in a can of tuna. Mix in your own berries to tame the tang or use it as a substitute for sour cream atop your favorite Mexican dish.

Red Bell Pepper
($1.99)

37 calories
0 g fat
2.5 g fiber
1 g protein

There's a reason red bell peppers cost more than green: They're nutritionally jacked. Compared to the green peppers, the red variety have twice the vitamin C and 10 times the vitamin A. Slice one up to use as a shoveling device for hummus or salsa, or add to penne pasta with grilled chicken, green beans and pesto.

Sirloin Steak
(8 oz, $2.50)

400 calories
11 g fat
(4 g saturated)
69 g protein

With far less fat than rib eye or porterhouse, sirloin gives you more protein for your dollar. The bonus is that it's loaded with zinc and vitamin B₁₂. Coat with crushed peppercorns and grill to your liking, or skewer steak chunks along with onions and bell peppers for a killer kabob.

Athenos Hummus Original
(7 oz, $3.49)

Per 1 oz:
50 calories
3 g fat
(0 g saturated)
1 g fiber
1 g protein

Little more than chickpeas, olive oil, sesame seeds, and garlic make this your go-to condiment. Smear it on sandwiches or set it out as a hunger-quashing dip with vegetables or crackers.

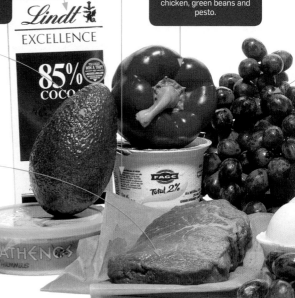

Red Grapes
($1.99 per pound)

Per cup:
105 calories
0 g fat
1.5 g fiber
1 g protein

The resveratrol found in grape skins has been shown to activate a longevity gene. Pop them straight from the bunch or put some in a cup of Greek yogurt for a protein-packed afternoon snack.

Garlic
(bulb, $0.50)

Per 3 cloves:
13 calories
0 g fat

The sulfur in these cloves can help expand blood vessels, keeping blood pressure in check. Allow chopped or minced garlic to sit for 10 minutes before cooking. According to research in the *Journal of Nutrition*, this preserves some of the healthful properties. Make a simple fresh salsa by mixing minced garlic with tomatoes, onions, cilantro, and fresh lime juice.

Apples
(5 small Gala, $2.00)

95 calories
0 g fat
4.5 g fiber

A flavonoid called quercetin reduces inflammation of all kinds, and the other polyphenols in apples have been shown to regulate blood sugar by inhibiting the enzymes that break down carbohydrates. Best part: You can throw it in your bag and, unlike peaches and pears, it won't turn mushy by day's end.

Yellow Onion
($0.60)

Per 1/4 onion:
10 calories
0 g fat
0.5 g fiber
0.5 g protein

Onions, like garlic, are in the allium family of vegetables, whose properties have been shown to decrease the risk of cancer. A 2002 study in the *Journal of the National Cancer Institute* specifically showed that they lowered the risk of prostate cancer for men, and choosing the yellow variety will save you cash at the register.

Eggs
(12 large, $1.79)

Per egg:
70 calories
4 g fat
(1.5 g saturated)
6 g protein

Eggs are welterweight fighters with nutritional knockout capabilities. Chief among their nutritional perks is choline, a vitamin B–like nutrient that studies say could help increase your brain's capabilities regarding learning and memory. Scramble them with spinach, mushrooms and goat cheese, or drop a fried egg on a turkey sandwich to break the lunchtime doldrums.

Odwalla Original Super Protein Bar
($0.99)

210 calories
4.5 g fat
(1 g saturated)
4 g fiber
14 g protein

With 14 grams of protein, 4 grams of fiber, and half a multivitamin's worth of nutrients, this bar is sure to keep you satisfied until your next meal. Keep one in your gym bag for postworkout recovery, or unwrap it at the office to combat waning energy.

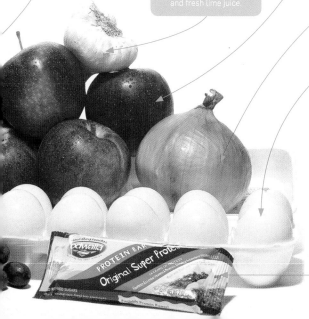

43

The World's Healthiest $50 Shopping Cart > Packaged Goods

Spinach
(frozen, 1 lb, $1.00)

Per 2 cups:
90 calories
1.5 g fat
9 g fiber
11 g protein

Spinach is among the world's best sources of folate, which protects against mental degeneration and age-related sexual issues. Fresh spinach is great, but it's pricey and a whole bunch wilts away into a small pile as soon as it touches a pan. Opt instead for frozen spinach—picked at the height of the season and flash frozen, it gives you more nutritional bang for your buck. Sauté a whole bag in olive oil with thinly sliced garlic and red pepper flakes, then use that as a side to grilled meat or fish, as a sandwich or pizza topping, or as a way to boost the benefits of a scrambled egg breakfast.

Bird's Eye Broccoli Florets
(frozen, 14 oz, $3.19)

Per cup:
30 calories
0 g fat
2 g fiber
1 g protein

For 30 calories, you get 2 grams of fiber, a gram of protein, a bevy of vitamins and minerals, and the phytonutrient sulforaphane, which research suggests has powerful antioxidant properties. Thaw, toss with olive oil and grated Parmesan cheese, and roast in a 450°F oven for 12 minutes. Spritz with lemon and serve.

Muir Glen Organic Diced Tomatoes
(28 oz, $2.59)

Per ½ cup:
30 calories
0 g fat
1 g fiber

A 10-year study from the University of California showed that organic tomatoes delivered nearly double the levels of two key flavonoids compared to conventionally grown. Add garlic and olive oil for marinara, or onion, cilantro and lime for salsa.

Quaker Quick-1 Minute Oats
(18 oz, $3.29)

Per ½ cup:
150 calories
3 g fat
(0.5 g saturated)
4 g fiber
5 g protein

Beta-glucan, a prominent fiber found in oatmeal, can help regulate blood sugar and keep you feeling full. Save cash by buying your Quaker unflavored and then adding berries, sliced almonds, and a small shot of maple syrup.

Blue Diamond Natural Oven Roasted Almonds Sea Salt
(8 oz, $4.29)

Per 1 oz, 24 nuts:
170 calories
15 g fat
(1 g saturated)
3 g fiber
6 g protein

An impressive 85 percent of almonds' calories come from protein, fiber, and heart-healthy unsaturated fats, and each serving contains a third of your daily vitamin E. Eat a handful by themselves or mix with raisins and dark chocolate for an antioxidant-rich treat.

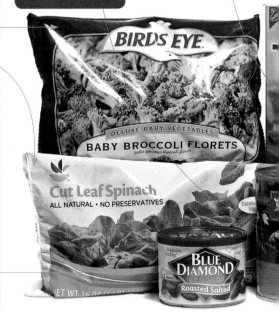

Triscuit Original
(9.5 oz, $2.99)

Per 28 g, 6 crackers:
120 calories
4 g fat
(0.5 g saturated)
3 g fiber
3 g protein

Triscuit is a cracker as a cracker should be: whole wheat with a touch of oil and salt. That gives you all the fiber and flavor you need to satisfy a snack craving. For more substantial hunger pangs, try dipping them in peanut butter or guacamole.

Dole Raspberries
(frozen, 12 oz, $4.49)

Per cup:
70 calories
1 g fat
9 g fiber
2 g protein

You pay the same amount for a 12 ounce bag of frozen raspberries that you would for 6 ounces of fresh. But the nutritional impact is the same—9 grams of fiber per serving and as many antioxidants as strawberries. Use them for giving a sweet-sour kick to yogurt or oatmeal.

Chicken of the Sea Pink Salmon Traditional Style
(14.75 oz, $3.69)

Per ¼ cup:
90 calories
5 g fat
(1 g saturated)
12 g protein

Each 90-calorie serving contains 625 percent of your recommended eicosapentaenoic acid (EPA) and docosa-hexaenoic acid (DHA) omega-3 fatty acids, and it costs at least 60 percent less than fresh fish. Replace the chicken in your chicken salad with salmon, or better yet, blend it with bread crumbs, onions, eggs, and parsley to form heart-healthy salmon burgers.

Bush's Black Beans
(15 oz, $1.39)

Per ½ cup:
105 calories
0.5 g fat
(0 g saturated)
6 g fiber

The antioxidant compound anthocyanin, which is responsible for this bean's dark exterior, has been linked to improved brain function and decreased erectile dysfunction in men. Cook with onions, bell peppers, garlic, and cumin for a tasty side dish.

TOTAL COST: $50.84

Ronzoni Healthy Harvest Whole Grain Spaghetti
(13.25 oz, $2.19)

Per 1.9 oz, 56 g:
180 calories
1 g fat
(0 g saturated)
6 g fiber
7 g protein

Still skittish about whole-grain pasta? Get over it: This box packs in 6 grams of fiber while slashing 20 to 30 calories off the typical pasta load. Toss a boxful with a few generous scoops of bottled pesto and a pint of cherry tomatoes for an easy weeknight dinner.

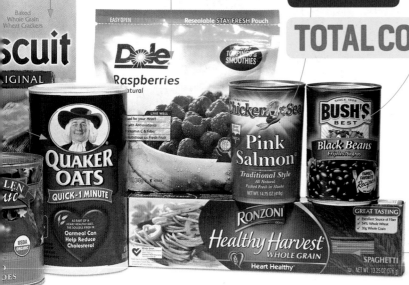

The Ultimate Brand Smackdown

WE SET 20 DISCRIMINATING TASTERS LOOSE ON THE LARGEST LABELS IN AMERICA TO ANSWER THE AGE-OLD QUESTION: DOES MORE EXPENSIVE FOOD TASTE BETTER?

You get what you pay for. At least, that's what we've been told since we were old enough to own wallets. But in an increasingly complicated, convoluted world—one where tomatoes come from Chile, asparagus from Peru, and cereals from chemists' labs—is it safe to equate quality with price? In these tough economic times, the question is more important than ever, and in order to answer it once and for all, we've pitted the top three category brand leaders against three top generic store brands—Wal-Mart's Great Value, Safeway, and Kroger—in a blind taste test of 10 of the most common supermarket staples. In it, we asked participants to rank each item on a scale between 1 and 10, which we then averaged for a final score. What did we find out? Our surprising results show exactly where it pays off to pay up—and where you can afford to cut a few corners.

Peanut Butter

	1	2	3	4	5	6
	FIRST PLACE					LAST PLACE
		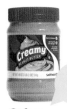		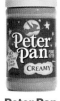		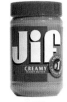
	WINNER!		**TIE!**			
	Kroger Creamy Peanut Butter	**Safeway Creamy Peanut Butter**	**Skippy Creamy**	**Peter Pan Creamy**	**Great Value Creamy Peanut Butter**	**Jif Creamy**
PRICE	$2.16 (18 oz)	$2.00 (18 oz)	$3.50 (16.3 oz)	$2.19 (16.3 oz)	$1.88 (18 oz)	$2.49 (18 oz)
COMMENTS	This peanut butter, thought to be Jif by one taster, was praised for its "nutty," "robust," and "roast-y" flavor.	Testers appreciated the smooth, "fluid" texture and "not too sweet" taste.	This boring butter was largely considered "mediocre," "standard," and "not overwhelmingly good... but not terrible either."	Tasters took offense to the "sticky" consistency and "average" quality.	Unimpressed tasters pronounced this butter "nothing special," and complained that it lacked a "real peanut-y taste."	The lowest ranking peanut butter, Jif was criticized as "too salty" and "muddy-tasting."
SCORE	7.1	6.5	6.5	6.2	5.5	5.2

Ketchup

	1	2	3	4	5	6
	FIRST PLACE					LAST PLACE

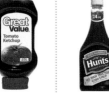

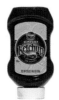

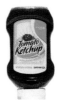

WINNER!

Great Value Tomato Ketchup	Hunt's Tomato Ketchup	Kroger Tomato Ketchup	Annie's Naturals Organic Ketchup	Safeway Tomato Ketchup	Heinz Tomato Ketchup
PRICE					
$1.18	$1.69	$1.79	$4.99	$1.99	$1.75
COMMENTS					
Wal-Mart's ketchup came in first, thanks to its "tomato-ey tanginess."	Hunt's product was described as "creamy" and "tart."	This middling, "standard" ketchup was thought to have a "bland" taste.	Though one bold taster lauded it as "spicy in a good way," this organic option generally received low scores.	Safeway's ketchup was found to be "way too sweet," with one taster complaining that it tasted "like artificial sweeteners."	In possibly the biggest upset of the test, Heinz's "way too vinegary" ketchup came in dead last.
SCORE					
6.8	6.7	6.0	5.7	3.0	2.7

Baked Beans

1	2	3	4	5	6
FIRST PLACE					LAST PLACE

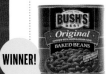

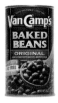

WINNER!

Bush's Original Baked Beans	Van Camp's Original Baked Beans	Great Value Baked Beans	Kroger Baked Beans	B&M's Original Baked Beans	Safeway Baked Beans

PRICE

$1.29	$1.99	$1.38	$1.19	$1.39	$1.50

COMMENTS

Many tasters were able to accurately identify these "flavorful," "non-mushy" beans as Bush's.	Van Camp's product earned points for being both "smoky" and "sweet."	Participants considered this can "pretty regular" and "run-of-the-mill," but "not barbecue quality."	Tasters found fault with the "tin-can taste" of these average beans.	Testers complained that these "nasty" beans suffered from an "odd," "off" flavor.	Safeway struck out with these "weak," "soupy" beans.

SCORE

6.2	6.0	5.8	5.7	5.0	4.8

Oatmeal

1	**2**	**3**	**4**	**5**	**6**
FIRST PLACE					LAST PLACE
WINNER!		TIE!			
Great Value 100% Whole Grain Old Fashioned Oats	**Safeway Quick Oats**	**McCann's Steel-Cut Irish Oatmeal**	**Bob's Red Mill Old Fashioned Rolled Oats, Whole Grain**	**Quaker Oats, Old Fashioned**	**Kroger Quick Oats**

PRICE

$1.58	**$1.99**	**$7.79**	**$2.69**	**$1.99**	**$1.89**

COMMENTS

Great Value's "solid" grains are "the way oatmeal should taste," according to our testers.	These oats had "good flavor," but lost points for "thinness" and "flakiness."	McCann's oats were praised for their "rich," "hearty texture."	These oats were deemed "unimpressive" and "papery."	Quaker's popular oats were commended for their "hearty," "solid" texture, but lost points for being "not at all creamy."	Kroger held the lowest score thanks to having "not a lot of flavor" and a "soupy consistency."

SCORE

7.5	**6.5**	**6.5**	**6.0**	**5.3**	**4.3**

Jelly

				5	
FIRST PLACE					LAST PLACE
		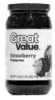			
WINNER! Kroger Strawberry Jam	Safeway Strawberry Preserves	Great Value Strawberry Preserves	Smucker's Strawberry Preserves	Welch's Strawberry Spread	Bonne Maman Strawberry Preserves

PRICE

$2.89	$2.50	$1.88	$2.39	$3.39	$4.69

COMMENTS

Kroger triumphed, thanks to "lots of fruit chunks" and a "full," "deep taste."	Safeway was applauded for their "yummy" preserves, which "tasted homemade" and like the "real deal."	Tasters complained that these preserves were "very sweet," but would maybe be "good for PB&J."	Tasters disapproved of the "bland" taste, but were mainly concerned by the "suspiciously consistent texture."	This spread was faulted for being "too sweet" and "tasting fake."	The most expensive jar we tested, Bonne Maman came in dead last thanks to being "way too sweet."

SCORE

7.4	6.6	6.1	5.7	5.0	4.6

Almonds

1 FIRST PLACE

WINNER!

Planters Roasted Almonds

2

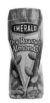

Emerald Dry Roasted Almonds

3

Kroger Almonds

4

Safeway Whole Almonds

5

Blue Diamond Almonds Whole Almonds

6 LAST PLACE

Great Value Whole Natural Almonds

PRICE					
$6.98	$5.99	$1.89	$2.29	$2.79	$5.98

COMMENTS					
Planters was praised for its "deep roasted flavor" and "nice crunch," and especially for being "not too salty."	Tasters applauded these almonds for their "mellow," "nutty" flavor.	Most took no offense to Kroger's almonds, but some criticized them as having a "harsh flavor" and "gummy texture."	Safeway's "basic" nuts were cited as "plain-tasting" with "little flavor."	Tasters reported that these "had a nice crunch," but were "dull-tasting" and "stale."	Testers found that Great Value's nuts were "dry" and "very stale."

SCORE					
6.3	6.2	5.8	5.5	5.1	4.6

Tuna

1	**2**	**3**	**4**	**5**	**6**
FIRST PLACE					LAST PLACE
WINNER!	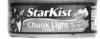				
Great Value Solid White Albacore Tuna in Water	**StarKist Chunk Light in Water**	**Kroger Chunk Light in Water**	**Chicken of the Sea Chunk White in Water**	**Safeway Chunk Light in Water**	**Bumble Bee Chunk Light in Water**

PRICE					
$1.18	$0.83	$0.69	$1.55	$0.50	$0.75

COMMENTS					
Wal-Mart trounced the competition with this "clean-tasting," "not fishy" can.	Tasters reported "good flaky texture" and a "nice fish flavor."	Kroger's can was deemed "unremarkable" and "dull," and had a "pulpy texture."	Tasters found fault with this "dry" can that "lacked body."	Safeway's "dry" tuna failed to impress, thanks to its "dull," "tasteless" flavor.	Tasters skewered this as "awful," with one even proclaiming it to be "probably the worst thing I've tasted in the last month."

SCORE					
8.0	6.0	4.8	4.2	3.6	2.5

Tomatoes

1 FIRST PLACE	**2**	**3**	**4**	**5**	**6** LAST PLACE
Del Monte Diced Tomatoes	**Muir Glen Organic Diced Tomatoes**	**Safeway Diced Peeled Tomatoes**	**Hunt's Petite Diced Tomatoes**	**Great Value Diced Tomatoes**	**Kroger Petite Diced Tomatoes**

TIE!

PRICE					
$1.09	$1.79	$0.80	$1.09	$0.68	$0.70

COMMENTS					
Tasters reported that these had a "strong tomato flavor," but were "not distractingly pungent."	These organic tomatoes were found to be "pleasant" and "sweet," with one taster commenting that they would be "great for sauce."	Most of our tasters found these to be "acceptable," but complained that they tasted "too salty."	Tasters took exception with the "fruity," "funny" taste of these tomatoes.	These "tin-like" tomatoes were panned as "tasting old" and "musty."	Tasters were "not loving" this can, which they criticized as "tasteless."

SCORE					
5.7	5.7	5.6	4.6	3.6	3.4

Pasta

1	**2**	**3**	**4**	**5**	**6**
FIRST PLACE					LAST PLACE

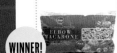

Kroger Elbow Macaroni	Great Value Elbows	Barilla Elbows	Safeway Elbow Macaroni	De Cecco Zita Cut	Ronzoni Elbows
			PRICE		
$1.19	$1.06	$2.39	$1.49	$2.59	$1.89
			COMMENTS		
Our tasters raved about this "rich," "springy" macaroni that "would taste great with just butter."	Great Value scored points with these "firm," "chewy" noodles that tasters praised as "lighter-tasting than the others."	Barilla's elbows were deemed "substantial," "solid," and "flavorful."	While our tasters found Safeway's pasta to be "decent enough" overall, most agreed that it "tasted cheap."	Despite being "chewy," De Cecco was considered by most to be "not horrible, but not great."	Tasters protested Ronzoni's "way too chewy," "gummy" texture.
			SCORE		
5.7	5.6	5.1	4.8	4.6	4.1

WINNER!

Coffee

1	**2**	**3**	**4**	**5**	**6**
FIRST PLACE					LAST PLACE
Safeway Breakfast Blend	**Starbucks Breakfast Blend**	**Maxwell House Breakfast Blend**	**Private Selection** (Kroger) Gourmet Coffee, Breakfast Blend	**Sam's Choice (Great Value) Breakfast Blend**	**Folger's Breakfast Blend**

WINNER!

PRICE					
$7.99	$7.49	$4.29	$8.19	$5.48	$3.79

COMMENTS					
Tasters praised Safeway's blend as "not bitter at all," citing it as "great for a dinner coffee."	The iconic coffeehouse's bagged blend was found to be "mild and pleasant," but "a tad bitter" by tasters.	Maxwell's "boring" beans were considered "aftertaste-y" and "bland."	Kroger's blend, while "inoffensive," was called out as "weak."	This "very weak," "plastic-y" coffee prompted a taster to ask, "Who put brown food coloring in my water?"	Tasters universally panned this low-priced option.

SCORE					
6.0	4.5	4.1	2.5	2.1	1.6

10 Amazing Meals for Under $10

Among the dozens of excuses people offer up when asked why they don't cook ("I'm too tired after work," "It's too complicated," "My dog ate my spatula"), the most puzzling is one we've been hearing all too often these days: It's too expensive.

Clearly a bit of context is needed: Four Big Mac Extra Value Meals will run you about $22 and will collectively provide thousands of relatively nutrition-devoid calories. Dinner at Outback or Olive Garden will cost about four times as much and deliver twice as many calories (if you're lucky).

To prove to people just how easy it is to cook fast, healthy, affordable meals at home, we've created 10 delicious recipes, all of which can be done in under 20 minutes, all of which cost less than $10 total. And all of which are a firm reminder that the best place to save money and shed pounds is in the kitchen.

Eat This!
Green Eggs & Ham

Anthony Bourdain famously wrote in his restaurant tell-all *Kitchen Confidential* that the hollandaise used to top eggs Benedict is a breeding ground for bacteria. "Nobody I know has ever made hollandaise to order. And how long has that Canadian bacon been festering in the walk-in?" If that's not enough to dissuade you, how about the fact that the sauce is made from pure egg yolks and melted butter? We've shaken Benedict up a bit, replacing the bacon with prosciutto, adding roasted red peppers for sweetness, and, most crucially, ditching the hollandaise in favor of a pesto-yogurt sauce to drizzle over the top.

Main Ingredients

 + + 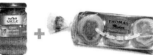 +

8 slices prosciutto, cooked ham, or cooked Canadian bacon:
Save money on prosciutto by opting for more affordable domestic brands and asking the counter person to slice it superthin—its flavor still shines.

2 Tbsp prepared pesto:
One of the best instant flavor boosters you can keep in your fridge. Toss a few tablespoons with cooked pasta and cherry tomatoes, or mix with mayonnaise for a bold sandwich spread.

4 Thomas' Light Multi-Grain English Muffins, toasted:
No muffin in the market packs more fiber (8 grams) in fewer calories (100), instantly converting this decadent breakfast into a potent hunger killer.

¼ cup bottled roasted red peppers, sliced:
Or roast your own red bell peppers in a 400°F oven until the skin blackens, about 30 minutes. Once cool, peel off the blistered skin and use as needed. Keeps for up to 10 days.

$(\Psi + \mathbf{l})^2$

MEAL MULTIPLIER

The creamy texture of Greek yogurt serves as the perfect base for savory sauces, and the sharp lactic tang proves more flavorful than traditional sauce bases like mayo, cheese, and oil. Try mixing a cup of plain Greek yogurt with any of the following ingredients for a killer on-the-spot sauce.

- Minced garlic, chopped parsley, olive oil, lemon juice (great with grilled chicken; see page 64)
- Sun-dried tomatoes, olives, fresh basil, olive oil (doubles as a sauce and a dip for pitas)
- Blue cheese, chives, lemon juice (a low-cal replacement for blue cheese dressing)

How to Make It:

- Bring 3" of water to a boil in a large sauté pan or saucepan. Turn down the heat to maintain a bare simmer and add the vinegar. One at a time, crack each egg into a shallow cup and gently slide it into the water. Cook the eggs until the whites are just firm and the yolks are still runny, about 3 minutes, then use a slotted spoon to move the eggs to a plate.

- In a small bowl, mix together the pesto and yogurt. Top each English muffin half with a slice of meat, a few red pepper slices, and a poached egg. Season with a bit of salt and cracked black pepper. Divide the pesto-yogurt sauce among the eggs. Makes 4 servings.

You'll Also Need:
8 eggs
1 Tbsp white vinegar
2 Tbsp plain Greek yogurt
Salt and cracked black pepper to taste

TOTAL COST $8.36

390 calories
18 g fat (6 g saturated)
960 mg sodium

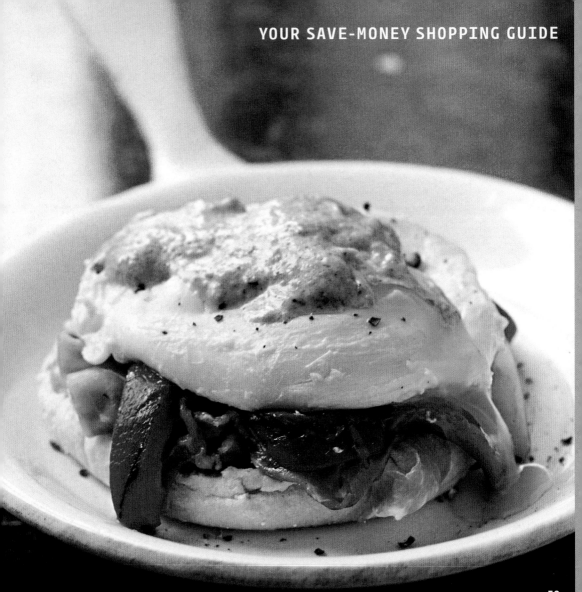

Penne alla Vodka

This Italian-American staple differs from a classic bowl of pasta marinara in two ways: First, the addition of cream, giving the sauce its orangish hue and rich taste. Some recipes call for up to a cup of fatty dairy, but we find that too much cream kills the bright tomato taste (and any chance of a healthy dinner). The second difference, of course, is the reliance on a couple of slugs of hooch to liven things up. Don't drink? Don't worry. All of the alcohol burns off, leaving behind a delicious whisper of grainy goodness.

Main Ingredients

 + + +

12 oz Ronzoni Smart Taste Penne Rigate:
Most whole-wheat pastas have the taste and texture of sand, but Ronzoni manages to pack 5 grams of fiber into a serving of penne that tastes just like the noodles you're used to.

1 can (28 oz) Muir Glen Organic Crushed Tomatoes:
Our team of crack tomato tasters in our Ultimate Brand Smackdown (see page 54) singled out Muir Glen as being especially great for tomato sauce.

¼ cup vodka:
High-end vodkas with huge price tags have flooded the American market, but a blind tasting panel from the New York Times found that humble, $10 Smirnoff beat out the other 20 bottles "hands down."

Parmesan cheese:
Ditch that cheeselike powder in the green can and pick up a hunk of Parmigiano-Reggiano, real Italian Parmesan aged for a minimum of 12 months. It's pricey, but a $10 block will last for months.

Upgrade ★

How to Make It:

- Bring a pot of water to a boil and cook the pasta according to the package directions, until al dente.

- While the water boils, heat the olive oil in a large saucepan over medium heat. Add the onion and garlic and sauté until lightly browned, about 3 to 4 minutes. Stir in the tomatoes and the red pepper and turn the heat down so the sauce lightly simmers. Add the vodka and continue simmering.

- Drain the pasta. Stir the heavy cream and basil into the sauce and season with salt and black pepper to taste. Add the pasta directly to the sauce and toss to combine. Serve with the cheese. Makes 4 servings.

You'll Also Need:

1 Tbsp olive oil

1 small onion, finely chopped

4 cloves garlic, minced

Pinch of crushed red pepper

2 Tbsp heavy cream

½ cup chopped fresh basil

Salt and ground black pepper to taste

NUTRITIONAL

Pasta dishes falter most often not because of an excess of calories, but because of a lack of substantive nutrition. To get more out of red sauce dishes like this, consider adding any of the following ingredients to the mix to power up your next plate of pasta.

- 8 ounces of grilled or shredded rotisserie chicken

- 8 ounces of sliced button or cremini mushrooms added to the pan along with the onions and garlic at the beginning of cooking

- 8 cups of baby spinach in place of the basil, stirred in with the pasta and sauce at the final moment until just wilted

TOTAL COST $8.17

490 calories
10 g fat
(3 g saturated)
580 mg sodium

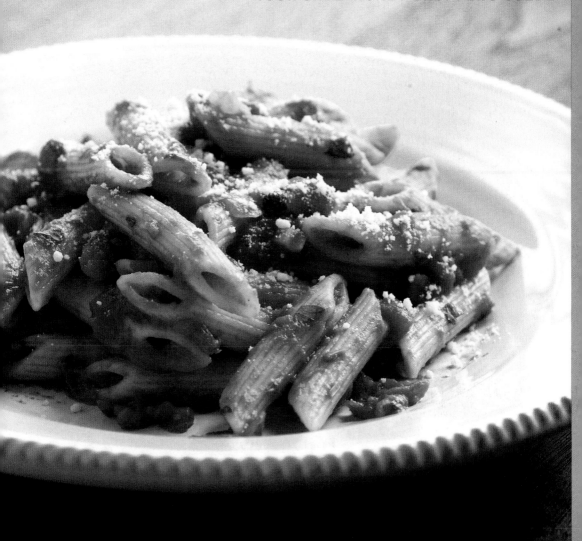

Eat This!
Chicken & Sweet Potato Stir-Fry

If the popularity of takeout staples like General Tso's, sweet and sour pork, and orange chicken has shown us anything, it's that Americans like their Chinese food with a heavy hit of sweetness. Nothing wrong with that, as long as that sweetness comes from reputable sources and is balanced with plenty of fresh vegetables. In this unconventional but hugely satisfying stir-fry, orange juice and sweet potatoes contribute a perfect amount of natural sugar while a squeeze of chili sauce and a shake of soy balance the sweet-spicy-salty interplay.

Main Ingredients

 + + +

1 large sweet potato, peeled and sliced into ⅛" rounds:
While not a typical stir-fry ingredient by any means, sliced sweet potatoes add a nice touch of natural sugar, plus hits of fiber and beta-carotene, to the mix.

¾ cup orange juice:
Fresh OJ makes a good base for sauces because it boasts a lovely balance of sweetness and acidity.

1 Tbsp cornstarch:
Whereas European chefs typically thicken sauces by reducing, Chinese cooks mix their stir-fry liquids with cornstarch to create a sauce that clings perfectly to proteins and vegetables.

½ Tbsp chili sauce, such as sriracha:
In the 5 years since we started writing these books, sriracha has gone from being an obscure condiment to a ubiquitous staple in the international sections of major supermarkets.

You'll Also Need:

½ pound green beans, trimmed

1 Tbsp low-sodium soy sauce

1 Tbsp canola or peanut oil

1 medium onion, chopped

2 cloves garlic, minced

1 Tbsp minced fresh ginger

1 lb boneless, skinless chicken thighs, cut into ½" pieces

How to Make It:

- Bring a large saucepan of salted water to boil. Add the sweet potato and cook for 3 minutes. Add the green beans and continue cooking for another 3 to 4 minutes, until the potatoes and green beans are just tender. Drain and set aside.

- In a small mixing bowl, combine the orange juice, cornstarch, soy sauce, and chili sauce and whisk to thoroughly incorporate. Reserve.

- Heat the oil in a wok or large sauté pan over high heat until the oil is lightly smoking. Add the onions, garlic, and ginger and cook until lightly browned, using a metal spatula to keep the ingredients in near-constant motion. Add the chicken and cook until lightly browned on the outside and nearly cooked through, about 3 minutes. Add the green beans, potatoes, and orange juice mixture to the wok and cook until the liquid thickens and clings lightly to the chicken and vegetables. Taste, adding a pinch of salt and pepper if necessary. Serve over steamed rice. Makes 4 servings.

TOTAL COST $7.67

300 calories
13 g fat
(2.5 g saturated)
310 mg sodium

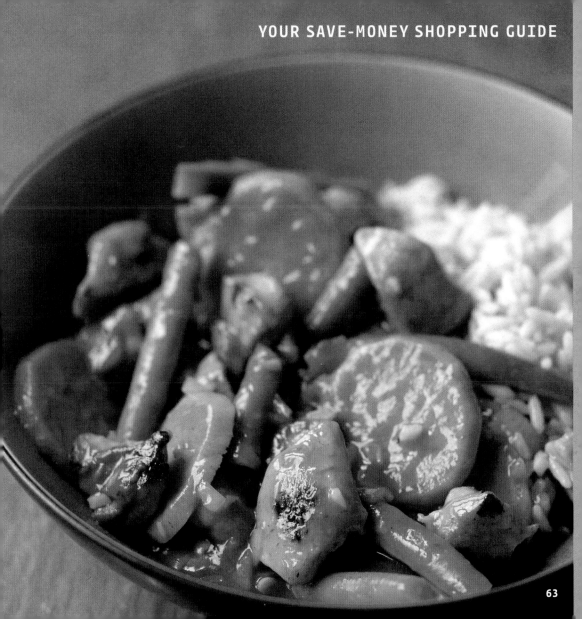

Grilled Chicken Gyro

From the bustling avenues of Midtown Manhattan to the back-alley food stalls of Istanbul, gyros have long been one of the world's most beloved street foods. It's hard to argue that the popularity isn't due: warm pitas overflowing with grilled meat and crisp vegetables, all tied together with a slew of vibrant sauces. This recipe will give you the core components needed for a serious gyro, but we implore you to load your pita up with plenty of fixings: fresh sliced tomatoes and onions, a shake of hot sauce, a swipe of hummus—it's hard to go wrong.

Main Ingredients

 + 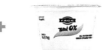 +

1 lb boneless, skinless chicken thighs, cut into ½" pieces:
Chicken breasts work just fine here, but we prefer thighs for two reasons: First, they emerge juicier and more flavorful from the high-heat grilling. Second, they cost about half as much as the more popular breasts.

1 ½ cups Greek yogurt:
Yogurt does double-duty here, serving as the base for the cucumber sauce used to top the pitas as well as the foundation for the marinade. Yogurt is popular as a marinade for meat in the Middle East because the natural lactic acids help break down tough muscle fiber.

4 Food for Life Ezekiel 4:9 Prophet's Pocket Breads:
Of course, any solid whole-wheat pita will do, but we love Food for Life's because each pocket packs 7 grams of protein and 4 grams of fiber into just 100 calories—an impressive nutritional feat unmatched by other national bread makers.

You'll Also Need:

3 cloves garlic, minced

1 tsp cumin

½ tsp dried oregano

Juice of 1 lemon

Salt and ground black pepper

1 Tbsp olive oil

½ Tbsp red wine vinegar

1 cup peeled, seeded, and finely chopped cucumber

Recommended condiments

choose as many or as few as you see fit:

- Hummus
- Hot sauce
- Sliced tomatoes
- Chopped romaine
- Chopped cucumber
- Sliced onions
- Fresh chopped herbs like parsely, oregano, and basil

How to Make It:

- Combine the chicken with ½ cup of the yogurt, two-thirds of the minced garlic, and the cumin, oregano, and lemon juice, plus a few pinches each of salt and pepper, in a large mixing bowl. Cover with plastic and marinate in the refrigerator for at least 2 hours and up to 8.

- Preheat a grill or grill pan to medium. While it's heating, combine the remaining yogurt and garlic with the olive oil, vinegar, cucumber, and salt to taste in a medium bowl. Set it aside.

- Grill the chicken until it's lightly charred on each side and cooked all the way through, about 8 minutes on a hot grill. Remove it to a plate and set it aside. While the grill is still hot, lightly toast the pitas on it. After the chicken has rested for 5 minutes, slice it into strips and stuff it into the toasted pitas along with the yogurt sauce and any other condiments you choose. Makes 4 servings.

TOTAL COST $9.12

370 calories
10 g fat
(2.5 g saturated)
470 mg sodium

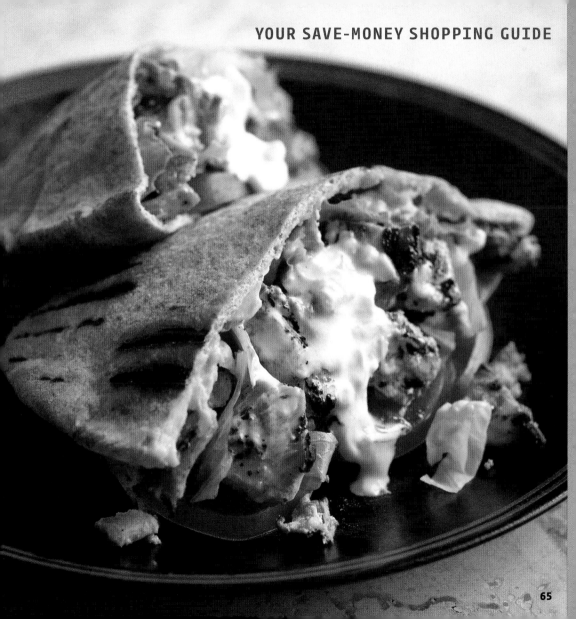

Grilled Mexican Pizza

The words Taco Bell and genius seldom meet in the same sentence, but it's hard to deny that the executive behind the invention of the Mexican Pizza was a savant of some kind. Its convergence of melted cheese, creamy beans, and peppery hot sauce represents one of the great creations of this modern fast-food era, but it also happens to be one of the Bell's most calorie- and sodium-saddled entrées. We lighten the load here by ditching the superfluous extra layer of tortilla, trading that weird crumbled beef for chunks of chicken chorizo, and going long on the good stuff like black beans and salsa.

Main Ingredients

 + + +

4 whole-wheat flour tortillas (8"):
We're not normally fans of the flour tortilla, but solid, fiber-packed flotillas are available nationwide these days. Look for anything made by La Tortilla Factory or Tumaro's Gourmet Tortillas, the top producers of healthy tortillas and wraps.

1 can (16 oz) refried black beans:
Refried black beans have a lovely earthy flavor and creamy texture that play perfectly on this pizza, but the more common pinto beans will do here as well. Add extra layers of flavor by stirring in a pinch of smoky cumin and squeezing in the juice of a lime.

2 links Al Fresco Chipotle Chorizo Chicken Sausage, diced:
We love the lean, precooked chicken chorizo links from Al Fresco, but raw chorizo will do, too. Just be sure to first remove it from its casing and sauté until it's cooked through, about 5 minutes.

Pickled jalapeño chili peppers (optional):
The perfect balance of sweet and heat. Save a few bucks by pickling them yourself: Combine thinly sliced chilies with equal parts water and apple cider vinegar, plus a few good pinches of salt and sugar. They're ready in 30 minutes.

You'll Also Need:

2 cups shredded low-fat pepper jack cheese

2 scallions, chopped, green and white parts separated

½ cup low-fat sour cream

Juice of 1 lime

1 cup bottled salsa

TOTAL COST $8.90

380 calories
13 g fat
(6 g saturated)
980 mg sodium

How to Make It:

- Preheat the oven to 400°F. Add a few tablespoons of water to the beans to thin them slightly, then divide them among the tortillas, spreading them out so they cover the surfaces evenly like tomato sauce on a pizza crust. Divide the cheese, chorizo, and scallion whites among the pizzas. Place the pizzas on baking sheets and cook until the bottoms are well toasted and the cheese is fully melted, about 12 to 15 minutes.

- In a small bowl, combine the sour cream with the lime juice and the scallion greens. Cut each pizza into six slices, drizzle with the sour cream, and serve with salsa and pickled jalapeños, if using. Makes 4 servings.

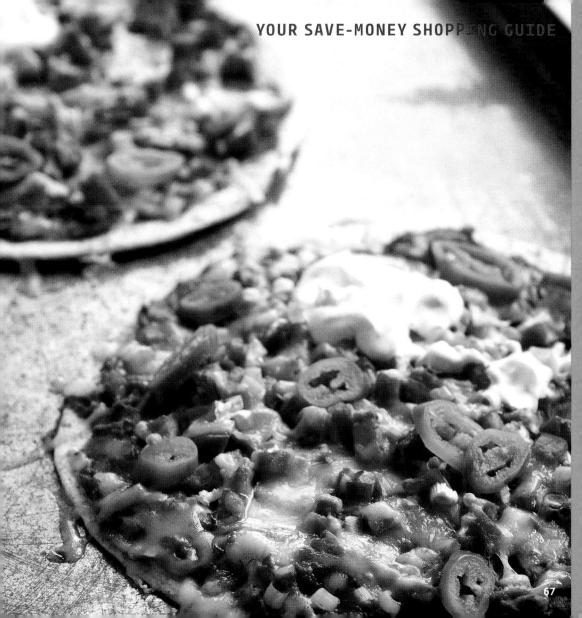

Bulgogi Skirt Steak

For decades, Chinese and Japanese foods have flourished in the United States while one of the great cuisines of Asia, Korean, has remained relatively obscure to most American diners. Thankfully, that's changing, as many a delicious Korean cornerstone is starting to find a home on menus across America. Bulgogi is one of those cornerstones, a Korean barbecue staple normally made with thinly sliced beef marinated in a heady bath of soy and sesame. We love the intense flavors, but we also love a more substantial cut of beef we can grill to a rosy medium-rare—hence the skirt steak.

Main Ingredients

 + **+**

1 lb skirt steak:
No cut of beef packs more flavor for less money than skirt. The acidic marinade help break down tough muscle fibers, turning skirt steak into an ideal cut of tender, beefy goodness. If you can't find skirt, try flank steak.

½ Tbsp sesame oil:
The toasted notes of sesame oil play a pivotal role in many Asian cuisines. Try a splash in your next stir fry, or combine 2 parts soy sauce with 1 part each sesame oil and rice wine vinegar for an all-purpose dipping sauce.

4 scallions, white and green parts separated and chopped:
The beauty of scallions is that a single 99-cent bunch gives you two unique components to play with: the sharp, oniony whites at the base, best for cooking process, and the mild green tops, best for garnishing.

How to Make It:

- Combine the skirt steak, sesame oil, garlic, soy sauce, vinegar, brown sugar, sesame seeds, scallion whites, and a few pinches of pepper in a sealable plastic bag. Marinate in the refrigerator for at least 2 hours and up to 12.

- Preheat a grill. When it is very hot, remove the steak from the marinade and place it on the grill. Cook until it is lightly charred on the outside but still tender through, about 3 minutes per side. Let the beef rest for at least 5 minutes before slicing it thinly across the natural grain of the meat. Serve it garnished with sesame seeds and scallion greens and alongside steamed rice and grilled vegetables. Makes 4 servings.

You'll Also Need:

4 cloves garlic, minced

2 Tbsp soy sauce

1 Tbsp rice wine vinegar

2 Tbsp brown sugar

½ Tbsp sesame seeds + additional for garnish

Ground black pepper to taste

TOTAL COST $8.18

230 calories
12 g fat
(4 g saturated)
240 mg sodium

LEFTOVER LOVE

In a strange turn of events, Korean-Mexican cuisine has helped fuel the recent American street food craze. And no Kore-Mex-fusion food truck would be complete without a roster of bulgogi-fueled treats. We suggest using any leftovers to make one or more of them.

- **Quesadilla:** Top a flour tortilla with shredded jack cheese, chopped scallions, and bulgogi. Fold and toast in a pan.

- **Tacos:** Combine bulgogi, sesame seeds, and a spoonful of kimchi (fermented cabbage) in warm corn tortillas.

- **Sliders:** Combine sliced bulgogi, cucumbers, and chili sauce on small buns slathered with hoisin sauce.

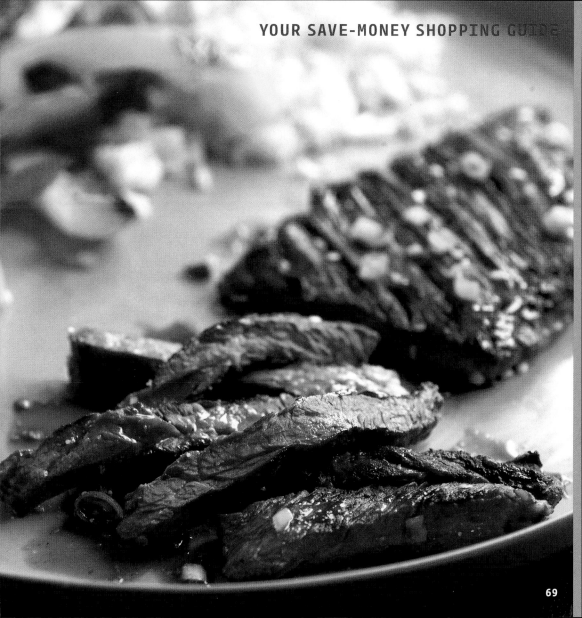

Eat This!

Blackened Tilapia with Garlic-Lime Butter

Ever eaten any blackened food that wasn't delicious (besides those steaks your dad scorches every year at the Fourth of July barbecue)? Neither have we. Consider it a bonus that blackening is actually an incredibly healthy way of cooking, giving the fish or meat a body armor of potent disease-fighting antioxidants in the form of tantalizing spices. Truth be told, the flavored butter here is the icing on the cake; if you have a great piece of fresh fish, just coat it with a bit of blackening spice, follow the cooking instructions, and maybe squeeze a lemon over the top.

Main Ingredients

 + +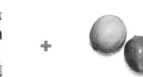

4 tilapia fillets (about 6 oz each):
Few fish are as versatile, widely available, and affordable as tilapia. According to the Monterey Bay Aquarium Seafood Watch, it's also one of the most ecologically responsible fish choices you can make.

1 Tbsp blackening seasoning:
Store-bought blackening spice is fine, but you can save money by making up your own at home. Mix equal parts salt, ground black pepper, cayenne, paprika, cumin, ground oregano, and garlic powder; it will keep for 3 months in your spice rack.

1 tsp lime zest + juice of 1 lime:
The zest of citrus fruits is rich with essential oils, meaning that it packs serious flavor—even more than the juice itself. Use the smallest holes on a cheese grater, or better yet, a Microplane to separate the zest from the pith (the white part) of the fruit.

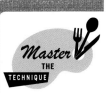

Master THE **TECHNIQUE**

Blackening

You can blacken fish or meat on the grill, but the best—and most traditional—way to get the full sear you want is in a scorching-hot cast-iron skillet. Heat a thin film of oil in the skillet over the highest possible heat (and turn on the hood or kitchen fan). When wisps of smoke begin to rise from the oil, carefully add the fish or meat. Don't touch it—whatever it may be—for at least 2 minutes; you want a dark crust to set in over the protein, and fiddling with the food will prevent this from happening. Cook for 75 percent of the time on one side, then flip and finish on the other.

How to Make It:

- Combine the butter, cilantro, garlic, lime zest, and lime juice in a small mixing bowl and stir to thoroughly blend. Set it aside.
- Heat the oil in a large cast-iron skillet or sauté pan over high heat. Rub the tilapia all over with the blackening spice. When the oil in the pan begins to lightly smoke, add the fish and cook, undisturbed, for 3 to 4 minutes on the first side, until the spice rub becomes dark and crusty. Flip and continue cooking for 1 to 2 minutes, until the fillets flake with gentle pressure from your finger.
- Transfer the fish to 4 serving plates and immediately top each with a bit of the flavored butter. Makes 4 servings.

You'll Also Need:

2 Tbsp butter, softened at room temperature

2 Tbsp chopped fresh cilantro

2 cloves garlic, finely minced

1 Tbsp canola oil

TOTAL COST $9.28

300 calories
14 g fat
(6 g saturated)
510 mg sodium

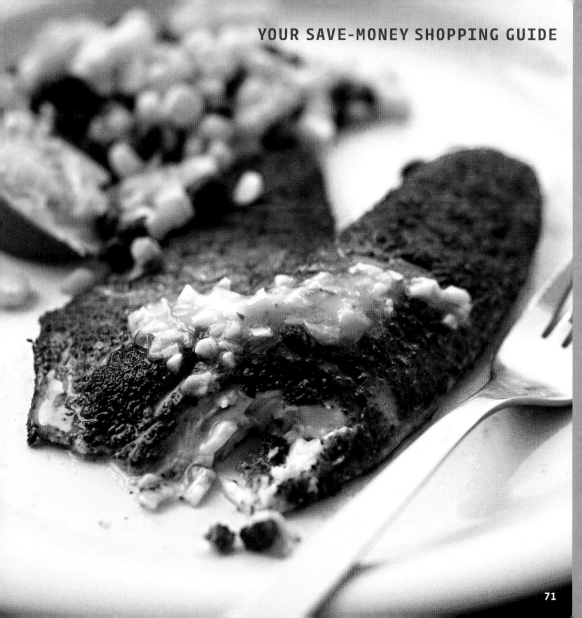

Eat This!
Chicken Tacos with Salsa Verde

Perhaps the greatest part about the modern supermarket is the ubiquity of rotisserie chicken. Juicy, healthy, and about $6 a pop, these beautiful birds make a great dinner served alongside roasted vegetables, but we also love to use the meat as the base for other inventions. Tossed with a good dose of bright, mildly spicy salsa verde, it makes the perfect filling for tacos, burritos, and even enchiladas. Indeed, there might not be a better use of a rotisserie chicken.

Main Ingredients

+
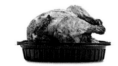
+

8 corn tortillas:
Traditionally made from just stone-ground corn and water, these tiny tortillas are vastly superior to their floppy flour- and-lard- constructed cousins.

3 cups shredded rotisserie chicken (about ¾ of a store-bought chicken):
Be sure to remove the skin first. As delicious as it may be, its finer points will be lost in the salsa-strewn meat itself, so you may as well save the calories.

1 ½ cups bottled salsa verde:
Salsa appears in hundreds of interpretations up and down Mexico, many with nary a tomato in sight. Salsa verde, made with tart tomatillos, relatives of the gooseberry, has a bright, acidic flavor and mild spice that pairs beautifully with grilled chicken and fish.

$$(\text{♜}+\text{♟})^2$$

MEAL MULTIPLIER

This two-ingredient mixture is simply too delicious to confine to tacos. Here are a few other ways to let it sing:

- Make enchiladas by rolling it into warm corn tortillas. Top with more salsa and Jack cheese and bake in a 400°F oven for 20 minutes.

- Grill romaine hearts until lightly wilted and top with the chicken mixture, toasted corn, and chopped tomatoes.

- Follow this recipe, but top with a fried egg and eat with a knife and fork— preferably for breakfast after a long night out.

How to Make It:

- Heat the tortillas in a large skillet or sauté pan until lightly toasted.
- Combine the chicken with the salsa in a large mixing bowl, then divide it evenly among the tortillas. Top with cheese, onion, and cilantro. Serve with the lime wedges. Makes 4 servings.

You'll Also Need:

½ cup crumbled Cotija or feta cheese

1 medium onion, finely chopped

1 cup chopped fresh cilantro

2 limes, quartered

TOTAL COST
$9.32

345 calories
12 g fat
(4.5 g saturated)
800 mg sodium

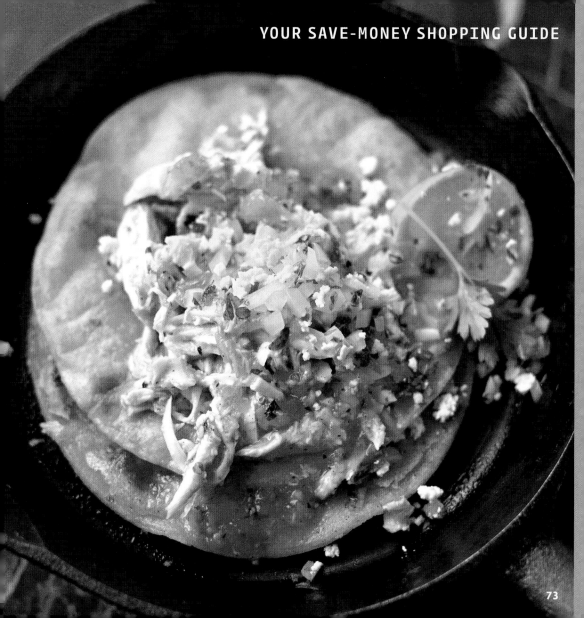

Poor Man's Steak with Garlicky Gravy

This country has fallen on lean times in recent years, but unfortunately the figurative belt-tightening doesn't seem to be accompanied by a literal one. That's because the most potent sources of calories and seasoning (oil, butter, sugar, salt) are still cheap and more common in restaurant cooking than ever. All the more reason to take to the kitchen! Here we turn inexpensive lean ground sirloin and cover it with a soy-spiked sauce good enough to make your doormat taste delicious. Serve this hot, decadent mess over a bed of mashed potatoes, or for a healthier sidekick, try spinach sautéed in olive oil and garlic.

Main Ingredients

1 lb ground sirloin, shaped into 4 equal patties:
Ground sirloin benefits from being both lean (it contains about 10 percent fat) and long on big, beefy flavor. Don't limit its use to standard burgers, though; it's also perfect for Italian meat sauces, chili, and, as seen here, a great steak alternative.

+

4 oz button or cremini mushrooms, stems removed, sliced:
Cremini mushrooms are also known as baby portabellas. They are nearly as cheap and widely available as standard white button mushrooms, but they have a deeper, earthy flavor that stands up well in this lusty gravy.

+

2 tsp Worcestershire sauce:
Outside of Bloody Marys, Worcestershire makes far too few appearances in the kitchen. It packs a huge dose of umami, that elusive "fifth" flavor group best described as savoriness. Try basting a steak or a burger with a 50-50 mix of Worcestershire and butter right after you pull it off the grill.

You'll Also Need:

½ Tbsp canola oil

Salt and ground black pepper to taste

1 yellow onion, sliced

2 cloves garlic, minced

½ Tbsp flour

½ cup beef or chicken stock

1 Tbsp ketchup

1 Tbsp low-sodium soy sauce

How to Make It:

- Preheat the oven to 200°F.

TOTAL COST $7.24

220 calories
9 g fat
(3 g saturated)
470 mg sodium

- Heat a large cast-iron skillet or sauté pan over medium-high heat. Season the patties all over with salt and pepper. Add the oil to the pan and cook until a nicely browned crust forms on the patties, about 3 to 4 minutes, then flip and continue cooking for another 3 to 4 minutes for medium-rare. Move the patties to a baking sheet and place in the oven to keep warm.

- Add the onion, garlic, and mushrooms to the same pan and cook until the vegetables begin to brown, about 5 to 7 minutes. Sprinkle the flour over the vegetables, stir so it coats them evenly, then add the stock and continue stirring to keep lumps from forming. Stir in the ketchup, soy sauce, and Worcestershire sauce and continue cooking until the gravy thickens, another 2 to 3 minutes. Serve the patties on beds of mashed potatoes or sautéed spinach (or both) with the gravy drizzled over the top. Makes 4 servings.

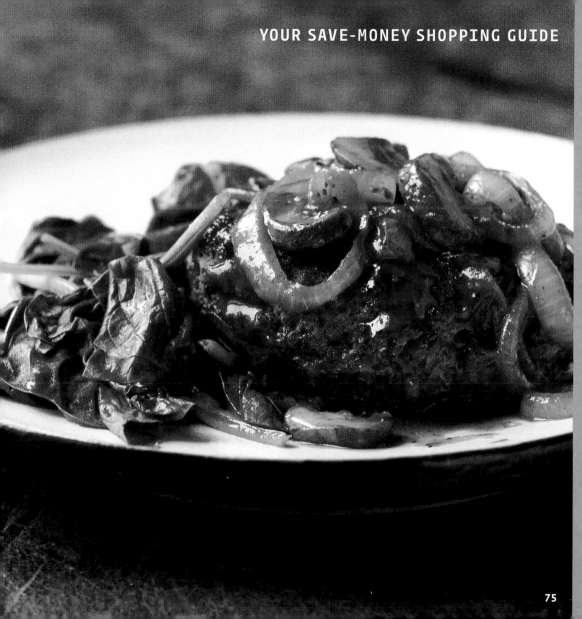

Eat This!
Vietnamese Pork Salad

Not all salads are built with a pile of lettuce. In Vietnam, where rice and rice-based products play a central role in all meals, a bed of thin, springy noodles often serves as the base for a mixture of juicy grilled pork, crisp vegetables, and fresh herbs. What you end up with is something akin to an Asian pasta salad, a low-calorie, high-nutrient bowl loaded with an incredible range of flavors and textures.

Main Ingredients

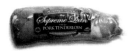 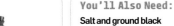

1 lb pork tenderloin:
Nearly as lean as boneless, skinless chicken breast, but with considerably more flavor. Add to that a reasonable price tag (about $5 a pound) and you can see why pork tenderloin is one of our favorite cuts of meat.

+

6 oz rice noodles, prepared according to package instructions:
Thicker noodles may be sold as pad thai noodles, the thinner, lighter noodles as vermicelli. In a pinch, angel hair will even do. Whatever your noodles may be, after cooking, keep them submerged in cold water until just before serving.

+

1 Tbsp chunky peanut butter:
Peanuts play the base for many a memorable sauce throughout Asia. Here, it's combined with sweet (honey), salty (soy), spicy (chili sauce), and sour (vinegar)—a full spectrum of flavors that tastes just as good slathered on grilled chicken as it does dressing this salad.

You'll Also Need:

Salt and ground black pepper to taste

1 Tbsp fish sauce or low-sodium soy sauce

2 Tbsp rice wine vinegar

1 Tbsp honey

1 tsp chili sauce, such as sriracha

1 medium cucumber, peeled, seeded, and sliced into half moons

2 medium carrots, cut into matchsticks

½ cup chopped fresh mint

Chopped peanuts for garnish (optional)

How to Make It:

- Preheat a grill or grill pan set over medium heat. Season the pork all over with salt and pepper. When the grill is hot, place the pork on the grates and cook for 5 to 6 minutes per side, until it's firm and springy to the touch. (A thermometer inserted into the thickest part of the loin should read 145°F). Allow the pork to rest for at least 5 minutes before slicing.

- While the pork is resting, whisk together the peanut butter, fish or soy sauce, vinegar, honey, and chili sauce in a medium bowl. If the mix is too thick, add a table-spoon or two of water to thin it out until it has the consistency of ranch dressing.

- Slice the pork into thin pieces. In a large bowl, combine the pork, noodles, cucumber, carrots, mint, and peanut dressing. Toss until all the ingredients are evenly coated. Divide among 4 plates or bowls and garnish with the chopped peanuts, if you like. Makes 4 servings.

TOTAL COST $9.84

340 calories
4.5 g fat (1 g saturated)
340 mg sodium

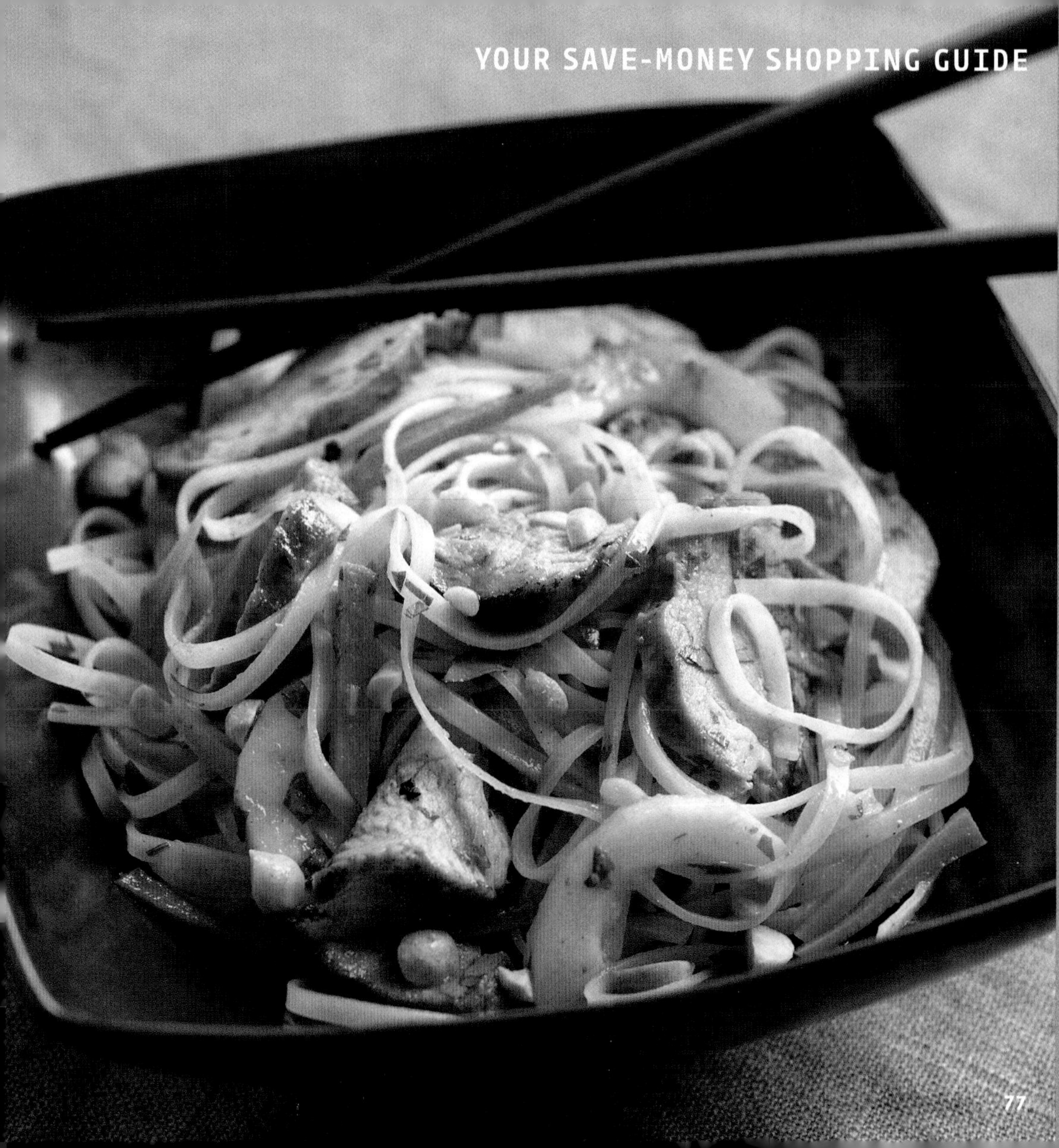

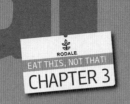

THE PRODUCE SECTION

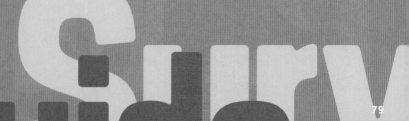

EAT THIS NOT THAT!

SUPERMARKET
SURVIVAL GUIDE

Pity the Poor Potato

Spuds have gotten nothing but bad press for years: They're still being held accountable for the Irish famine of the 1800s. (Totally not their fault, blame the British.) Their top media celebrity is a toy that can't keep track of his own facial features. And worst of all, their once-revered position in America's culinary heritage, playing the brains to beef's brawn on a plate of steak and potatoes, has been reduced to a greasy, ignominious existence inside a cardboard fast-food holder—or, more likely, somewhere under your car seat, covered in dust.

Indeed, so far has the mighty potato fallen that today, 51 percent of all taters grown in the United States are sliced up into french fries.

And that's too bad. Because a potato, when treated with proper respect, offers almost twice as much vitamin C as a tomato, and nearly as much potassium as a banana. Eat the skin and you get 4 grams of fiber as well, more than 10 percent of your recommended daily intake.

But like so many other fruits and vegetables on offer in the produce aisle, potatoes are having a tough time. In this era of prepackaged, precooked, practically predigested convenience foods, the produce aisle is more like the Island of Misfit Toys, piled high with unwanted gems sadly waiting for someone, anyone, to come by and show them some love.

Be that hero. Embrace a potato—or a squash, a radish, a head of cauliflower, even a handful of brussels sprouts if you have the urge. And embrace them in their natural forms. If you want to lose weight, cutting calories isn't enough: In one study, researchers compared people on a low-fat diet with those who ate low-fat but also increased their consumption of fruits and vegetables. Those in the high-produce group lost 33 percent more weight in the first 6 months!

That's right: Just eating more fruits and vegetables will strip a third more pounds off your belly! Another study at Harvard looked at how changes in eating habits affected weight loss over a 4-year period. The number one most-effective change in one's diet? Eating more fruits and vegetables.

The absolute worst thing you can do, according to the same study? Eat potato chips. (Wow, it really does suck to be a potato.)

Sure, eating more fruits and vegetables might not be as instantaneously gratifying as downing the newest tricked-out McCalorie burger at the local drive-thru. And fresh produce doesn't come in brightly colored boxes with Cap'n Kohlrabi on the label. But the rewards you'll reap from mastering the produce aisle are greater than anywhere else in the supermarket. In another Harvard study of 110,000 men and women, those who ate 8 or more servings of fruits and vegetables a day were 30 percent less likely to have a heart attack or stroke than those who ate less than 1.5 servings a day. And even eating just 5 servings a day reduces your risk by up to 20 percent.

You can do that, right? Some orange juice and a banana in your cereal at breakfast, an apple for a snack, a salad or a bowl of vegetable soup at lunch, a side of broccoli at dinner. Done! If you see fruits or vegetables, put them in your mouth: It's like a Get Out of Fat Jail Free card! And just look at some of the additional benefits you'll get.

YOU'LL LOWER YOUR BLOOD PRESSURE.

One study found that people with high blood pressure who ate a diet rich in fruits, vegetables, and dairy products reduced their systolic blood pressures by 11 points and their diastolic blood pressures by 6 points—as much as medications can achieve.

YOU'LL REDUCE YOUR HEART DISEASE RISK.

If heart disease runs in your family, focus on apples and broccoli. In a study in the *American Journal of Clinical Nutrition,* women who regularly ate broccoli were found to have a 25 to 30 percent lower risk of coronary disease; those who ate apples cut their risk by 13 to 22 percent.

YOU'LL FEEL LESS HUNGRY.

In a study at Pennsylvania State University, people who ate whole fruits with their meals reported being more satiated by what they ate than those who ate processed fruit products like applesauce or juice. The whole-fruit crowd felt fuller, even though they consumed 15 percent fewer calories!

YOU'LL BUILD A LEANER BODY.

Calcium (from kale and broccoli), potassium (from Swiss chard, lima beans, winter squashes, and avocados), and magnesium (from almonds, spinach, potatoes, and beans) are just three of the essential muscle-building nutrients you can get from vegetables. And the fiber that's packed into most produce will keep you fuller longer—which means you'll stay slimmer longer.

YOU'LL HAVE FEWER SICK DAYS.

Sure, an apple a day keeps the doctor away. But the essential antioxidant vitamins E (from almonds, spinach, broccoli, and peanuts), C (from broccoli, bell peppers, strawberries, papayas, cauliflower, kale, and brussels sprouts), and A (from carrots, cantaloupes, and apricots) will protect you against everything from wrinkles to heart disease.

The produce aisle is where you're in charge like nowhere else. That bright red bell pepper, that dusky handful of grapes, that Incredible Hulk—colored watermelon— they're pure, unadulterated nutrition. No food scientist has added high-fructose corn syrup or trans fatty acids or butylated hydroxyanisole to them. Treat them well, and they'll treat you even better.

The Antioxidant Superhero Scorecard

Antioxidants are the nutrients in fruits and vegetables that help us ward off every disease from cancer to type 2 diabetes to dengue fever. Any molecule that protects your cells from oxidation—basically, the aging process—is technically an antioxidant. But which fruits and vegetables have the most potent punches? Below are the scores for some of the most powerful disease-fighting foods known to man, based on their ORAC scores—oxygen radical absorbance capacity.

FOOD	ORAC SCORE PER 100 G
Apple, Red Delicious, skin on	4,275
Artichoke, raw	6,552
Banana, raw	795
Beans, black, raw	8,494
Beans, navy, raw	1,861
Blueberries	4,669
Broccoli, raw	1,510
Cocoa, dry, unsweetened	55,653
Corn, raw	728
Cranberries	9,090
Elderberries	14,697
Garlic, raw	5,708
Lentils, raw	7,282
Oranges, raw	2,103
Spinach, raw	1,513

THE TRUTH ABOUT CALORIES

You can't go anywhere without being confronted by calories. Restaurants now print calorie counts on menus. You go to the supermarket and there they are, stamped on every box and bottle. You hop on the treadmill and watch your "calories burned" click upward.

But just what are calories? The more calories we take in, the more flab we add—and if we cut back on them, then flab starts to recede too, right? After all, at face value, calorie counts seem to be the factor by which all foods should be judged. But if that were true, 500 calories of parsnips would equal 500 calories of Double Stuf Oreos.

Only that's not quite right. Learn the distinctions and lose the lard.

Calories Fuel Our Bodies

ACTUALLY, THEY DON'T

A calorie is simply a unit of measure for heat; in the early 19th century, it was used to explain the theory of heat conservation and steam engines. The term entered the food world around 1890, when the USDA appropriated it for a report on nutrition. Specifically, a calorie was defined as the unit of heat required to raise 1 gram of water 1°C.

To apply this concept to foods like sandwiches, scientists used to set food on fire (really!) and then gauge how well the flaming sample warmed a water bath. The warmer the water, the more calories the food contained. (Today, a food's calorie count is estimated from its carbohydrate, protein, and fat content.) In the calorie's leap to nutrition, its definition evolved. The calorie we now see cited on nutrition labels is the amount of heat required to raise 1 kilogram of water by 1°C.

Here's the problem: Your body isn't a steam engine. Instead of heat, it runs on chemical energy, fueled by the oxidation of carbohydrates, fats, and protein that occurs in your cells' mitochondria. "You could say mitochondria are like small power plants," says Maciej Buchowski, PhD, a research professor of medicine at Vanderbilt University Medical Center. "Instead of one central plant, you have several billion, so it's more efficient."

YOUR MOVE > Track carbohydrates, fats, and protein—not just calories—when you're evaluating foods.

All Calories Are Created Equal

NOT EXACTLY

Our fuel comes from three sources: protein, carbohydrates, and fats. "They're handled by the body differently," says Alan Aragon, a *Men's Health* nutrition advisor. So that old "calories in, calories out" formula can be misleading, he says. "Carbohydrates, protein, and fats have different effects on the equation."

Example: For every 100 carbohydrate calories you consume, your body expends 5 to 10 to digest it. With fats, you expend slightly less (although thin people seem to break down more fat than heavy people do). The calorie-burning champion is protein: For every 100 protein calories you consume, your body needs 20 to 30 for digestion, Buchowski says. Carbohydrates and fats give up their calories easily: They're built to supply quick energy. In effect, carbs and fats yield more usable energy than protein does. *YOUR MOVE >* If you want to lose weight, make protein a priority at every meal.

A Calorie Ingested Is a Calorie Digested

IT'S NOT THAT SIMPLE

Just because the food is swallowed doesn't mean it will be digested. It passes through your stomach and then reaches your small intestine, which slurps up all the nutrients it can through its spongy walls. But 5 to 10 percent of calories slide through unabsorbed. Fat digestion is relatively efficient—fats easily enter your intestinal walls. As for protein, animal sources are more digestible than plant sources, so a top sirloin's protein will be absorbed better than tofu's. Different carbs are processed at different rates, too: Glucose and starch are rapidly absorbed, while fiber dawdles in the digestive tract. In fact, the insoluble fiber in some complex carbs, such as that in vegetables and whole grains, tends to block the absorption of other calories. A study in the *Journal of Nutrition* found that a high-fiber diet leaves roughly twice as many calories undigested as a low-fiber diet does. And fewer calories means less flab. *YOUR MOVE >* Maximize fiber intake by increasing fruit and vegetable consumption and by loading your pantry with whole-grain staples like bread, cereal, brown rice, and quinoa.

Exercise Burns Most of Our Calories

NOT EVEN CLOSE

Even the most fanatical fitness nuts burn no more than 30 percent of their daily calories at the gym. Most of your calories are burned to maintain your body's constant simmer, fueling the automated processes that keep you alive. If you want to burn fuel, hit the gas in your everyday activities. "Some 60 to 70 percent of our total caloric expenditure goes toward normal bodily functions," says Wanda Howell, PhD, a professor of nutritional sciences at the University of Arizona. This includes replacing old tissue, transporting oxygen, mending shaving wounds, and so on. NEAT, or nonexercise activity thermogenesis, consists of the countless daily motions you make outside the gym—the calories you burn while making breakfast, window shopping, or chasing the bus. Brandon Alderman, PhD, director of the exercise psychophysiology lab at Rutgers University, says emerging evidence suggests that "a conscious effort to spend more time on your feet might net a greater calorie burn than 30 minutes of daily exercise."
YOUR MOVE > Take frequent breaks from your desk (and couch) to move your body and burn bonus calories.

Low-Calorie Foods Help You Lose Weight

NOT ALWAYS

Processed low-calorie foods can be weak allies in the weight-loss war. Take sugar-free foods, for example. Omitting sugar is perhaps the easiest way to cut calories. But food manufacturers generally replace those sugars with calorie-free sweeteners, such as sucralose or aspartame. And artificial sweeteners can backfire. One University of Texas study found that consuming as few as three diet sodas a week increases a person's risk of obesity by more than 40 percent. And in a 2008 Purdue University study, rats that ate artificially sweetened yogurt took in more calories at subsequent meals, resulting in more flab. The theory is that the promise of sugar—without the caloric payoff—may actually lead to overeating. "Too many people are counting calories instead of focusing on the content of food," says Alderman. "This just misses the boat."
YOUR MOVE > Avoid artificial sweeteners and load up your plate with the bona fide low-calorie saviors: fruits and vegetables.

—*Additional reporting by* Men's Health

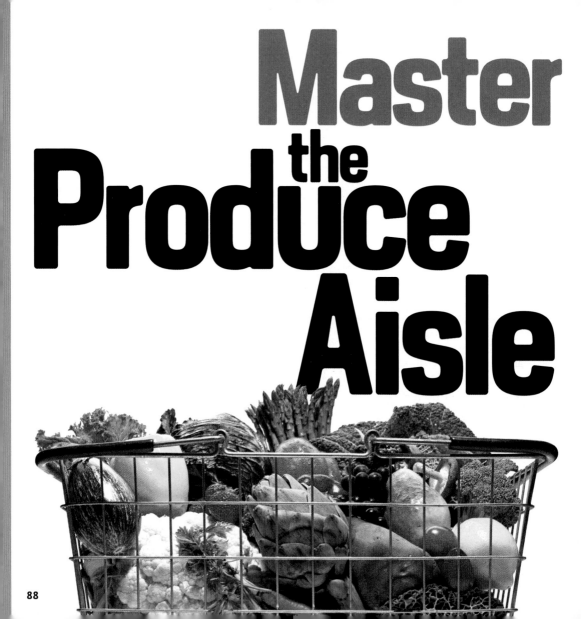

Master
the
Produce
Aisle

One of the reasons why Italians eat so well is that every last one of them believes it is their fundamental right to walk out of the market with the very best ingredients. They won't settle for a wrinkled eggplant, a withering artichoke, or an apple that tastes like Styrofoam. And neither should you.

Problem is, finding the best, ripest, most jaw-droppingly tasty fruits and vegetables isn't as intuitive as you might think. It's a task that requires the attention of all five senses in order to pick up on the subtleties and nuances behind ultimate ripeness and utmost quality.

Regardless of what you're shopping for, start with these three rules.

1. BEAUTIFUL DOESN'T MEAN DELICIOUS.

Sub-par conventional produce is bred to look waxy, glistening, and perfectly symmetrical, while prime fruits and vegetables are often irregularly shaped, with slight visual imperfections outside but a world of flavor waiting inside.

2. USE YOUR HANDS.

You can learn more about a fruit or vegetable from picking it up than you can from staring it down. Heavy, sturdy fruits and vegetables with taut skin and peels are telltale signs of freshness.

3. SHOP WITH THE SEASONS.

In the Golden Age of the American supermarket, Chilean tomatoes and South African asparagus are an arm's length away when our soil is blanketed in snow. Sure, sometimes you just need a tomato, but there are three persuasive reasons to shop in season: it's cheaper, it's better, and it's better for you. So mark your calendar.

To dig even deeper in our hunt for perfect produce, we asked Aliza Green, author of *Field Guide to Produce,* and Chef Ned Elliott, formerly of Portland's Urban Farmer restaurant, for the dirt on scoring the best of the bounty. Use the tips and tricks that follow and you'll bring home the best fruits and vegetables every time, just like an Italian grandma.

PRODUCE	PERFECT PICK	PEAK SEASON	HANDLE WITH CARE	THE PAYOFF
Apples	**Firm and heavy for its size with smooth, matte, unbroken skin and no bruising.** The odd blemish (read: worm hole) or brown "scald" streaks do not negatively impact flavor. The smaller the apple, the bigger the flavor wallop.	September to May	Keep apples in a plastic bag in the crisper away from vegetables. Here, they should remain edible for several weeks.	Quercetin, a flavonoid linked to better heart health, plus the soluble fiber pectin, which keeps cholesterol in check.
Artichokes	**Deep green and heavyset with undamaged, tightly closed leaves.** The leaves should squeak when pinched together. One that is starting to open is past its best days.	March to May	Store in the fridge in a plastic bag for up to 5 days.	A higher total antioxidant capacity than any other common vegetable, according to USDA tests.
Arugula	**Emerald green leaves that are not yellowing or limp.** The smaller the leaf, the less pungent its bite.	March to November	Enclose roots in a damp paper towel and place the leaves in a plastic bag. Store in the fridge for 2 to 3 days.	Vitamin K, which may improve insulin sensitivity, offering protection against diabetes.
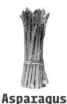 **Asparagus**	**Vibrant green spears with tight purple-tinged buds.** Avoid spears that are fading in color or wilting. Thinner spears are sweeter and more tender.	March to June	Trim the woody ends and stand the stalks upright in a small amount of water in a tall container. Cover the tops with a plastic bag and cook within a few days.	Folate, a B vitamin that protects the heart by helping to reduce inflammation.

PRODUCE	PERFECT PICK	PEAK SEASON	HANDLE WITH CARE	THE PAYOFF
Avocados	**Firm to the touch without any sunken, mushy spots.** They should not rattle when shaken—a sign the pit has pulled away from the flesh.	Year-round	To ripen, place avocados in a paper bag and store at room temperature for 2 to 4 days. To speed up this process, add an apple to the bag, which emits ripening ethylene gas.	Plenty of cholesterol-lowering monounsaturated fat.
Bananas	**Ripe bananas have uniform yellow skins or small brown freckles indicating they are at their sweetest.** Avoid any with evident bruising or split skins.	Year-round	Store unripe bananas on the counter, away from direct heat and sunlight (speed things up by placing green bananas in an open paper bag). Once ripened, refrigerate.	Vitamin B_6, which helps prevent cognitive decline, according to scientists at the USDA.
Beets	**Smooth, deep-red surface that's unyielding when pressed.** Smaller roots are sweeter and more tender. Attached greens should be deep green and not withered.	June to October	Remove the leaves (which are great sautéed in olive oil) and store in a plastic bag in the fridge for no more than 2 days. The beets will last in the crisper for up to 2 weeks.	Nitrate, which may help lower blood pressure.
Bell Peppers	**Lots of heft for their size with a brightly colored, wrinkle-free exterior.** The stems should be a lively green.	July to December	Refrigerate in the crisper for up to 2 weeks.	All bell peppers are loaded with antioxidants, especially vitamin C. Red peppers lead the pack, with nearly three times the amount of vitamin C found in oranges.

PRODUCE	PERFECT PICK	PEAK SEASON	HANDLE WITH CARE	THE PAYOFF
Blue-berries	**Plump, uniform indigo berries with taut skin and a dull white frost.** Check the bottom of the container for juice stains indicating berries have been crushed. Those with a red or green tinge will never fully ripen.	June to August	Transfer, unwashed, to an airtight container and refrigerate for 5 to 7 days. Blueberries spoil quickly if left at room temperature.	More disease-fighting antioxidants (especially in wild berries) than most commonly consumed fruits, according to Cornell University researchers.
 **Broccoli**	**Rigid stems with tightly formed floret clusters that are deep green or tinged purple.** Pass on any with yellowing heads—they will inevitably be more bitter.	October to May	Place in a plastic bag and store in the refrigerator for up to 1 week.	Sulforaphane, which activates enzymes that seek out and destroy cancerous cells.
Brussels Sprouts	**Compact, tight, and unshriveled heads that are vibrant green and feel overweight for their size.** Select ones of similar size for ease of cooking, knowing that smaller sprouts pack sweeter flavor.	October to November	Place in a plastic bag and store in the refrigerator for up to 1 week.	Nitrogen compounds called indoles, which have cancer-protecting efficacy.
Cabbage	**Tightly packed, crisp, deeply hued leaves free of blemishes.** Should feel dense when lifted; it's best that the stem not have any cracks at its base.	Year-round	Tightly enclose cabbage in a plastic bag and store in the fridge for up to 10 days.	More than half your vitamin K requirement in just 1 cup.

PRODUCE	PERFECT PICK	PEAK SEASON	HANDLE WITH CARE	THE PAYOFF
Cantaloupe	**The stem end should have a smooth indentation.** Look for a sweet aroma, slightly oval shape, and a good coverage of netting. The blossom end should give slightly to pressure. Avoid those with soft spots—an indication of an overripe melon.	May to September	Ripe cantaloupes should be stored in plastic in the fridge for up to 5 days, after which they begin to lose flavor.	Loads of vitamin C, which may offer protection against having a stroke.
Carrots	**Smooth and firm with bright orange color.** Avoid those that are bendable or cracked at the base, or that have patches of frosty white on their skin. Bunches with bright green tops still in place are your freshest choice.	Year-round	Store carrots with the greens removed in the crisper in a plastic bag for up to 3 weeks.	Beta-carotene, the source of vitamin A, which helps fight off infections.
Cauliflower	**Ivory white and compact florets with no dark spotting on them or the leaves.** The leaves should be verdant and perky.	September to November	Refrigerate, unwashed, in a plastic bag for up to 1 week. If light brown spots develop on the florets, shave off with a paring knife before cooking.	Detoxifying compounds called isothiocyanates, which offer protection against aggressive forms of prostate cancer.
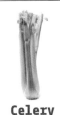 Celery	**Solid, tight stalks with only a few, if any, cracks and vivid green, not yellowing leaves.** The darker the celery, the stronger the flavor.	Year-round	Sturdy celery can be stored in the fridge in a plastic bag for 2 weeks.	Luteolin, a flavonoid linked to reduced brain inflammation, a risk factor for Alzheimer's.

PRODUCE	PERFECT PICK	PEAK SEASON	HANDLE WITH CARE	THE PAYOFF
Eggplant	Good weight to them with tight, shiny, wrinkle-free skin. When they're pressed, look for them to be springy, not spongy. The stem and cap should be forest green, not browning	August to September	Store eggplants in a cool location (not the fridge) for 3 to 5 days. Eggplants are quite sensitive to the cold.	Chlorogenic acid, a phenol antioxidant that scavenges disease-causing free radicals.
Fennel	Bulbs should be uniform in color, with no browning and a clean, fragrant aroma. Smaller bulbs have a sweeter flavor similar to licorice. Leave bulbs with wilted tops, called fronds, behind.	Year-round	Separate the greens and bulbs and keep each, unwashed, in plastic bags in the refrigerator for 3 to 5 days. Wilted fennel can be revived in ice water.	Anethole, a phytonutrient that may lessen inflammation and cancer risk.
Figs	Plump with deeply rich color; soft but not mushy to the touch. Avoid those with bruises or a sour odor.	July to September	Place fresh figs on a plate lined with a paper towel and eat them as they ripen. They bruise easily, so gentle handling is prudent. They also ripen quickly, so eat within a few days.	Phytosterols, which help keep cholesterol levels in check.
Garlic	The bulb should feel heavy for its size, with tightly closed cloves in the bulb that remain firm when gently pressed. The skin can be pure white or have purple-tinged stripes and should be tight fitting.	Year-round	Place bulbs in a cool, dark, well-ventilated location for up to 1 month.	The cancer-fighting compound allicin, which can cut down *Helicobacter pylori*— the bacteria strain responsible for the development of stomach ulcers.

PRODUCE	PERFECT PICK	PEAK SEASON	HANDLE WITH CARE	THE PAYOFF
Grapefruit	**Opt for a heavy fruit (a sign of juiciness) with thin skin that is a tad responsive to a squeeze.** Small imperfections in color and skin surface are not detrimental to the sweet-tart flavor. Yet, avoid any that are very rough or have soft spots. The same criteria apply for oranges.	October to June	Store refrigerated for 2 to 3 weeks.	The anticancer phytonutrient lycopene and 120 percent of daily vitamin C needs in 1 cup.
Grapes	**Plump, wrinkle free, and firmly attached to the stems.** There should be no browning at the stem connection, but a silvery white powder ("bloom") keeps grapes, especially darker ones, fresher longer. Green grapes with a yellowish hue are the ripest and sweetest.	June to December	Loosely store, unwashed, in a shallow bowl in the fridge for up to 1 week.	Resveratrol, a potent antioxidant in red/purple grapes that offers protection against cardiovascular disease.
Green Beans	**Vibrant, smooth surface without any visible withering.** They should "snap" when gently bent and appear moist on the inside.	April to October	Refrigerate, unwashed, in an unsealed bag for up to 1 week.	Fiber (4 grams in 1 cup), which can reduce all-cause mortality, according to Dutch researchers.
Kale	**Dark blue-green color with moist, jaunty leaves.** The smaller the leaves, the more tender the kale. Avoid wilted foliage with discolored spots.	Year-round	Peppery kale is best kept in the fridge tightly wrapped in a plastic bag pierced for aeration, where it will last 3 to 4 days.	Lutein, an antioxidant in the retina that protects against vision loss.

PRODUCE	PERFECT PICK	PEAK SEASON	HANDLE WITH CARE	THE PAYOFF
Kiwi	**A ready-to-devour kiwi will be slightly yielding to the touch.** Steer clear of those that are mushy, wrinkled, or bruised with an "off" smell.	June to August	Store at room temperature to ripen. To quicken the process, place in a paper bag with an apple. Once ripened, place in the fridge in a plastic bag for up to 1 week.	Only 56 calories for a large kiwi and 20 percent more of the antioxidant vitamin C than an orange.
Leeks	**Green, crisp tops with unblemished white root ends.** Gravitate toward small- to medium-size leeks, which are less woody and tough than larger ones. Those with spotted or yellowing leaves should be ignored.	Year-round	Stored loosely wrapped in plastic in the fridge, they'll keep fresh for a week.	Good amounts of eye-protecting lutein, manganese, and vitamins A, C, and K.
Lemons/ Limes	**Brightly colored, well-shaped with smooth, thin skin.** They should feel sturdy but give ever so slightly when squeezed. Small brown splotches on limes do not affect flavor (although they are a sign of deterioration and those with splotches should be consumed first).	Lemons, year-round; limes, May to October	Store at room temperature, in a dark location, for about 1 week or refrigerate for up to 2 weeks.	Phytonutrient liminoids, which appear to have anticancer, antiviral properties.
Lettuce: Romaine	**The ideal Caesar salad staple has crisp leaves that are free of browning edges and rust spots.** The interior leaves are paler in color with more delicate flavor.	Year-round	Refrigerate romaine for 5 to 7 days in a plastic bag.	Vitamin K, which is needed for blood clotting and bone health.

PRODUCE	PERFECT PICK	PEAK SEASON	HANDLE WITH CARE	THE PAYOFF
Mangoes	**Mangoes to be eaten shortly after purchase should have red skin with splotches of yellow, and the soft flesh should give with gentle pressure.** Mangoes for later use will be firmer with a tight skin, a duller color, and green near the stem.	April to August	Ripen at room temperature until fragrant and giving. Ripe mangoes can be stored in the fridge for up to 5 days.	A good showing of vitamins A, B_6, and C, plus fiber.
Mushrooms: Cremini	**Tightly closed, firm caps that are not slimy or riddled with dark soft spots.** Open caps with visible gills indicate consumption should be a priority.	November to April	Place meaty mushrooms on a flat surface, cover with a damp paper towel, and refrigerate for 3 to 5 days.	Immune-boosting, tumor-suppressing, complex-carbohydrate polysaccharides.
Onions	**Nicely shaped with no swelling at the neck and dry, crisp outer skin.** Lackluster onions have soft spots, green sprouts, or dark patches.	Year-round	Keep onions in a cool, dark location away from potatoes for 3 to 4 weeks.	GPCS, a peptide shown to reduce bone loss in rats, plus the cancer-fighting compound quercetin.
Papayas	**Beginning to turn yellow and somewhat-yielding flesh when lightly squeezed.** Avoid papayas that are awash in green, have dark spots, or are shriveled. Blotchy papayas often have the most flavor.	Year-round	Once ripe, eat immediately or refrigerate for up to 3 days. Unripe, greener papayas should be ripened at room temperature in a dark setting until yellow blotches appear.	A complete nutritional package, including plenty of fiber and vitamins C, A, E, and K.

PRODUCE	PERFECT PICK	PEAK SEASON	HANDLE WITH CARE	THE PAYOFF
Peaches	**Fruity aroma with a background color that is a yellow or a warm cream color.** Those destined for immediate consumption yield to gentle pressure along their seams without being too soft. For future intake, opt for those that are firm but not rock hard.	June to September	Store unripe peaches at room temperature open to air. Once ripe, transfer to the refrigerator and consume within 2 to 3 days.	Vitamin C, the antioxidant beta-carotene, fiber, and potassium.
Pears	**Pleasant fragrance with some softness at the stem end.** The skin should be free of bruises, but some brown discoloration (russeting) is fine. Firmer pears are preferable for cooking use.	August to February	Ripen at room temperature in a loosely closed brown paper bag. Refrigerate once they're ripe and consume within a couple days.	Belly-busting fiber and vitamin C—as long as you eat them with the skin on.
Pineapple	**Look for vibrant green leaves with a bit of softness and a sweet, fragrant aroma from the stem end.** Avoid spongy fruit with brown leaves and/or a fermented odor.	March to July	Keep a pineapple with a weak aroma at room temperature for 2 to 3 days until it softens slightly. Then refrigerate for up to 5 days.	Bromelain, an enzyme with potent anti-inflammatory powers.
Pome- granates	**Pick pomegranates that are weighty for their size with glossy, taut, uncracked skin that is deep red.** Gently press the crown end—if a powdery cloud emanates, the fruit is past its prime.	August to December	Stored in a cool, dry location, pomegranates keep fresh for several weeks (up to 2 months in the fridge).	Hefty amounts of antioxidants shown to improve sperm quality, thus boosting fertility.

PRODUCE	PERFECT PICK	PEAK SEASON	HANDLE WITH CARE	THE PAYOFF
Potatoes: Sweet or White	**Unyielding, with smooth undamaged skin.** Avoid if bruised, cracked, or green tinged. Loose spuds tend to be better quality than bagged.	Sweet, September to December; white, year-round	Outside of the fridge, in a cool, dark place separated from onions, white potatoes will last for months. Sweet potatoes, however, should be used within a week.	Potassium, which may help preserve muscle mass as we age.
Raspberries	**Plump and dry, with good shape and intense, uniform color.** Examine the container carefully for mold or juice stains at the bottom. Raspberries with hulls attached are a sign of underripe, overly tart berries.	May to November	Place highly perishable raspberries, unwashed, on a paper towel in a single layer. Cover with a damp paper towel and refrigerate for no more than 2 to 3 days.	More fiber (8 grams per cup) than any other commonly consumed berry. Plus, the anticancer chemical ellagic acid.
Spinach	**Opt for bunches with leaves that are crisp and verdant green, with no spots, yellowing, or limpness.** Thin stems are best, as thick ones are a sign of more bitter, overgrown leaves.	March to May	Pack unwashed spinach bunches loosely in plastic bags and store in the fridge for 3 to 4 days.	Chromium, which is involved in carbohydrate and fat metabolism and may reduce hunger and food intake.
Squash: Butternut	**Should feel dense for its size with a rind that is smooth, hard, uniformly tan, and free of splits.** Being able to easily push a fingernail into the rind or scrape bits off indicates an immature, less flavorful squash.	September to November	Butternut should be stored outside the fridge in a cool, well-ventilated, dark place, where it will stay edible for up to 3 months.	Huge amount of vitamin A to ramp up your immune system.

PRODUCE	PERFECT PICK	PEAK SEASON	HANDLE WITH CARE	THE PAYOFF
Straw-berries	**Seek out unblemished berries with a bright red color that extends all the way to the stem.** Good berries should have a strong fruity smell and be neither soft and mushy nor hard and firm. Smaller strawberries often have more flavor than the oversized megamart versions.	June to August	Place unwashed strawberries in a single layer on a paper towel in a covered container. They will last for 2 to 3 days in the fridge.	The most vitamin C of any of the commonly consumed berries.
Tomatoes	**Look for heavy tomatoes that are rich in color and free of wrinkles, cracks, or bruises.** They should have some give, unlike the rock-solid ones bred for transport. Too soft, though, and the tomato is likely overripe. Off-season, select smaller types like Roma and cherry tomatoes.	May to August	Never store tomatoes in the fridge; the cool temps destroy flavor and texture. Keep them at room temperature out of direct sunlight for up to 1 week.	Lycopene, a carotenoid antioxidant that helps fend off prostate cancer.
Watermelon	**Dense, symmetrical melons that are free of cuts and sunken areas.** The rind should appear dull, not shiny, with a rounded, creamy-yellow underside that shows where ground ripening took place. A slap should produce a hollow thump.	May to August	Store whole in the fridge for up to 1 week. The cold prevents the flesh from drying out and turning fibrous.	Citrulline, an amino acid that's converted to arginine, which relaxes blood vessels, thus improving blood flow.
Zucchini	**Purchase heavy, tender zucchini with unblemished deep-green skins that are adorned with faint gold specks or strips.** Smaller zucchini are sweeter and more flavorful.	June to August	Refrigerate in the crisper in a plastic bag for up to 5 days.	Riboflavin, a B vitamin needed for red blood cell production and for converting carbohydrates to energy.

Your Organic Primer

THE 5 MOST IMPORTANT QUESTIONS ABOUT ORGANIC FOOD ANSWERED

Is organic worth the extra cost?

The short answer is yes, but it's complicated. As anyone who's been to Whole Foods (endearingly nicknamed Whole Paycheck by detractors and fans alike) can tell you, organic products cost more—according to a 2006 study in the *Journal of Food Science,* an average of 10 percent to 40 percent more for typical items. And while a thinner wallet is a small price to pay for protecting yourself from pesticides and fertilizers, some organic food is almost nutritionally identical to its conventional counterpart.

Take, for example, an onion: According to an extensive analysis by the Environmental Working Group, it's got the lowest pesticide load of all the 45 fruits and vegetables they tested. Also on the produce honor roll are avocados and asparagus. Really torn on whether or not to spend your hard-earned cash on organic? To see how your favorite fruit fares under the pressures of industrial agriculture, check out the table to the right.

IS ORGANIC BETTER FOR ME?

Yes and no. For every study that says organic food has higher concentrations of nutrients, there's another one that denies it. Researchers at the University of California at Davis found that organic kiwis had substantially more disease-fighting polyphenols than conventionally grown kiwis. Problem is, the same team of researchers found the opposite to be true of organic tomatoes—that organically grown tomatoes may have lower levels of antioxidants.

IS ORGANIC BETTER FOR THE EARTH?

In many respects, this may be the biggest reason to go organic. In fact, the certification criteria of the National Organic Standards Board specifically outline that organic food must be grown with methods that promote biodiversity, minimize pollution, and use cultural, biological, and mechanical methods of agriculture in place of synthetic materials. This goes beyond cutting out pesticides and fertilizers that can be harmful to people and animals; it involves methods that actually improve the soil—for those agrophiles out there, this means using cover crops, manure, and crop rotations to fertilize; grazing animals on mixed forage pastures; using renewable resources; and conserving soil and water.

But there are two sides to that coin. Researchers at the University of Alberta found that the environmental cost of greenhouse gas emitted to transport organically grown produce was comparable to the environmental cost to transport conventional fruit and vegetables. Your best bet: Head to the farmers' market (find one in your area at ams.usda.gov/farmersmarkets). While smaller farms don't always have the means to obtain official organic certification, you'll often find, after chatting with the farmers, that they use sustainable, healthy, environmentally friendly growing and transporting methods that are as good for the planet as they are for your palate.

Should You Splurge on Organic Fruit?

KNOW WHICH PRODUCE IS HARDEST HIT BY PESTICIDES

Sometimes the extra trip to the farmers' market is worth it. That's because buying organic produce can help you avoid pesticides, which may be more prevalent than you think. Case in point: The Environmental Working Group recently released its list of the pesticide levels of common fruits, ranked from 1 (lowest pesticide load) to 100 (highest load). The rankings, based on nearly 43,000 tests for pesticides conducted by the USDA, are surprising. Take a look:

*Environmental Working Group score based on pesticide load

YES

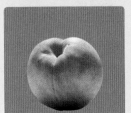

Peaches
100*
Peaches have the highest pesticide load of any fruit or vegetable.

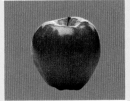

Apples
89
Apples are the second-most pesticide ridden.

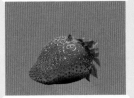

Strawberries
82
We think organic strawberries taste better anyway.

YES

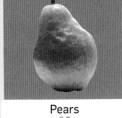

Pears
65
One of the top 10 dirtiest fruits.

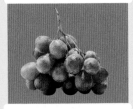

Grapes
43
Better to play it safe when buying grapes.

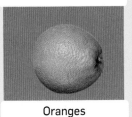

Oranges
42
42 is borderline; go organic when you can.

NO

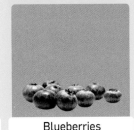

Blueberries
24
A 24 means conventional blueberries are relatively safe.

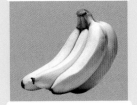

Bananas
16
Made the list of top 10 cleanest fruits.

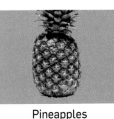

Pineapples
7
Pineapples are the fourth cleanest.

The 21st-Century Produce Aisle

THE LATEST IN VALUE-ADDED PRODUCE

Far from Frankenfoods, these natural crossbreeds of traditional fruits and vegetables represent the finest in genetic ingenuity. Find these brighter, more nutritious hybrids in a grocery store or farmers' market near you.

BROCCOLINI

A hybrid of broccoli and Chinese kale
It has a peppery sweet edge that isn't overly bitter. Four stalks boost immunity with 65 percent of your day's vitamin C.

PLUOTS

A crossbreed of plums and apricots
So sweet yet so good for you. They pack a punch of vision-protecting vitamin A.

SCARLET CORN

Bred from heirloom corn seeds
Good ol' Midwestern sweet corn raised to have high levels of anthocyanin, a red-hued flavonoid that helps fight disease.

ORANGE CAULIFLOWER

A white variety mixed with an orange-tinted one from Canada
It's creamier, more tender, and bursting with cancer-fighting beta-carotene.

RAINBOW CARROTS

Kaleidoscopic carrots from heirloom yellow, purple, and red seeds
They're sweeter than the classic. Yellow heaps eye-healthy lutein, while red and purple add cancer-fighting lycopene.

ROSSO BRUNO TOMATOES

A brown hybrid from a mix of wild varieties
A juicier, richer flavor than typical tomatoes. They also have double the fiber to help keep blood sugar stable.

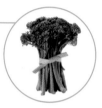
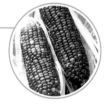
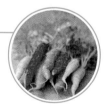
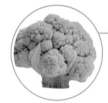
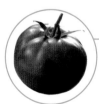

ARE ORGANIC PACKAGED FOODS BETTER FOR ME?

When it comes to packaged and processed foods, "organic" does not equal "healthy." As Michael Pollan quips in his "eater's manifesto," *In Defense of Food,* "Organic Oreos are not a health food"—they're still heavily processed cookies filled with fat and sugar, and your body metabolizes organic fat and sugar the same way it does conventional. In fact, some clever companies use organic as a marketing smoke screen, only to load up a cup of yogurt or a box of crackers with unhealthy amounts of organic high-fructose corn syrup (yes, HFCS made from organic corn fits under the FDA guidelines for organic).

DOES ORGANIC TASTE BETTER?

This is perhaps the most important question to discerning cooks the country over. Most chefs and organic enthusiasts would undoubtedly say so, but there is little research to back that up thus far. Part of the problem is the vast array of quality within the organic subset; while an heirloom tomato grown 10 miles from your house by a local farmer may be transcendent, an organic Roma tomato shipped in from China could leave a lot to desire. Your best bet is to find a store or a local farmer with reliably delicious products and stick to it.

Crack the Color Code

HERE ARE THE GUIDELINES, COURTESY OF THE USDA

The pigment of produce can provide you with information about its nutritional value. Check out how each of the five different color categories of fruits and vegetables can benefit your health. Then mix and match for a total of five servings every day. One serving equals 1 cup raw or ½ cup cooked.

 BLUES AND PURPLES Blueberries, blackberries, purple grapes, plums, raisins, eggplant. *Benefits:* Keep memory sharp and reduce risk of many types of cancer, including prostate cancer

 GREENS Kiwi, honeydew, spinach, broccoli, romaine lettuce, brussels sprouts, cabbage. *Benefits:* Protect bones, teeth, and eyesight

WHITES Pears, bananas, mushrooms, cauliflower, onions, garlic. *Benefits:* Lower LDL cholesterol and reduce risk of heart disease

 REDS Watermelon, strawberries, raspberries, cranberries, cherries, tomatoes, radishes, red apples. *Benefits:* Help prevent Alzheimer's disease and improve blood flow to the heart

 YELLOWS AND ORANGES Oranges, grapefruit, peaches, cantaloupe, mangoes, pineapple, squash, carrots. *Benefits:* Boost immune system and help prevent eye disease

FRANKENFACT VS. FRANKENFICTION

WHAT YOU NEED TO KNOW ABOUT GENETICALLY MODIFIED ORGANISMS

Over the past 2 decades, genetically modified foods have radically transformed the American farm system—and as a result, your supermarket's aisles. As these foods proliferate, the debate escalates about their long-term effects on our health and the environment. Ignore the hype. Here's the reality.

GENETICALLY MODIFIED FOODS ARE STILL A RELATIVELY SMALL FRACTION OF THE NATION'S FOOD SUPPLY.

FALSE

Just a decade ago, that was true. But in 2011, according to the USDA, a staggering 88 percent of the country's corn crops were from genetically modified seeds. Similarly, 94 percent of all soybean crops in the United States are now engineered. Because syrups and oils from those two plants are ubiquitous in packaged goods, the Grocery Manufacturers Association estimates that up to 75 percent of boxed foods contain genetically altered ingredients.

YOU CAN AVOID GENETICALLY MODIFIED FOODS IF YOU JUST READ LABELS.

FALSE

A 2004 study showed that 92 percent of Americans wanted to know if they were eating genetically modified foods, but, unlike in much of the rest of the first world, our FDA doesn't require these foods to be labeled as such. "We use product-based labeling in this country, not process-based labeling, like in Europe," says molecular geneticist Alan McHughen. Once modified crops like corn and soy enter the supply chain, they find their way into most of our processed foods.

THE UNITED STATES ALLOWS ONLY PLANT-BASED GENETICALLY MODIFIED FOODS TO ENTER THE MARKET.

TRUE

But that could change. In 2010, an FDA panel considered approving a salmon that grows twice as fast as the natural variety. Opponents call it the "frankenfish" and say that if it were to escape to open waters, it could ruin native salmon populations. Some FDA experts, on the other hand, believe that the fish may not be "materially" different from its wild counterpart. If the new rule were to go through as it's currently written, labels on the designer salmon wouldn't differ from conventional salmon.

THERE IS A WORLDWIDE CONSENSUS ON THE POTENTIAL OF GENETICALLY MODIFIED FOODS.

FALSE

Most notably, the European Union has given the cold shoulder to genetically engineered foods. While in 2011 the EU took the new step of allowing animal feed with trace amounts of genetically modified crops into the supply, it has largely steered clear of the planting of such crops. Why? Because the United States and other large GMO crop producers only follow the "scientific analysis from one side, the producer of this GMO," says Dacian Ciolos, the EU's agriculture commissioner. Even the USDA expressed some reservations when it said recently that "there is an ongoing controversy over the benefits and risks of this technology and concerns about unforeseen consequences of its use."

GENETICALLY MODIFIED FOODS COULD KILL YOU.

FALSE

Oft-cited studies linking these foods to medical problems in rodents have been widely discredited. Critics charge that the FDA isn't giving genetically modified foods nearly enough scrutiny, but, says Christine Bruhn, PhD, of the Center for Consumer Research at the University of California at Davis, "even though we don't have 12 generations of human studies, there's no indication of ill effects."

GENETICALLY MODIFIED CROPS ARE HARMING THE ENVIRONMENT.

?

Consumer-advocacy groups claim that genetically modified crops require more pesticides, while many scientists believe the opposite. Both sides cite myriad studies to support their stances. So who's right? "We don't know enough," says Charles Margulis of the Center for Food Safety. "And it could take another 50 years before we do."

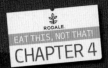

EAT
THIS
NOT
THAT!
SUPERMARKET
SURVIVAL GUIDE

THE MEAT & FISH COUNTERS

Life used to be a lot simpler. And so, too, was eating meat.

Back when our grandparents were young; back before "carbon footprints"; before 1,097 channels of basic cable; before librarians, accountants, and middle-age checkout clerks sported "edgy" tattoos on their backsides, grilling a hamburger was a pretty simple task. You went to the meat counter, bought some ground chuck, brought it home, and threw it on the grill. Just add ketchup.

Nowadays, however, it seems like just making ourselves burgers involves tense negotiation among scientific, ethical, and nutritional philosophies. Do we get the 95 percent lean, or the 85 percent lean? Is it grass fed, free range, and organic, or was this cow raised in the livestock equivalent of Alcatraz? (And exactly how many cows went into making that burger in the first place?) And should we make a turkey burger, or maybe a bison burger, or even a veggie burger instead? In a world where half the country wants to join PETA and the other half wants to join Sarah Palin on a caribou hunt, it's hard to know how to talk to a butcher—and whether to whisper when doing so.

All that confusion is too bad, because meat is perhaps our best source of protein, the nutrient essential for building healthy bones and muscle, providing the body with long-burning energy and self-healing powers. Protein is made of amino acids, which can be split into two types: essential and nonessential. A lot of foods, from broccoli to pasta to potatoes, include some of these amino acids. But the best forms of protein include all nine essential amino acids that your body can't produce naturally, compounds it needs to maintain muscles and battle fat. Beef, pork, poultry, and fish—as well as dairy, eggs, nuts, quinoa, and oats—are the best sources.

But too much meat—and too much of the wrong kinds of meat—can wreak havoc on our bellies, our blood pressures, and our poor, hardworking arteries. Processed meats in particular—stuff like ham, sausage, pepperoni, and other things that you might apply to the top of a pizza or the interior of a hero—are usually saltier than a Chris Rock monologue and packed with more lard than an appropriations bill. And even smart choices like poultry, fish, and lean beef can pack on the posterior pounds if they're breaded and fried or slathered with sugary sauces.

In this chapter, we'll show you exactly what you're buying when you're buying what you buy and help you get the most from your food dollar—hey, meat is expensive nowadays! But first, let us lay out some guiding principles worth keeping in mind the next time you approach the butcher or the fishmonger.

PLAY 20 QUESTIONS.

Nowhere does your ability to choose wisely matter more than at the fish and meat counters. End up with a chewy steak or a 3-day-old scrap of salmon and you've wasted a meal and a good chunk of change. Make friends with the butcher: Ask him about his favorite cuts of meat, the freshest protein in the case, his favorite Woody Allen films—whatever it takes for him to open up and share the goods on the mountains of meat he lords over day and night. Play your cards right and he'll save special steaks for you, dish out his favorite recipe for braised veal shanks, and generally help you navigate your way through one of the most critical—and confusing—sections of the supermarket. And if your butcher isn't the talkative type, or, worse yet, your supermarket has replaced the butcher with a shrink-wrap machine, well, then it's time to shop somewhere else.

WHEN GOING FISHING, THINK SMALL.

Fish build up stores of mercury and pesticides in their fat and muscle tissue. Then larger fish eat them, adding all of those contaminants to those already in their bodies. Then even larger fish eat those fish, and so on. The higher a fish is on the food chain, the more pesticides and other nasty nibbles it has stored in its tissues. Sardines, anchovies, and Atlantic mackerel will generally be lower on the contamination scale than the big predators like swordfish, shark, and tilefish.

DON'T FEAR THE BACON.

Regularly skipping breakfast increases your risk of obesity by 450 percent. And breakfast is one meal it's hard to cook up too many calories for, especially protein calories. In a 2008 study, researchers at Virginia Commonwealth University found that people who regularly ate a protein-rich, 610-calorie breakfast lost significantly more weight in 8 months than those who consumed only 290 calories and a quarter of the protein. The big-breakfast eaters lost an average of 40 pounds and had an easier time sticking to their diets, even though both groups were prescribed the same number of daily calories. And bacon is one of the best ways to pack protein into your morning—four strips will give you 12.5 grams of the muscle-building stuff for fewer than 200 calories.

ALWAYS EAT PROTEIN BEFORE AND AFTER EXERCISING.

Syracuse University researchers found that when you down protein before and after strenuous activity, you blunt the effects of cortisol, the stress hormone that tells your body to store fat. As a result, you burn more fat, not only during your workout, but also for an additional 24 hours after. And Finnish scientists who had weight lifters down protein before and after a workout discovered that their subjects produced more of a molecule called cyclin-dependent kinase 2. This compound signals your muscles to produce more stem cells, which aid in the process of building muscle and improve your body's ability to heal after exercise.

SNARF A STEAK TO STOP HUNGER.

A British study found that high-protein foods trigger the release of a hormone that stifles hunger. If it's going to be a while before you eat again, go for the meat—it will tide you over longer than a salad will.

GET IN TOUCH WITH YOUR WILD SIDE.

Researchers at the University of Wisconsin suggest that people who want to cut down on calories, saturated fat, and cholesterol—while still indulging their inner carnivores—might want to play games. No, wait, that's not it. They say people might want to prey on game. Ah, yes. Meats like ostrich, bison, venison, and elk typically contain as much protein and iron as beef or pork, but have less fat and fewer calories.

In other words, don't let the confusion stop you. Follow the tips on the upcoming pages and you'll be on your way to enjoying the muscle-making, bone-building, flab-fighting, stress-stopping benefits of biting into a juicy burger, just like your grandparents did.

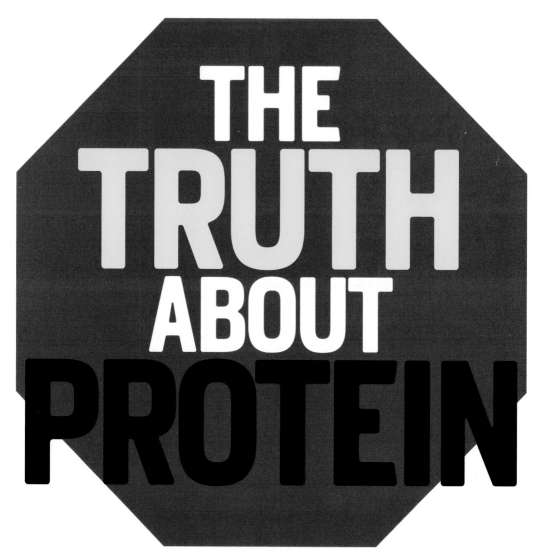

THE TRUTH ABOUT PROTEIN

If you are what you eat, what does that make a vegan? A green bean? Of course not—and there are more than a few meat-free muscleheads out there to prove it. But most people eat animal products. And we really do become what we eat. Our skin, bones, hair, and nails are composed mostly of protein. Plus, animal products fuel the muscle-growing process called protein synthesis. That's why Rocky chugged eggs before his a.m. runs. Since those days, nutrition scientists have done plenty of research. Read up before you chow down.

You Need More

Think big. Most adults would benefit from eating more than the recommended daily intake of between 46 and 56 grams, says Donald Layman, PhD, a professor emeritus of nutrition at the University of Illinois. The benefit goes beyond muscles, he says: Protein dulls hunger and can help prevent obesity, diabetes, and heart disease.

How much do you need? Step on a scale and be honest with yourself about your activity level. According to Mark Tarnopolsky, MD, PhD, who studies exercise and nutrition at McMaster University in Hamilton, Ontario, highly trained athletes thrive on 0.77 gram of daily protein per pound of body weight. That's 139 grams for a 180-pound man.

Of course, most of us aren't highly trained athletes. Men who work out for 45 minutes 3 to 5 days a week need about 0.45 gram per pound; women with the same activity level need 0.35 gram per pound. So a 180-pound guy who works out regularly needs about 80 grams of protein a day. For a 140-pound woman, that translates to nearly 50 grams of protein daily.

Now, if you're trying to lose weight, protein is still crucial. The fewer calories you consume, the greater the proportion of calories that should come from protein, says Layman. And no, that extra protein won't wreck your kidneys: "Taking in more than the recommended dose won't confer more benefit. It won't hurt you, but you'll just burn it off as extra energy," Dr. Tarnopolsky says.

It's Not All the Same

Many foods, including quinoa, nuts, and beans, can provide good doses of protein. But the best sources are dairy products, eggs, meat, and fish, Layman says. Animal protein is complete— it contains the right proportions of the essential amino acids your body can't synthesize on its own.

It's possible to build complete protein from plant-based foods by combining legumes, nuts, and grains at one meal or over the course of a day. But you'll need to consume 20 to 25 percent more plant-based protein to reap the benefits that animal-derived sources provide, says Dr. Tarnopolsky. And beans and legumes have carbs that make it harder to lose weight.

So if protein can help keep weight off, is a chicken wing dipped in blue cheese dressing a diet secret? Not quite: Total calories still count. Scale down your fat and carbohydrate intakes to make room for lean protein: eggs, low-fat milk, yogurt, lean meats, and fish.

But remember, if you're struggling with your weight, fat itself is not the culprit; carbs are the likely problem. Fat will help keep you full, while carbs can put you on a blood sugar roller coaster that leaves you hungry later.

Timing Is Everything

"At any given moment, even at rest, your body is breaking down and building protein," says Jeffrey Volek, PhD, RD, a nutrition and exercise researcher at the University of Connecticut.

But when do you eat most of your protein? At dinner, right? That means you could be fueling muscle growth for only a few hours a day, and breaking down muscle the rest of the time, Layman says. Instead, spread out your protein intake.

Your body can process only so much protein in a single sitting. A recent study from the University of Texas found that consuming 90 grams of protein at one meal provides the same benefit as eating 30 grams. It's like a gas tank, says study author Douglas Paddon-Jones, PhD: "There's only so much you can put in to maximize performance; the rest is spillover."

Eating protein at all three meals—plus snacking on protein sources such as cheese, jerky, and milk—will help you eat less overall. People who start the day with a protein-rich breakfast consume 200 fewer calories a day than those who opt for a carb-heavy breakfast, like a jam-smeared bagel. Ending the day with a steak doesn't have the same appetite-quenching effect, Layman says.

—*Additional reporting by* Men's Health

The Eat This, Not That! Fish Finder

You know you should be eating more fish, but do you know which kind is healthiest? Fresh or frozen, wild or farmed, local or imported: The challenges and nuances of the industrial food complex have made choosing the right fish more complicated than string theory. To simplify matters, we've analyzed a dozen of the most popular fish choices and ranked them from first to worst. Our favorite sea creatures are rich in omega-3s; relatively low in mercury, PCBs, and dioxins; and ecologically sustainable.

HERE'S THE CATCH:

A high level of mercury in your fish will undo any heart-health benefit the fish might provide, according to Finnish scientists. That's because mercury impairs arterial flexibility.

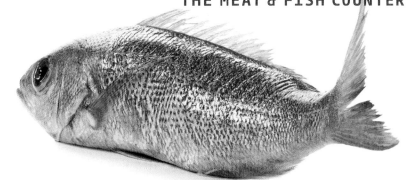

FISH	Omega-3s (mg per 3 oz serving)	Protein (g per 3 oz serving)	Contaminants *	Eco-Friendly **
Wild Alaskan Salmon	1,253	18	low	
Farmed Rainbow Trout	838	18	low	
Pacific Halibut	444	18	low	
Farmed Catfish	391	13	medium	
Farmed Tilapia	185	17	low	
Yellowfin Tuna	207	20	medium	
Farmed Salmon	1,705	17	high	
Mahimahi	104	16	low	
Swordfish	701	17	high	
Grouper	227	16	medium	
Atlantic Cod	166	15	medium	
Chilean Sea Bass	570	16	medium	

*Based on Environmental Defense's analysis of mercury and PCB data
**Based on each fish's sustainability, as monitored by Monterey Bay Aquarium's Seafood Watch

Making Sense of Meat

When it comes to picking a protein, you'll find there's a lot to digest before you sit down to eat. Nearly everything you buy at the supermarket comes with a story, a collection of proclamations that are as ambiguous as they are bold. The USDA has its hands full trying to regulate these claims, leaving a gaping hole for manufacturers to fill with fluff. So whether you're planning to feast on fowl or binge on beef, be on high alert when meandering the meat section of your local market. The next four pages are filled with clues to the most important—and commonly abused—terms in the industry.

BELL & EVANS AIR CHILLED BONELESS, SKINLESS CHICKEN THIGHS

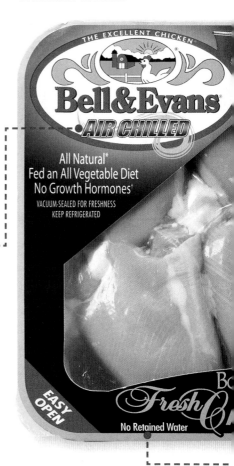

THE EXCELLENT CHICKEN

Bell & Evans

AIR CHILLED

All Natural*
Fed an All Vegetable Diet
No Growth Hormones†
VACUUM-SEALED FOR FRESHNESS
KEEP REFRIGERATED

EASY OPEN

Fresh

No Retained Water

The Claim:
"AIR CHILLED"

The Truth:
Standard practice for chicken processing includes dunking the birds in a frigid bath to keep bacteria at a minimum. Air chilling skips the cold-water treatment in favor of placing chickens in cooling chambers. Manufacturers have proclaimed its cleansing superiority, but some studies do not support the theory. Both air chilling and immersion are comparable at reducing bacteria before packaging. Flavor, however, may indeed be superior, as the slow chilling can yield a more tender, less water-saturated chicken.

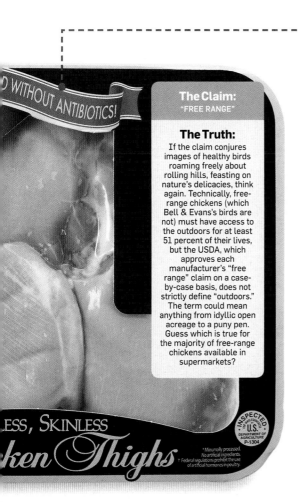

The Claim:
"RAISED WITHOUT ANTIBIOTICS"

The Truth:
Unlike the beef industry, big chicken producers have begun to curtail the use of antibiotics in recent years, addressing concerns that bacteria dangerous to humans could be developing drug resistance. Still, Tyson, Perdue, and others have been unable to wean their birds entirely off antibiotics, so this claim is worth something. A couple extra bucks a pound? That's for you to decide.

The Claim:
"FREE RANGE"

The Truth:
If the claim conjures images of healthy birds roaming freely about rolling hills, feasting on nature's delicacies, think again. Technically, free-range chickens (which Bell & Evans's birds are not) must have access to the outdoors for at least 51 percent of their lives, but the USDA, which approves each manufacturer's "free range" claim on a case-by-case basis, does not strictly define "outdoors." The term could mean anything from idyllic open acreage to a puny pen. Guess which is true for the majority of free-range chickens available in supermarkets?

The Claim:
"ORGANIC"

The Truth:
The organic chicken industry has grown wildly in recent years. Big Agriculture has seen the potential profit boon of charging an average of 100 percent more for organic chickens, and they have secured the coveted (and often pricey) USDA stamp for what some activists argue are less-than-reputable practices. Look for two certification stamps—the Secretary of Agriculture seal and the USDA Organic seal—confirming that the animals were fed organic feed and had access to pasture. The chicken here was conventionally raised.

The Claim:
"NO RETAINED WATER"

The Truth:
When immersed in their cold-water baths after slaughter, poultry can absorb up to 8 percent of their body weight, diluting taste and nutrition. On top of added water, conventional poultry can be "enhanced" with salt. The USDA has ignored petitions to consider salt a food additive; in turn, some manufacturers have jacked up the sodium content of their chickens.

NATURE'S PROMISE USDA CHOICE BEEF

The Claim:
"NO ANTIBIOTICS ADMINISTERED"

The Truth:
Crowded feedlots are breeding grounds for bacteria, illness, and disease, which is one reason why most beef cattle are pumped full of antibiotics. The other reason: corn. Cows' stomachs are designed to digest grass, but with cheap, subsidized corn in high supply, most cows in this country live on a diet consisting of 75 percent corn, 10 percent roughage, and 15 percent animal by-products. To fight off the ulcers, heartburn, and potentially fatal liver abscesses caused by this diet, the beef industry turns to antibiotics. It's bad not only for the cow, but also for you: Corn-fed beef is nearly twice as fatty as grass-fed beef and has lower concentrations of omega-3 fatty acids.

The Claim:
"NO GROWTH STIMULANTS OR ADDED HORMONES"

The Truth:
A good thing, to be sure, and decidedly rare in the world of industrial beef. About two-thirds of cows in the United States are treated with growth hormones to speed growth and ultimately maximize profit. While the USDA has deemed growth hormones safe for cattle and the humans who consume them, the European Union (EU) isn't quite so sure. Over the years, researchers have raised concern over possible links between growth hormones and issues like early puberty in girls, lower sperm count in men, and breast cancer, but the jury is still out on the final effects. The EU prohibits the use of growth hormones in the raising of cattle and has banned hormone-injected beef since 1988.

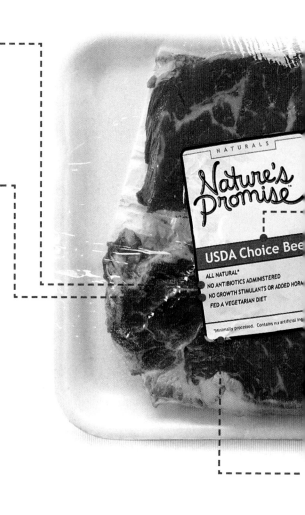

NATURALS

Nature's Promise™

USDA Choice Bee

ALL NATURAL*
NO ANTIBIOTICS ADMINISTERED
NO GROWTH STIMULANTS OR ADDED HORM
FED A VEGETARIAN DIET

*Minimally processed. Contains no artificial ing

The Claim:
"USDA CHOICE BEEF"

The Truth:
Not all steaks taste the same. The USDA grades beef based on marbling and the age of the animal, which affect the quality of your sizzling steak. The higher the degree of marbling—which is to say, the fattier—the more tender and flavorful (and caloric) the meat. You'll probably never see a lower grade than Select at the supermarket, which is leaner than Prime and Choice grades, respectively the highest and second-highest grades. Pricey Prime is a rare supermarket find, too, considering just 2 percent of all beef is graded Prime and most of that goes to restaurants.

The Claim:
"PRODUCT OF USA"

The Truth:
A required label as of September 2008, this country-of-origin labeling informs consumers about the origins of their T-bones. Fish and most produce already required an origin label. For meat, it indicates where the animal was raised, which sometimes includes multiple countries or an indication that the animal was brought to the United States for slaughter. The food industry fought the legislation for many years to avoid the burden and expense of the extra label, and some importers fear that US consumers may be less likely to buy imported beef labeled as such. Considering that we import about 2.5 billion pounds of beef a year, expect vested interests to continue to duke it out.

The Claim:
"ALL NATURAL*
*MINIMALLY PROCESSED.
CONTAINS NO ARTIFICIAL
INGREDIENTS"

The Truth:
You'll see the word "natural" all over meat packaging, both beef and poultry. The meat industry became very fond of the term "natural" with the rising popularity of organic foods. Producers of nonorganic foods worried that consumers would assume that conventional meat would translate into "chemical ridden," which spurred almost all meat manufacturers to emblazon their products with the phrase "all natural." It's easy enough, since the USDA doesn't carefully regulate the term—making it all but meaningless to the consumer.

PRODUCT OF USA

The Meat Matrix

Not all meat was created equal. From the lean, mean bison sirloin to a heavily marbled dry-aged rib eye, the protein spectrum is populated by a vast array of characters that vary greatly in con-siderations both culinary and nutritional. To simplify matters a bit, we've put every major cut of beef, pork, poultry, and alternative meats through a rigorous equation to assess its core nutritional value. The criteria? We started with protein-to-fat ratio; because all the calories in your steak or your chicken breast will come from one or the other, you want to choose cuts based on as high a protein-to-fat ratio as possible. Next, we considered the density of 10 essential nutrients commonly found in proteins, from vitamins B_6 and B_{12} to zinc. We rounded out the equation by factoring in saturated fat concentrations and cholesterol levels. The result is a chart that lets you compare chicken breast with duck leg, porterhouse with pork chops, and ultimately allows you to indulge your carnivorous side with a little more strategy.

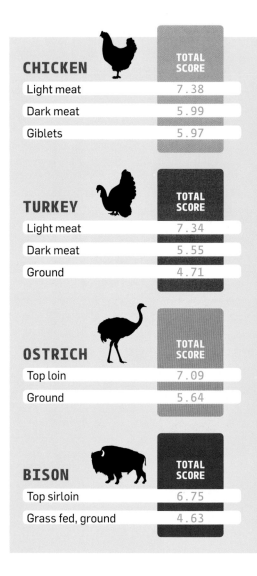

CHICKEN

	TOTAL SCORE
Light meat	7.38
Dark meat	5.99
Giblets	5.97

TURKEY

	TOTAL SCORE
Light meat	7.34
Dark meat	5.55
Ground	4.71

OSTRICH

	TOTAL SCORE
Top loin	7.09
Ground	5.64

BISON

	TOTAL SCORE
Top sirloin	6.75
Grass fed, ground	4.63

BEEF

	TOTAL SCORE
Kidney	6.79
Liver	6.22
Heart	5.82
Round	4.91
Flank	4.73
Top loin	4.25
Grass fed, ground	4.13
T-bone	3.92
Top sirloin	3.90
Ground 90% lean	3.87
Tongue	3.77
Porterhouse	3.75
Brisket, whole	3.71
Rib eye, small end	3.60
Tenderloin	3.45
Ground 80% lean	3.38
Rib roast, whole	3.20

PORK

	TOTAL SCORE
Tenderloin	6.90
Top loin/loin chops	5.92
Center loin/center rib	5.39
Sirloin	5.13
Ribs	4.72
Spareribs	4.09
Blade chops/roast	4.02
Ham, whole	3.24
Bacon (cured)	3.03

DUCK

	TOTAL SCORE
Domesticated	5.22

LAMB

	TOTAL SCORE
Sirloin chops, Australian	4.95
Ground	3.15

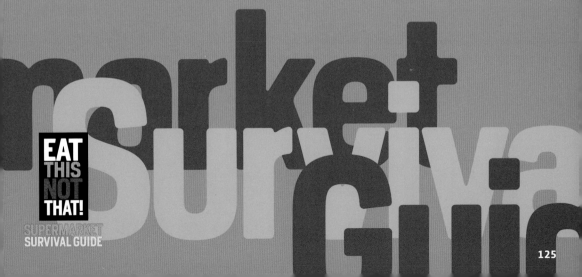

THE REFRIGERATOR SECTION

EAT
THIS
NOT
THAT!
SUPERMARKET
SURVIVAL GUIDE

The refrigerator is the Twilight Zone of your kitchen.

It's where most of the paranormal activity in the house takes place. While all seems fine at first glance, a lot of mysterious things are happening in the shadows. Way in the back, hidden by an old bottle of long-flat soda, something that once was meat—or maybe cake, it's hard to tell—has taken on new life forms. Yogurt containers have become penicillin factories, and at the bottom of the crisper, asparagus spears have metastasized into limp, black lances of biohazardous waste.

Seriously, cleaning the fridge can be as daunting as trying to tidy up the set of a *Saw* movie.

Why does so much good food go into our refrigerators, only to go out in the trash weeks—or, let's face it, months—later? A lot of times, it's because we buy food on impulse, without really having a plan for how we'll use it. Those heirloom tomatoes might have looked luscious in the produce aisle, but if you have to keep them for more than a few days, you'll probably stick them in the fridge—where they'll just get cold and mealy. And unlike the freezer or the pantry, where things tend to hang around for years without doing anything at all (sort of like the guys on *Jersey Shore*), the fridge is the home of the short shelf life.

Saving money while also eating great usually comes down to one essential skill: Knowing what you want to buy, and sticking to that list. That's what this book is designed to help you do. (Of course, it's important to always be trying new foods, especially in the produce department, but use this shopping trick: Each time you go to the market on a big shopping trip, buy no more than two items that weren't on your list. You'll be more selective if you have a limit on what you can put in your cart.)

The refrigerated section might be the place where buying wisely can save you the most money; it's also the place where choosing the right foods can have the biggest impact on your ability to meet your weight-loss goals. The reason is simple: Protein and calcium—both of which you find in abundance in the dairy case—are two of the most potent weight-loss nutrients around. In fact, the very act of ingesting and digesting dairy foods can actually burn away calories.

You see, food contains energy in the form of chemical bonds, but your body can't use that energy until it first breaks those bonds. Scientists call the energy that we expend breaking those bonds the "thermic effect" of eating—basically, the calorie-burning sideshow to digestion. And your body expends almost twice as many calories trying to digest protein as it does carbohydrates—about 25 calories for every 100 you eat, compared to only 10 to 15 calories for carbs. In fact, when Arizona State University researchers compared the benefits of a high-protein diet with those of a high-carbohydrate diet, they found that women who ate a high-protein diet burned about twice as many calories in the hours after their meals as those who ate a high-carb diet.

There's a second way in which the contents of your fridge can help you achieve the body you want. See, our bodies are constantly building up and breaking down muscle tissue, and muscle is an important player in the weight-loss game. That's because it takes more energy to maintain muscle tissue than it does fat tissue; in fact, muscle burns about 6 calories per pound every day, about three times as much as fat does. (So if you're carrying around 70 pounds of muscle, you're burning 420 calories a day just to maintain it; if that 70 pounds were just flab, you'd only burn 140 calories a day to maintain it. And that 280-calorie-a-day difference is enough to add another pound of flab every 12.5 days, or more than 29 pounds in a year!) That's why the greater your percentage of muscle, the greater your protection against fat.

And eating protein gives us the raw material to build muscle with. In fact, every time you eat 10 or more grams of protein—about what you'd find in a fruit-and-granola parfait, half a pouch of chunk light tuna, or 8 ounces of low-fat milk—you trigger a burst of what's called "protein synthesis." In other words, you start building and strengthening your lean muscle tissue, and taking aim at flab.

Indeed, there are a ton of health and fitness advantages to be found in the refrigerated section. Consider this:

- A study in the *International Journal of Obesity* found that dieters who ate a breakfast of eggs (yolks and all) at least five times a week for 5 weeks lost 65 percent more weight than those who ate bagels for breakfast.

- Meanwhile, researchers in Sweden found that conjugated linoleic acids (CLA), which are found in dairy and beef fat, can decrease waist size.

- Research published in the journal *Molecular Systems Biology* found that yogurt-based bacteria may actually help your body avoid absorbing fat!

- In a British study, men who drank milk at least once a day had a 16 percent lower risk of heart disease and were 20 percent less likely to have a stroke. And just one glass of milk per day decreases the risk of colorectal cancer by 12 percent, according to a study in the *Journal of the National Cancer Institute*.

- Nutrients in dairy products, including calcium, may reduce the risk of insulin resistance syndrome, a precursor to diabetes, according to research in the *Journal of the American College of Nutrition*.

But as we said, choosing wisely is critical. You'd think that screwing up milk, cheese, and yogurt would be hard to do, but modern food manufacturers have found near-miraculous ways to ruin even the healthiest foods, mostly by adding unnecessary sugars. As you peruse the dairy case and other refrigerated foods, keep this one principle in mind: Sugar is more dangerous than fat. Sugar is digested quickly, causing your blood glucose level to spike and forcing your body to store those calories in the form of fat. Dietary fat is digested slowly, meaning that your blood sugar doesn't spike, and those calories can be burned off at a steady pace, protecting you from rapid weight gain.

And it's in many of the "healthy," low-fat foods that you'll find more of the totally unhealthy, make-you-fat sugars. A quick look at the USDA National Nutrient Database for Standard Reference reveals a very interesting fact: 8 ounces of whole-fat plain yogurt has about 11.5 grams of sugar and 149 calories. Plain low-fat yogurt has about 17 grams of sugar and 154 calories. Yes, you read that right: Low-fat yogurt has more calories than whole fat does, and about 47 percent more sugar, too.

That's why your trip through the refrigerator case requires more care than you might have thought. Choose wisely, though, and you'll be on your way to a lifetime of lean!

What's Really in...
Ball Park Franks

MECHANICALLY SEPARATED TURKEY

What makes mechanically separated turkey different than the legs and thighs you covet at Thanksgiving? Well it comes from the same animal, but it's the waste you typically set out for the garbage truck. See, in the '60s, someone in the meat industry began to question whether there was any use for the gristly pieces of meat left clinging to carcasses after the recognizable cuts had been removed. To answer the question, processors began siphoning animal remains—bones and all—through pressurized sieves that extracted all the edible pieces and churned them into a bright pink paste. The goal was to wring every last dollar out of every last carcass, and a British chief trading standards officer estimated the cuts to be 10 times cheaper than traditional cuts. Today, mechanical separation is commonplace, and the extracted sludge is typically pressed into hot dogs, jerky, and other processed deli meats.

TOTAL FAT 15 G

You might think that all the poultry being pumped into hot dogs has made them leaner over the years, but the numbers don't lie. According to the USDA, in 1937 the average hot dog was composed of 19 percent fat and 19.6 percent protein. The humble frankfurter has plumped up quite a bit in the last 75 years; today, hot dogs contain about 28 percent fat to just 11.7 percent protein. Ball Park, one of America's iconic dogs, fares even worse. In its best, most unadulterated form, a hot dog can still be a solid meal option, but you must choose wisely. For our dollar, Applegate Natural Beef Hot Dogs are the best in class: Made from grass-fed beef and little else, they hark back to a day when meat wasn't such a mystery.

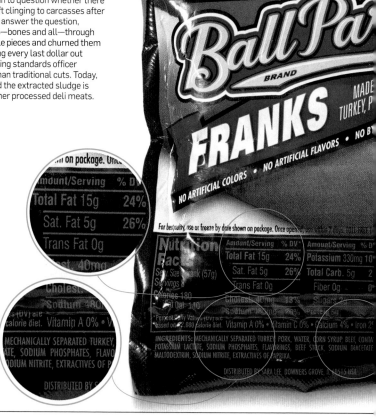

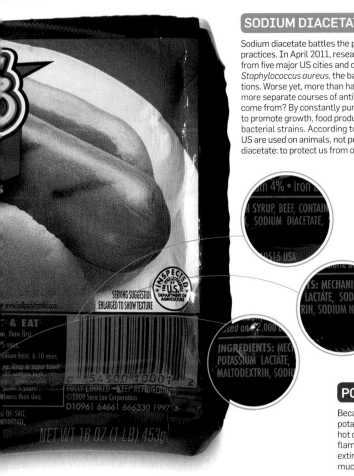

SODIUM DIACETATE

Sodium diacetate battles the pathogens introduced by unscrupulous farming practices. In April 2011, researchers in Arizona tested meat and poultry samples from five major US cities and discovered that 47 percent were contaminated with *Staphylococcus aureus,* the bacterial strain responsible for most staph infections. Worse yet, more than half of these staph bugs refused to die after three or more separate courses of antibiotics. Where did these drug-resistant superbugs come from? By constantly pumping farm animals full of bacteria-fighting drugs to promote growth, food producers have encouraged the growth of stronger bacterial strains. According to the FDA, 80 percent of the antibiotics sold in the US are used on animals, not people, and that's why we need additives like sodium diacetate: to protect us from our own food system.

SODIUM NITRITE

The most controversial additive on this ingredient list, nitrites and nitrates are unsettlingly common in the deli cooler, and they play roles in curing and preserving the pinkish color of meats and fish. Trouble is, once digested, nitrites can bond with amines to form cancer-causing nitrosamines. But see the sodium erythorbate on this ingredients list? It's been shown to hinder the reaction, in theory protecting you from the risk of cancer.

POTASSIUM LACTATE

Because it inhibits mold and fungus growth, potassium lactate is a commonly used preservative in hot dogs and deli meats. Interestingly, it also inhibits flame growth, which is why it often appears in fire extinguishers. Looks like you don't have to worry too much about your Ball Park catching fire.

131

I Can't Believe It's Not

"70% LESS SATURATED FAT THAN BUTTER"

Butter lost favor during the low-fat fad of the '90s, and that opened the door for trans fatty margarine. As enthusiasm for trans fats turned into fear of cardiovascular disease, manufacturers turned to highly saturated palm oils. Researchers at Tufts University fed subjects large amounts of palm oil, partially hydrogenated oil (trans fats), soybean oil, or canola oil for more than a month, and they discovered that those consuming palm oil and partially hydrogenated oil saw similar jumps in LDL cholesterol levels.

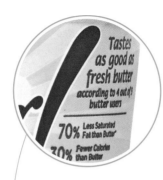

"TASTES AS GOOD AS FRESH BUTTER"

We don't fashion ourselves the grand arbiters of taste, but it's hard to imagine a 16-ingredient science experiment tasting as good as something made from just sweet cream. At 70 calories per tablespoon, I Can't Believe It's Not Butter saves you only 20 to 30 calories over the 90 or so in the same amount of regular butter. What you give up in return—healthy fat, vitamins and antioxidants, the joy of simple, whole foods—might not be worth the handful of calories.

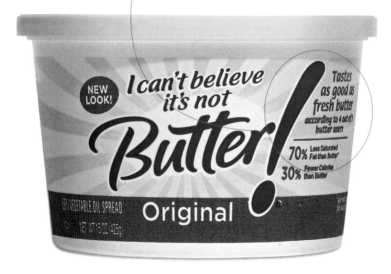

Butter

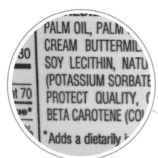

SOY LECITHIN

In butter, naturally occurring proteins act as emulsifiers by binding together fat and water, but vegetable oils, once refined, don't have a similar emulsifying component. That's where lecithin comes into play. It's a fatlike compound found in the cells of all living things, and it's the reason I Can't Believe It's Not Butter doesn't slosh around inside its tub. So think about it: I Can't Believe It's Not Butter contains soybean oil, and it also contains soy lecithin. At one point, those two ingredients were part of the same plant, but they were separated through a process known as "degumming" and eventually reunited in this tub. Never underestimate the irony of processed foods.

BETA-CAROTENE

This one should sound familiar—it's the orange pigment found in carrots and sweet potatoes, and it's a precursor to vitamin A. It's used here to give the spread a golden, butterlike hue. We commend the use of natural ingredients over artificial colors, but keep in mind that coloring of any sort is used to hide unappetizing characteristics. Without beta-carotene, I Can't Believe It's Not Butter would look a lot like Crisco shortening, and that's something you might not want to spread on your pancakes.

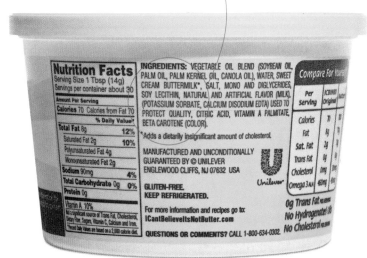

Yogurts
Eat This

It takes Fage more than a pound of raw milk to make one container of this yogurt, which is why it's so thick and loaded with protein. Equally as commendable is the fact that Fage eschews preservatives and artificial thickeners.

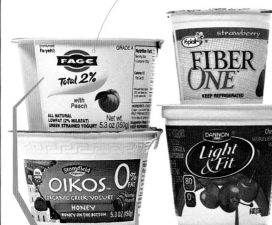

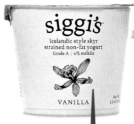

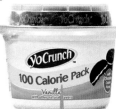

Yoplait Fiber One Nonfat Strawberry
(4 oz, 1 container)

50 calories
0 g fat
4 g sugars
3 g protein

Fiber One has fewer than half the calories and nearly double the fiber of Dannon.

Fage Total 2% with Peach
(5.3 oz, 1 container)

130 calories
2.5 g fat
(1.5 g saturated)
17 g sugars
10 g protein

Stonyfield Oikos Organic Greek Yogurt Honey
(5.3 oz, 1 container)

120 calories
0 g fat
17 g sugars
13 g protein

Oikos uses honey to turn this into a lightly sweetened treat, not ice cream.

Dannon Light & Fit Cherry
(6 oz, 1 container)

80 calories
0 g fat
11 g sugars
5 g protein

We prefer a yogurt with more protein, but it's tough to argue against a yogurt with just 80 calories per serving.

Siggi's Vanilla
(5.4 oz, 1 container)

100 calories
0 g fat
9 g sugars
14 g protein

In Iceland, yogurt is made by skimming away the watery whey. The result, called skyr, is a thick, creamy, protein-dense wonder.

Breyer's YoCrunch 100 Calorie Vanilla with Chocolate Cookie Pieces
(106 g, 1 container)

100 calories
1.5 g fat
(0.5 g saturated)
13 g sugars
3 g protein

A cookie-strewn nutritional bargain.

Not That!

Yoplait commits the cardinal sin of fruit-flavored yogurts by candying these peaches with more sugar than you'd find in a two-pack of Reese's Peanut Butter Cups. The only yogurts worth eating are those that are unflavored or that can claim to have more fruit than sugar.

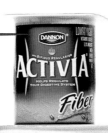
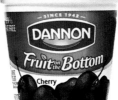
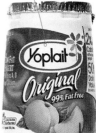
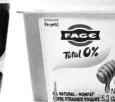

Yoplait Whips! Chocolate Mousse Style
(4 oz, 1 container)

160 calories
4 g fat
(2.5 g saturated)
22 g sugars
5 g protein

You'd be better off eating a small scoop of Breyers Chocolate ice cream.

Wallaby Organic Nonfat Vanilla Bean
(6 oz, 1 container)

140 calories
0 g fat
22 g sugars
6 g protein

Organic dairy is awesome, but not when there's this much sugar.

Dannon Fruit on the Bottom Cherry
(6 oz, 1 container)

140 calories
1.5 g fat
(1 g saturated)
24 g sugars
6 g protein

"Fruit" means a few cherries soaked in sugar and fructose.

Fage Total 0% with Honey
(6 oz, 1 container)

160 calories
0 g fat
29 g sugars
11 g protein

We are unabashed Fage junkies, but this sugar-loaded cup is a serious buzzkill.

Yoplait Original 99% Fat Free Harvest Peach
(6 oz, 1 container)

170 calories
1.5 g fat
(1 g saturated)
26 g sugars
5 g protein

Butter & Butter Sub

Eat This

The process of whipping butter introduces air, thus making it easier to spread and lighter in calories.

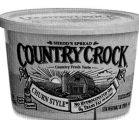

PAM Olive Oil Cooking Spray
(0.3 g, one ¼-second spray)

0 calories
0 g fat
0 mg sodium

Technically, the olive oil in this can still delivers calories, but with just a light misting, the impact is negligible.

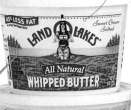

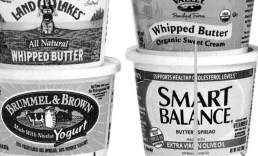

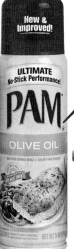

Land O'Lakes Whipped Butter
(7 g, 1 Tbsp)

50 calories
6 g fat
(3.5 g saturated)
50 mg sodium

Brummel & Brown Spread
(14 g, 1 Tbsp)

45 calories
5 g fat
(1.5 g saturated)
90 mg sodium

This ingenious tub replaces cream with fat-free yogurt to create one of the lowest-calorie spreads in the cooler.

Organic Valley Whipped Butter
(7 g, 1 Tbsp)

50 calories
6 g fat
(3.5 g saturated)
40 mg sodium

Hormones used to treat cattle tend to concentrate in butterfat, so buy organic to cut out the potential hormone-related risks.

Smart Balance Buttery Spread with Extra Virgin Olive Oil
(11 g, 1 Tbsp)

60 calories
7 g fat
(2 g saturated)
70 mg sodium

Studies show that the omega-3 fatty acids in this spread may protect against breast, prostate, and colon cancer.

Shedd's Spread Country Crock Churn Style
(14 g, 1 Tbsp)

60 calories
7 g fat
(2 g saturated)
85 mg sodium

Don't be fooled by the heavy-sounding "Churn Style." This spread is lighter than most.

stitutes

THE REFRIGERATOR SECTION

Not That!

**I Can't Believe
It's Not Butter!
Spray Original**
(0.2 g, 1 spray)

0 calories
0 g fat
0 mg sodium

The soybean oil
used in this spray
delivers only a third
as much heart-healthy
monounsaturated
fat as olive oil.

*How do they get vegetable oil
to solidify? Simple: by partially hydrogenating
the oil. The by-product of this process is
trans fats, the artificial fatty acids known
to spike bad cholesterol levels.*

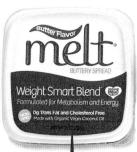

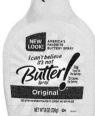

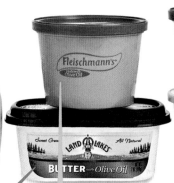

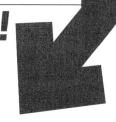

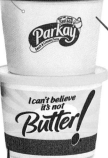

**Melt
Buttery Spread**
(14 g, 1 Tbsp)

80 calories
9 g fat
(4 g saturated)
85 mg sodium

Despite the marketing
pitch that it's a
healthier buttery
spread, it contains as
much as or more fat
than most of the
Country Crock versions.

**Land O'Lakes
Butter
with Olive Oil**
(14 g, 1 Tbsp)

90 calories
10 g fat
(4 g saturated)
90 mg sodium

Including olive oil
in the name is a sleight
of hand. The main
ingredient is cream,
which has nearly double
the saturated fat
as olive oil.

**Fleischmann's
Olive Oil Spread**
(11 g, 1 Tbsp)

60 calories
6.5 g fat
(1 g saturated)
45 mg sodium

Despite listing zero
trans fats in the
nutritional information,
Fleischmann's second
ingredient is partially
hydrogenated oil.
That's the primary
source of trans fats.

**I Can't Believe
It's Not Butter!
Original**
(14 g, 1 Tbsp)

70 calories
8 g fat
(2 g saturated)
90 mg sodium

Comprised of a
concerning mix of
oils and buttermilk,
this spread packs
60 percent more fat
than Brummel &
Brown's version.

Parkay
(14 g, 1 Tbsp)

80 calories
9 g fat
(1.5 g saturated,
1.5 g trans)
130 mg sodium

Cheeses

Eat This

Cheese adds a creamy texture to your foods and flab-fighting calcium to your diet. But to keep the calories in check, use it smartly—which is to say, sparingly.

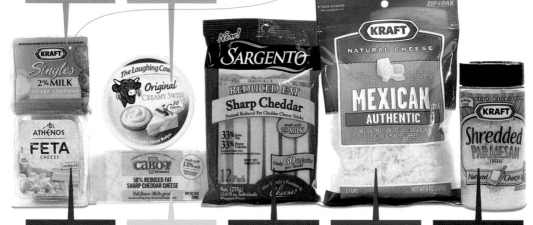

Kraft Singles 2% Milk Sharp Cheddar
(19 g, 1 slice)

45 calories
3 g fat
(1.5 g saturated)
250 mg sodium
4 g protein

The Laughing Cow Original Creamy Swiss
(21 g, 1 wedge)

50 calories
4 g fat
(2.5 g saturated)
210 mg sodium
2 g protein

Spreads every bit as easily as Alouette's, yet it cuts your calorie load by a third.

Athenos Traditional Crumbled Feta
(34 g, ¼ cup)

90 calories
7 g fat
(4 g saturated)
400 mg sodium
6 g protein

A reasonable fat-to-protein ratio makes feta the most reliable go-to crumbled cheese.

Cabot 50% Reduced Fat Sharp Cheddar
(28 g)

70 calories
4.5 g fat
(3 g saturated)
170 mg sodium
8 g protein

A smart approach: Cut half the fat, but leave enough to add a rich, creamy texture.

Sargento Reduced Fat Sharp Cheddar Sticks
(21 g, 1 stick)

60 calories
4.5 g fat
(3 g saturated)
135 mg sodium
5 g protein

Portable snacks don't get any better than this.

Kraft Authentic Mexican Style
(28 g, ¼ cup)

90 calories
7 g fat
(4 g saturated)
200 mg sodium
6 g protein

Bagged cheese blends tend to carry a heavy caloric toll, but this Mexican mix is a good option for all your melting needs.

Kraft Shredded Parmesan Cheese
(2 tsp)

18 calories
1 g fat
(0 g saturated)
68 mg sodium
1.5 g protein

Consider this the leanest way to add big flavor to your pastas and baked potatoes.

Not That!

These slices earn three-quarters of their calories from fat. And what does that earn you? Nothing but extra calories.

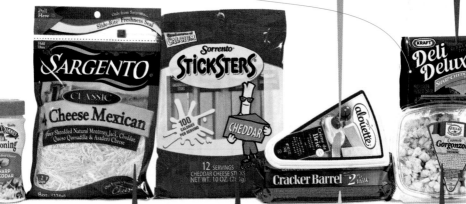

Alouette Crème de Brie Spreadable
(28 g, 2 Tbsp)

90 calories
8 g fat
(4.5 g saturated)
200 mg sodium
4 g protein

The portion-controlled approach used by The Laughing Cow helps prevent cheese overload.

Kraft Deli Deluxe Sharp Cheddar Slices
(28 g, 1 slice)

110 calories
9 g fat
(5 g saturated)
450 mg sodium
6 g protein

Land O'Lakes Sharp Cheddar Seasoning
(2 tsp)

20 calories
0 g fat
800 mg sodium
1 g protein

By "seasoning," Land O'Lakes means "sodium." Each serving contains a third of your day's intake.

Sargento 4 Cheese Mexican
(24 g, 1 stick)

110 calories
9 g fat
(6 g saturated)
200 mg sodium
6 g protein

The Blended Cheese Principle: The more varieites of cheese in a package, the more calories it will contain.

Sorrento Sticksters Cheddar Cheese Sticks
(24 g, 1 stick)

100 calories
8 g fat
(4.5 g saturated)
150 mg sodium
6 g protein

The rollerblading cheese stick on the label doesn't mean this is a kid-friendly snack.

Kraft Cracker Barrel Extra Sharp 2% Milk
(28 g)

90 calories
6 g fat
(3.5 g saturated)
240 mg sodium
7 g protein

Switch to Cabot's and you'll cut 320 calories from each pound of cheese you buy.

Stella Crumbled Gorgonzola
(28 g, ¼ cup)

100 calories
8 g fat
(6 g saturated)
380 mg sodium
6 g protein

Even with less cheese in each serving, you still end up with more calories and fat.

139

Deli Meats
Eat This

Applegate Farms eschews antibiotics, producing some of the most pristine, natural meats in the supermarket.

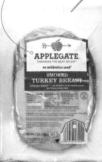

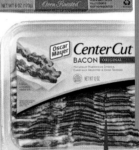

Applegate Smoked Turkey Breast
(56 g)

50 calories
0 g fat
360 mg sodium
12 g protein

Hormel Natural Choice Carved Chicken Breast Oven Roasted
(56 g)

60 calories
1.5 g fat
(0.5 g saturated)
340 mg sodium
12 g protein

This chicken is almost pure protein.

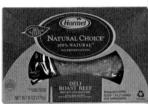

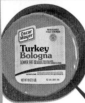

Hormel Natural Choice Deli Roast Beef
(56 g)

60 calories
2 g fat
(1 g saturated)
520 mg sodium
11 g protein

One of the few deli brands to forgo all nitrites, nitrates, and other preservatives.

Oscar Mayer Turkey Bologna
(28 g, 1 slice)

50 calories
4 g fat
(1 g saturated)
270 mg sodium
3 g protein

Turkey doesn't always mean healthier, but Oscar Mayer wields the lean white meat wisely, using it to soften the blow of traditional bologna.

Jones Naturally Hickory Smoked Canadian Bacon
(51 g)

60 calories
1.5 g fat
(0.5 g saturated)
460 mg sodium
11 g protein

The easiest swap in the supermarket; you get twice as much food for half the calories.

Oscar Mayer Center Cut Bacon
(2 slices)

70 calories
4.5 g fat
(1.5 g saturated)
270 mg sodium
7 g protein

If you want bacon, eat bacon. You won't take in any extra calories or fat grams and you'll actually cut sodium.

Not That!

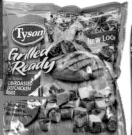
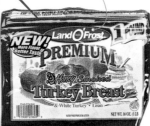
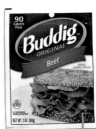
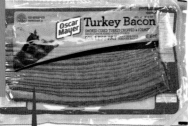
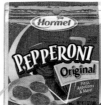
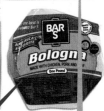

Land O'Frost Premium Honey Smoked Turkey Breast
(52 g)

90 calories
4.5 g fat
(1 g saturated)
670 mg sodium
8 g protein

Tyson Grilled & Ready Oven Roasted Diced Chicken Breast
(56 g)

73 calories
2 g fat
(1 g saturated)
220 mg sodium
13 g protein

It takes 15 ingredients to make this FrankenChicken.

Oscar Mayer Turkey Bacon
(2 slices)

70 calories
6 g fat
(2 g saturated)
360 mg sodium
4 g protein

More sodium than regular pork bacon, but also more than triple the number of ingredients.

Hormel Pepperoni
(28 g)

140 calories
13 g fat
(6 g saturated)
490 mg sodium
5 g protein

Pepperoni is the downfall of far too many pizzas served in America, and the blame rests entirely on its egregious load of fat.

Bar-S Bologna
(38 g, 1 slice)

100 calories
8 g fat
(2.5 g saturated)
350 mg sodium
3 g protein

You could eat two slices of Oscar Mayer's Turkey Bologna for the same calories from 1 Bar-S slice.

Buddig Original Beef
(56 g)

90 calories
5 g fat
(2 g saturated)
790 mg sodium
10 g protein

Most deli meats fail in one of two ways: too much fat or too much sodium. Buddig's products routinely fail in both ways.

Hot Dogs & Sausages
Eat This

*There's no reason to fear hot dogs.
A recent study from Kansas State University found
that microwave-cooked hot dogs have fewer cancer-causing
compounds than even rotisserie chicken.
Stick with low-calorie brands and you're never far from a quick,
healthy, and protein-packed meal.*

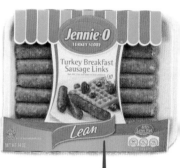

**Aidells
Cajun Style
Andouille**
(85 g, 1 link)

160 calories
11 g fat
(4 g saturated)
600 mg sodium
15 g protein

Remember Aidells.
It's one of the
most reliable purveyors
in the deli fridge.

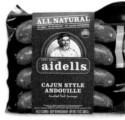

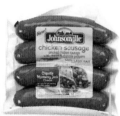

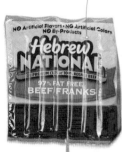

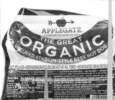

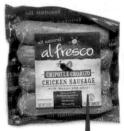

**Hebrew
National
97% Fat Free
Beef Franks**
(45 g, 1 frank)

40 calories
1 g fat
(0 g saturated)
520 mg sodium
6 g protein

**Applegate Farms
The Great Organic
Hot Dogs**
(56 g, 1 frank)

110 calories
8 g fat
(3 g saturated)
330 mg sodium
7 g protein

Applegate Farms has
re-created the famous
frank of New York, but it's
done so without resorting
to dubious waste cuts
or antibiotic-heavy meat.

**Johnsonville
Chicken Sausage
Chipotle
Monterey Jack
Cheese** (85 g, 1 link)

170 calories
12 g fat
(4 g saturated)
770 mg sodium
13 g protein

We're glad to see
the sausage behemoth
get on board with
the chicken variety.

**Al Fresco
Chipotle Chorizo
Chicken Sausage**
(85 g, 1 link)

140 calories
7 g fat
(2 g saturated)
420 mg sodium
15 g protein

Our love for
Al Fresco runs deep.
No company offers
a wider variety of
bold-flavored,
low-calorie sausages.

**Jennie-O
Turkey Breakfast
Sausage Links
Lean** (56 g, 2 links)

90 calories
5 g fat
(1.5 g saturated)
370 mg sodium
10 g protein

Cutting fat
doesn't just drop the
calorie count,
it also makes more
space for protein.

Not That!

*Hot dogs vary widely in terms of fat content,
so it's important to flip the package and scan the ingredients list.
Case in point: You could eat half a dozen of
the Hebrew National dogs on the opposite page and still
not reach the fat load of these "light" franks.*

Hillshire Farm Smoked Bratwurst
(76 g, 1 link)

240 calories
22 g fat
(8 g saturated)
780 mg sodium
8 g protein

More than 80 percent of this brat's calories come from fat.

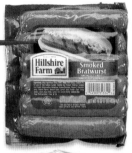

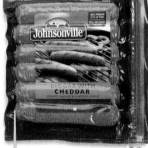

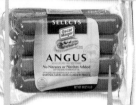

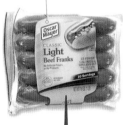

Jennie-O Breakfast Lover's Turkey Sausage
(56 g, 2 links)

130 calories
10 g fat
(3 g saturated)
310 mg sodium
8 g protein

With "turkey" on the label you should expect more from your breakfast sausage.

Hillshire Farm Polska Kielbasa
(56 g)

180 calories
16 g fat
(5 g saturated)
510 mg sodium
7 g protein

Both kielbasa and chorizo are spicy ethnic sausages, but opt for Al Fresco and you double up on protein while cutting calories, fat, and sodium.

Johnsonville Beddar with Cheddar
(66 g, 1 link)

200 calories
17 g fat
(6 g saturated)
620 mg sodium
8 g protein

More calories, less protein, and a hearty dose of MSG.

Oscar Mayer Selects Angus Hot Dogs
(57 g, 1 frank)

180 calories
17 g fat
(7 g saturated)
420 mg sodium
6 g protein

"Angus" beef is just as likely as regular beef to be loaded with fat, and whether it tastes any better is a subject for debate.

Oscar Mayer Classic Light Beef Franks
(45 g, 1 frank)

90 calories
7 g fat
(3 g saturated)
450 mg sodium
5 g protein

143

Meat Substitutes
Eat This

Boca
Ground Crumbles
(57 g, 1 cup)

60 calories
0.5 g fat
(0 g saturated)
270 mg sodium

Boca's regular soy blend is the best you can find. Nearly 90 percent of the calories come from protein.

Quorn
Classic Burgers
(60 g, 1 patty)

90 calories
3 g fat
(0.5 g saturated)
290 mg sodium

Quorn is made primarily from high-fiber mycoprotein, a fungus similar to mushrooms.

For a faux sausage of this size, one that packs 13 grams of soy protein, 140 calories is a bargain.

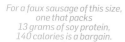

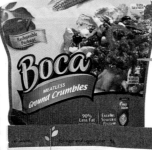

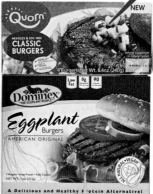

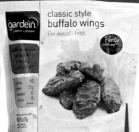

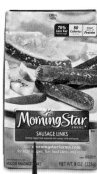

LightLife
Smart
Sausages
(85 g, 1 link)

140 calories
7 g fat
(1 g saturated)
500 mg sodium

LightLife
Smart Dogs
(42 g, 1 link)

45 calories
0 g fat
310 mg sodium

Protein accounts for more than 70 percent of the calories in this dog.

Gardein
Classic Style
Buffalo Wings
(90 g, 5 wings with sauce)

125 calories
2.5 g fat
(0 g saturated)
519 mg sodium

Each wing packs in more than 3 grams of protein.

Dominex
Eggplant
Burgers
(78 g, 1 patty)

90 calories
1 g fat
(0 g saturated)
450 mg sodium

This real eggplant patty will earn you 9 grams of protein and a hearty dose of chlorogenic acid, a potent antioxidant with cancer-fighting properties.

MorningStar
Farms
Veggie Sausage
Links
(45 g, 2 links)

80 calories
3 g fat
(0.5 g saturated)
300 mg sodium

The 9-gram protein boost in these links will help prevent you from overeating later in the day.

Not That!

Boca All American Classic Meatless Burgers Made with Non-GMO Soy
(71 g, 1 patty)

140 calories
5 g fat
(1.5 g saturated)
500 mg sodium

Even withous GMOs, this still falls flat.

LightLife Gimme Lean Smart Ground Beef Style
(57 g, 2 oz)

70 calories
0 g fat
350 mg sodium

These crumbles contain barely half the protein of Boca's.

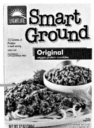

Amazingly enough, this fake Italian sausage packs nearly as many calories as the real stuff.

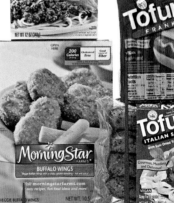
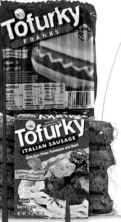
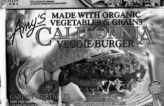
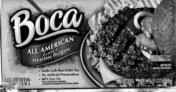
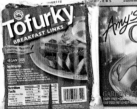

Tofurky Breakfast Links
(45 g, 1 link)

120 calories
6 g fat
(0 g saturated)
320 mg sodium

A heavy hand with vegetable oil adds more than 50 calories to each link.

Amy's California Veggie Burgers
(71 g, 1 patty)

150 calories
5 g fat
(0.5 g saturated)
500 mg sodium

More calories, fat, and sodium and less protein. The choice is simple.

MorningStar Farms Buffalo Wings
(85 g, 5 wings)

200 calories
8 g fat
(1 g saturated)
640 mg sodium

MorningStar's wings are no match for Gardein's—they have nearly double the calories and 220 percent more fat per serving.

Tofurky Franks
(45 g, 1 link)

80 calories
2 g fat
(0 g saturated)
370 mg sodium

For the same number of calories, you could switch over to Smart Dogs' Jumbo dog and get more protein for your caloric buck.

Tofurky Italian Sausage
(100 g, 1 sausage)

270 calories
13 g fat
(1.5 g saturated)
620 mg sodium

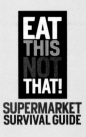

EAT
THIS
NOT
THAT!
**SUPERMARKET
SURVIVAL GUIDE**

THE PANTRY AISLES

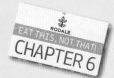

RODALE
EAT THIS, NOT THAT!
CHAPTER 6

Congratulations!

You have already taken an enormous step toward making your staple shopping a leaner, smarter process.

How? By choosing to read about the food you eat. And that puts you well ahead of most Americans.

In a 2007 report, the National Endowment for the Arts sounded a warning call: Americans simply aren't reading as much as we used to, and as a result, we aren't particularly good at it anymore. In fact, the report stated, "Reading scores for American adults of almost all education levels have deteriorated" and noted that even those of us who others might describe as "bookish" aren't spending enough time with our noses in the books. "From 1992 to 2003, the percentage of adults with graduate school experience who were rated proficient in prose reading [experienced] a 20 percent rate of decline."

Now, who do you think is happiest about this development?

• Gym teachers, who never thought book learnin' was all that important anyways

• TV studio heads, who don't even have to make sure their channel guides are spelled right anymore, as long as those *Deadliest Catch* guys keep hauling in the crabs

• The folks at Twitter, who are pretty sure 140 characters is all any of us can tolerate at one time

• Food manufacturers, who can stick words like "lite" and "natural" and "fortified" on their packages of nutritionally questionable noshes and laugh all the way to the bank

Chances are, they're all pretty happy. But my guess is that nobody's life has been made easier by our national reading decline than food producers. Because when it comes to packaged foods, the most important way to protect your waistline is to read the labels before you buy.

Most of us don't pay too much attention to our boxed, canned, and bagged foods. You might think that the big-ticket items are in the meat and produce aisles, but think again. In fact, a 2006 study found that we spend nearly 27 percent of our food budgets on nonperishable pantry goods—almost as much as meat (13 percent), produce (10.5 percent), and dairy (9 percent) combined! And when you consider how much of what's in that box or bag is nothing but air, the pantry is where the *cha-ching* really lies.

When it comes to packaged foods, the marketers have the upper hand. You can coax and cajole the butcher into giving you the best cut of meat and master the art of detecting a ripe peach among a pile of rock-hard Georgia baseballs. But you can't squeeze the cereal to see if it's fresh, or sniff the macaroni before you pop it into your cart. All you have to go on is what the manufacturers tell you, and so it's easy to fall back on that old mainstay of food shopping—blind trust. The soups, noodles, and canned hearts of palm that make their way into your cart are probably a mix of the products Mom used to buy and whatever's on sale, featured in a coupon, or just easily within reach. But unless you read the fine print, you may be bringing home a lot more fat, sodium, sugar, and calories than you ever imagined.

For example, let's say you wanted a fast-and-easy rice dish. Mom always made Rice-A-Roni, so you grab its Rice Pilaf and saunter down the aisle, crossing "box of rice" off your list. But if you had lingered and done a little homework, you might instead have reached for a very similar product, Near East Rice Pilaf Curry. Preparing the Rice-A-Roni according to the box's instructions will pile 310 calories, 9 grams of fat, and 1,060 milligrams of sodium on your plate, as a side dish to whatever that night's meat might be. But if you'd chosen the Near East version,

you would have saved 90 calories—and a swap like that once a day is worth a pound of weight loss every 39 days, or about 9 pounds a year. You'd have also reduced your fat intake by nearly two-thirds and cut more than 500 milligrams of blood-pressure-pushing sodium. And you didn't have to change your eating habits one bit!

And that's not even an extreme example. In the cereal aisle, you'll find that nice Quaker man smiling out at you from the box of Quaker Natural Lowfat Granola with Raisins. What can be bad about that? It's "natural" and "lowfat," and it even says things like "good source of fiber" and "0 g trans fat" right there on the box! But flip to the side nutrition label and you'll see what you're really buying in each cup: 315 calories, and 27 grams of sugar—more than you'd get in a pack of Peanut M&Ms! But you can cut the calories and sugar by almost half if you opt for a similar product, Fiber One Raisin Bran Clusters. Make that switch every morning and you're saving 145 calories a day, or a pound of weight every 24 days. By this time next year you'll weigh 15 pounds less!

What's great about mastering shopping for your pantry is a) it will make a huge impact, and b) you really only have to do it once. Spend more time reading labels on your next shopping trip and identify the products that have more fiber, less sugar, fewer calories, and—especially—fewer ingredients. Few ingredients means more real food, and that can only be good for you. You'll identify the healthiest items in the market, and you can go back to them time and time again. And while you're at it, look for some terrific products out there that you might have missed. Barilla, the pasta maker, recently launched a line of whole-grain pastas that, when cooked, taste and feel exactly like regular pasta, but have a nutritional punch. (Nice going, guys!) Products like these are everywhere in your supermarket.

You just have to be willing to read. Here are some other tips that can save you calories, and money, on your next trip to the market.

• Take longer looks at private label (store brand) canned and packaged goods when possible. In many cases, they're made by the same manufacturers, using the same ingredients, as your major-label brands. They almost always taste just as good, provide comparable nutritional content, and come at a fraction of the cost.

• Canned foods are wallet friendly and easy to cook with, but watch out for a couple of common belt-busting pitfalls: high sodium content and unhealthy packing materials like oil and syrup. When buying cans, look for low-sodium options and canned meats packed in water, not oil.

• Keep your pantry clean—crumbs and forgotten packages can attract pests, and you may waste money replacing items you forgot you already had. Once a month, take everything out of your pantry, toss stale and expired foods, vacuum up crumbs, take stock of what you have, and put it all back so it's organized.

• If you notice tiny flies or little wriggly creatures in your pantry, it's probably because a pest either got inside a package or laid eggs on the outside before it got shipped to the store. To prevent pests, repackage products that come in bags and boxes (especially beans and grains) in mason jars or sealed plastic containers. Or, if you have room, store grains in the fridge.

If there's anything that our series of blind taste tests proved—tests that pitted the most high-profile brands in the supermarket versus the lowly generic labels of national grocers—it's that brand recognition and quality don't always go together. (See the shocking results of The Ultimate Brand Smackdown for yourself on page 44.) And if there's anything that years of scouring the aisles, poring over ingredient labels with microscopes while dodging disgruntled supermarket stockers has taught us, it's that you're never more than a few simple swaps away from a leaner, healthier lifestyle. You'll find hundreds of examples proving just that in the pages to come.

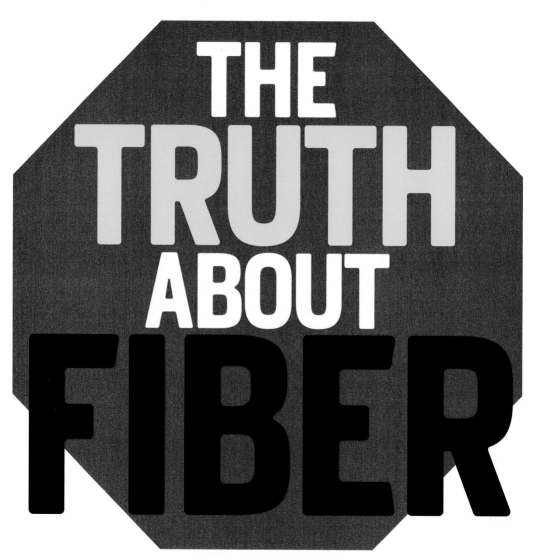

THE TRUTH ABOUT FIBER

You hear the advice constantly: You need fiber. It's crucial to your health. Fine, but how much fiber, and how crucial is it? Maybe you're even wondering, What is fiber, exactly?

Let's start with the basics. Fiber is a type of carbohydrate that makes up the structural material in the leaves, stems, and roots of plants. But unlike sugar and starch—the other two kinds of carbs—fiber stays intact until it nears the end of your digestive tract. This, it seems, is what makes fiber beneficial, and why you've probably heard you can't eat enough of it. Now read on to separate the facts from the fiction.

All Fiber Is Created Equal
FALSE

There are two basic types of fiber, and they have different functions. Insoluble fiber is found in wheat bran, nuts, and many vegetables. Its structure is thick and rough, and it won't dissolve in water, so it zips through your digestive tract and increases stool bulk. Soluble fiber is found in oats, beans, barley, and some fruits. It dissolves in water to form a gel-like material in your digestive tract. This allows it to slow the absorption of sugar into your bloodstream. What's more, soluble fiber, when eaten regularly, has been shown to slightly lower LDL (bad) cholesterol levels.

Fiber Has No Calories
FALSE

Fiber is essentially composed of a bundle of sugar molecules. These molecules are held together by chemical bonds that your body has trouble breaking. In fact, your small intestine can't break down soluble or insoluble fiber; both types just go right through you. That's why some experts say fiber doesn't provide any calories. However, this claim isn't entirely accurate. In your large intestine, soluble fiber's molecules are converted to short-chain fatty acids, which do provide a few calories. A gram of regular carbohydrates has about 4 calories, as does a gram of soluble fiber, according to the FDA. (Insoluble fiber has essentially zero calories.)

Fiber Can Help You Lose Weight

TRUE

Fiber's few calories are more than offset by its weight-control benefits. The conclusion of a review published in the journal *Nutrition* is clear: People who add fiber to their diets lose more weight than those who don't add it. Fiber requires extra chewing and slows the absorption of nutrients in your gut, so your body is tricked into thinking you've eaten enough, says review author Joanne Slavin, PhD, RD. And some fibers may also stimulate release of cholecystokinin (CCK), an appetite-suppressing hormone in the gut.

Fiber Is All-Natural Goodness

SORT OF

Fiber is showing up in everything these days—yogurt, grape juice, artificial sweetener. If this seems impossible, remember that these are molecules; you don't have to see or feel fiber for it to be present. Scientists now have a new class of fiber they refer to as "functional" fiber, meaning that it's created and added to processed foods. "You can make fiber from bacteria or from yeast," says Slavin. "And as long as you prove that it can lower cholesterol or feed the good bacteria in your gut or increase stool weight, it's fiber."

Supplemental Fiber Is Healthy

TRUE

But foods with added fiber don't necessarily provide the benefits you might expect. Inulin, for example, a soluble fiber extracted from chicory root, can be found in products like Fiber One bars. In addition to boosting fiber content, it's also commonly used to replace fat. Inulin is known as a prebiotic, which means it promotes the growth of healthy bacteria in your gut. That's good, of course. "But," says Slavin, "inulin doesn't have the same cholesterol-lowering effect as the fiber found in oat bran."

Food Companies Are Jumping on the Fiber Bandwagon

DUH

In 2007, the FDA declared that poly-dextrose can be called fiber. Polywhat? Polydextrose is made from glucose, sorbitol (a sugar alcohol), and citric acid. It's what puts the fiber in Fruity Pebbles. Polydextrose received FDA approval because it mimics some attributes of dietary fiber: It isn't absorbed in the small intestine, and it increases stool weight. Polydextrose mainly bulks up foods so they're not as high in calories. However, there's no research to prove that polydextrose is as beneficial as the fiber found in whole foods.

Men Need 38 Grams of Fiber a Day; Women Need 25

FALSE

Those are the recommendations from the Institute of Medicine. Scientists there crunched data from three studies and squeezed out the number 38 for men in 2005. It equals 9 apples, or 12 bowls of instant oatmeal. (Most people eat about 15 grams of fiber daily.) The studies found a correlation between high fiber intake and lower incidence of heart disease. But none of the high-fiber-eating groups in those studies averaged as high as 38 grams, and, in fact, people saw maximum benefits with a daily gram intake averaging from the high 20s to the low 30s. It's hard for even those who eat the healthiest diets to consume more than 25 grams of fiber. Aim high, of course, but you can afford to fall a bit short.

This Is Complicated

FALSE

A simple strategy: Eat sensibly. Favor whole, unprocessed foods. Make sure the carbs you eat are fiber rich—this means produce, legumes, and whole grains—to help slow the absorption of sugar into your bloodstream. "The more carbohydrates you eat, the more fiber becomes important to help minimize the wide fluctuations in blood sugar levels," says Jeff Volek, PhD, RD, a nutrition and exercise researcher at the University of Connecticut.

—*Additional reporting by* Men's Health

What's Really in...
Lucky Charms

These aren't the Lucky Charms you grew up with. Starting in 2005, General Mills began slowly moving whole grains into all its cereals, and today you'll find whole-grain corn, rice, oats, and wheat in cereals like Trix, Cocoa Puffs, Reese's Puffs, and Count Chocula. Considering that 95 percent of Americans fall short on their whole-grain intake, we applaud General Mills's effort, but unfortunately the move is a lot like sticking a small bandage on a machete wound. Consider this: With whole grains in the fold, Lucky Charms now contains 2 grams of fiber per serving, while other whole-grain General Mills cereals have only 1 gram. Post Shredded Wheat, by comparison, consists entirely of whole-grain wheat, and it packs 6 grams of fiber into each serving. But what Lucky Charms lacks in fiber it makes up for in sugar—10 grams per ¾ cup. It's not unlikely that a child would eat twice that much for breakfast, bringing the overall sugar load to almost a twin-wrapped package of Peanut Butter Twix. Thanks for the improvement, General Mills, but you'll have to do better before we'll sign off.

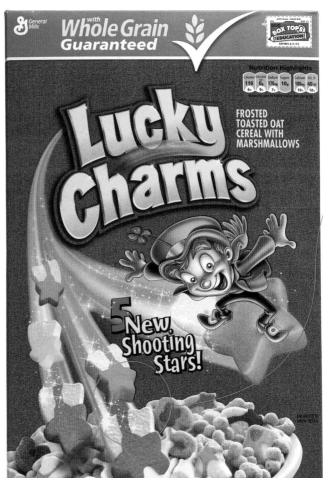

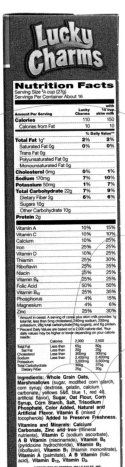

Nutrition Facts

Serving Size ¾ cup (27g)
Servings Per Container About 16

Amount Per Serving	Lucky Charms	with ½ cup skim milk
Calories	110	150
Calories from Fat	10	10

	% Daily Value**	
Total Fat 1g*	2%	2%
Saturated Fat 0g	0%	0%
Trans Fat 0g		
Polyunsaturated Fat 0g		
Monounsaturated Fat 0g		
Cholesterol 0mg	0%	1%
Sodium 170mg	7%	10%
Potassium 50mg	1%	7%
Total Carbohydrate 22g	7%	9%
Dietary Fiber 2g	6%	6%
Sugars 10g		
Other Carbohydrate 10g		
Protein 2g		

Vitamin A	10%	15%
Vitamin C	10%	10%
Calcium	10%	25%
Iron	25%	25%
Vitamin D	10%	25%
Thiamin	25%	30%
Riboflavin	25%	35%
Niacin	25%	25%
Vitamin B₆	25%	25%
Folic Acid	50%	50%
Vitamin B₁₂	25%	35%
Phosphorus	4%	15%
Magnesium	4%	6%
Zinc	25%	30%

* Amount in cereal. A serving of cereal plus skim milk provides 1g total fat, less than 5mg cholesterol, 240mg sodium, 250mg potassium, 28g total carbohydrate (16g sugars), and 6g protein.
** Percent Daily Values are based on a 2,000 calorie diet. Your daily values may be higher or lower depending on your calorie needs:

		Calories	2,000	2,500
Total Fat	Less than		65g	80g
Sat Fat	Less than		20g	25g
Cholesterol	Less than		300mg	300mg
Sodium	Less than		2,400mg	2,400mg
Potassium			3,500mg	3,500mg
Total Carbohydrate			300g	375g
Dietary Fiber			25g	30g

Ingredients: Whole Grain Oats, Marshmallows (sugar, modified corn starch, corn syrup, dextrose, gelatin, calcium carbonate, yellows 5&6, blue 1, red 40, artificial flavor), **Sugar, Oat Flour, Corn Syrup, Corn Starch, Salt, Trisodium Phosphate, Color Added, Natural and Artificial Flavor. Vitamin E** (mixed tocopherols) **Added to Preserve Freshness.**

Vitamins and Minerals: Calcium Carbonate, Zinc and Iron (mineral nutrients), **Vitamin C** (sodium ascorbate), **A B Vitamin** (niacinamide), **Vitamin B₆** (pyridoxine hydrochloride), **Vitamin B₂** (riboflavin), **Vitamin B₁** (thiamin mononitrate), **Vitamin A** (palmitate), **A B Vitamin** (folic acid), **Vitamin B₁₂, Vitamin D₃.**

DISTRIBUTED BY GENERAL MILLS SALES, INC.,
MINNEAPOLIS, MN 55440 USA

If you are not satisfied with the quality of this product, a prompt refund or adjustment of equal value will be made. Your comments and questions are

MARSHMALLOWS

In the cereal industry, brightly colored marshmallow pieces are called "marbits." We have another name for them: candy. Thanks to the sugar impact of these marshmallows, your child can fulfill the American Heart Association's added-sugar limit for the entire day by eating 1 cup of cereal. Starting the day like that sets a young eater up for a short-run sugar rush and a long-run propensity for calorically dense, sugar-loaded foods. And don't think you're exempt as an adult—America's sugar addiction extends past the generation gap. The average American eats up to 4 ½ times more than the recommended limit, adding up to a total sugar intake of 132 pounds annually for every man, woman, and child.

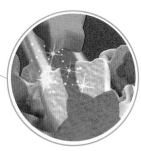

25g

hole Grain Oats,
, (sugar, modified corn
dextrose, gelatin, calcium
ellows 5&6, blue 1, red 4(
r), **Sugar, Oat Flour, Corn
Starch, Salt, Trisodium
Color Added, Natural an
r. Vitamin E** (mixed
ded to Preserve Fr
als: Calciu

25g

Whole Grain Oats,
ws (sugar, modified corn
dextrose, gelatin, calcium
yellows 5&6, blue 1, red
vor), **Sugar, Oat Flour, Co
rn Starch, Salt, Trisodium
Color Added, Natural a
vor. Vitamin E** (mixed
dded to Preserve
erals: Calc

YELLOWS 5 & 6

The average American child consumes approximately 121 milligrams of artificial food dye every day. That's a serious problem. Take the two colors listed here. Studies have indicted Yellows 5 and 6 as potential causes of behavioral problems, learning problems, and hyperactivity in children. Add to that a roller coaster–style spike in blood sugar and it's no wonder 5.4 million US kids have been diagnosed with ADHD. Bottom line: A daily cereal like Lucky Charms doesn't guarantee academic failure, but it sure doesn't improve the odds of success.

TRISODIUM PHOSPHATE

Trisodium phosphate has its share of critics, but most of them are in the plumbing community. Yes, the additive is a key ingredient in many toilet bowl cleaners, and it has taken heat for being corrosive to metal pipes. In foods, trisodium phosphate is used to balance acidity, and the moderate amounts in which it appears are unlikely to be dangerous. That said, there's something discomforting about the idea of filling your cereal bowl and toilet bowl with the same chemical.

What's Really in...
Chef Boyardee Beef Ravioli

HIGH-FRUCTOSE CORN SYRUP

Ettore "Hector" Boiardi always held dear the idea that the best meals begin with the best ingredients. The Italian immigrant moved to the United States when he was a teenager to pursue his dream of becoming a chef. He ascended through New York City's hotel restaurants and eventually catered President Woodrow Wilson's wedding reception. Then he launched his own food line: Chef Boyardee. Even as a mass producer, he remained devoted to his ingredients. He located the factory in a town near the tomato farmers, and in the damp basement of the plant he grew mushrooms for his sauce. Oh, how things have changed. Now the cans bearing the chef's likeness are filled with more engineered ingredients than actual foods. Chief among them is high-fructose corn syrup, a sweetener that requires a centrifuge to make. Whether or not it's the ultimate nutritional evil is a topic still up for debate, but what it represents is an industrial food system that has brought us far from the days when pasta was made with flour, tomatoes, and little else.

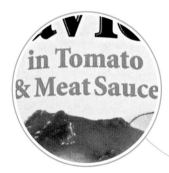

"BEEF"

Beef is the big tout, but the meat in here is cut with something called textured vegetable protein. The little orange, soy-based protein pellets probably weren't around in Boiardi's time. The food industry will tell you it helps retain the water the meat normally loses during cooking, but with an average cost of less than one-third that of beef it's easy to see why else it's used. How else could they charge $1 for a 1-pound can composed largely of beef when a pound of ground beef goes for nearly $4?

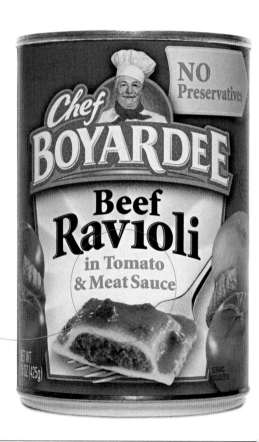

in Tomato & Meat Sauce

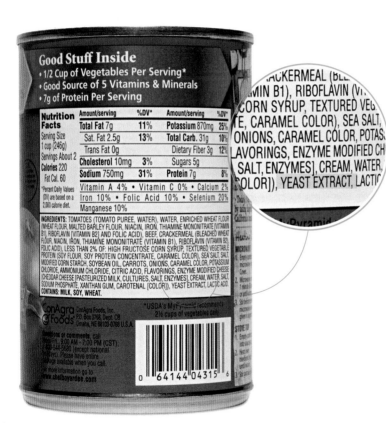

Good Stuff Inside
- 1/2 Cup of Vegetables Per Serving*
- Good Source of 5 Vitamins & Minerals
- 7g of Protein Per Serving

Nutrition Facts	Amount/serving	%DV*	Amount/serving	%DV*
Serving Size 1 cup (246g)	Total Fat 7g	11%	Potassium 870mg	25%
Servings About 2	Sat. Fat 2.5g	13%	Total Carb. 31g	10%
Calories 220	Trans Fat 0g		Dietary Fiber 3g	12%
Fat Cal. 60	Cholesterol 10mg	3%	Sugars 5g	
	Sodium 750mg	31%	Protein 7g	8%

*Percent Daily Values (DV) are based on a 2,000 calorie diet.

Vitamin A 4% • Vitamin C 0% • Calcium 2%
Iron 10% • Folic Acid 10% • Selenium 20%
Manganese 10%

INGREDIENTS: TOMATOES (TOMATO PUREE, WATER), WATER, ENRICHED WHEAT FLOUR [WHEAT FLOUR, MALTED BARLEY FLOUR, NIACIN, IRON, THIAMINE MONONITRATE (VITAMIN B1), RIBOFLAVIN (VITAMIN B2) AND FOLIC ACID], BEEF, CRACKERMEAL (BLEACHED WHEAT FLOUR, NIACIN, IRON, THIAMINE MONONITRATE (VITAMIN B1), RIBOFLAVIN (VITAMIN B2), FOLIC ACID), LESS THAN 2% OF: HIGH FRUCTOSE CORN SYRUP, TEXTURED VEGETABLE PROTEIN (SOY FLOUR, SOY PROTEIN CONCENTRATE, CARAMEL COLOR), SEA SALT, SALT, MODIFIED CORN STARCH, SOYBEAN OIL, CARROTS, ONIONS, CARAMEL COLOR, POTASSIUM CHLORIDE, AMMONIUM CHLORIDE, CITRIC ACID, FLAVORINGS, ENZYME MODIFIED CHEESE (CHEDDAR CHEESE [PASTEURIZED MILK, CULTURES, SALT, ENZYMES], CREAM, WATER, SALT, SODIUM PHOSPHATE, XANTHAN GUM, CAROTENAL [COLOR]), YEAST EXTRACT, LACTIC ACID. CONTAINS: MILK, SOY, WHEAT.

ConAgra Foods
ConAgra Foods, Inc.
P.O. Box 2768, Dept. CB
Omaha, NE 68103-0768 U.S.A.

Questions or comments, call Mon.-Fri., 9:00 AM - 7:00 PM (CST), 1-800-544-5680 (except national holidays). Please have entire package available when you call. For more information go to: www.chefboyardee.com

*USDA's MyPyramid recommends 2½ cups of vegetables daily

0 64144 04315 6

CRACKERMEAL (BLE... ...MIN B1), RIBOFLAVIN (VI... ...CORN SYRUP, TEXTURED VEG... ...E, CARAMEL COLOR), SEA SALT, ...ONIONS, CARAMEL COLOR, POTAS... ...LAVORINGS, ENZYME MODIFIED CH... ...SALT, ENZYMES]), CREAM, WATER, ...OLOR]), YEAST EXTRACT, LACTIC...

One year after Hector Boiardi sold his company in 1946, monosodium glutamate was introduced to American consumers. You might not see MSG on this ravioli's ingredients list, but its troublesome compound, glutamic acid, is found inside a couple of ingredients that are there, including yeast extract. After years of bad publicity surrounding MSG, considered a "flavor enhancer" in food-additive terminology, many manufacturers stopped including it and instead slipped through an FDA loophole: They don't have to mention glutamic acid if it's hidden in other ingredients. So what's the big deal about glutamic acid? A review compiled for the FDA recently concluded that the substance triggers some people to have reactions, including migraine headache, nausea, changes in heart rate, and difficulty breathing. It's easy to imagine that Boiardi never would have allowed such an ingredient in his carefully cultivated sauces. But Chef Boyardee's narrative is the same as that of so many other iconic American foods: McDonald's hamburgers, Heinz ketchup, KFC chicken. They were all simple ideas that have been corrupted by seismic shifts in the industrial food complex that dictated replacing costlier raw ingredients with cheaper versions and "flavor enhancers."

Sweet Cereals
Eat This

It's still far from a healthy choice, but the denigrated Froot Loops actually have more fiber than the Kashi.

General Mills Cinnamon Burst Cheerios
(1 cup)

110 calories
2 g fat
(0 g saturated)
5 g fiber
9 g sugars

As fiber-rich as sweet cereal gets.

General Mills Kix
(1 cup)

88 calories
1 g fat
(0 g saturated)
2.5 g fiber
2.5 g sugar

Kix just might be the safest of all the sweetened kids' cereals. Try it with blueberries.

Special K Red Berries
(1 cup)

110 calories
0 g fat
3 g fiber
9 g sugars

This cereal employs wheat bran to up the fiber count and dried strawberries for natural sweetness.

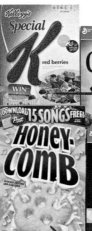

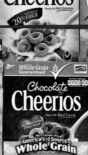

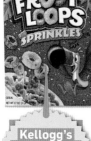

Kellogg's Froot Loops with Sprinkles
(1 cup)

110 calories
1 g fat
(0.5 g saturated)
3 g fiber
12 g sugars

Kellogg's Apple Jacks
(1 cup)

100 calories
0.5 g fat
(0 g saturated)
3 g fiber
12 g sugars

The whole-grain corn flour adds just enough fiber to offset the sugar.

General Mills Cocoa Puffs
(1 cup)

133 calories
2 g fat
(0 g saturated)
2.5 g fiber
13.5 g sugars

General Mills has slowly added more whole grains to all of its Big G cereals.

Post Honeycomb
(1 cup)

87 calories
0.5 g fat
(0 g saturated)
0.5 g fiber
7 g sugars

We'd love more fiber, but at least they keep the sugar and calories down.

General Mills Chocolate Cheerios
(1 cup)

133 calories
2 g fat
(0 g saturated)
3 g fiber
12 g sugars

Two of the first five ingredients are whole grains.

Kellogg's Corn Pops
(1 cup)

120 calories
0 g fat
3 g fiber
10 g sugars

Following the lead of General Mills, Kellogg's began bulking up its fiber profile in 2009.

160

Not That!

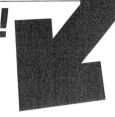

This is one of Kashi's biggest flops. Strawberry Fields features white rice instead of the 7 Whole Grain Blend found in many of its cereals.

Quaker Life (1 cup)

160 calories
2 g fat
(0 g saturated)
2.5 g fiber
8 g sugars

Life isn't the worst cereal on the shelf, but it does pack in more than three times as much sugar as fiber.

General Mills Cinnamon Chex (1 cup)

160 calories
3 g fat
(0 g saturated)
<1 g fiber
11 g sugars

This cereal delivers more than 130 calories of pure carbohydrates.

Post Honey Bunches of Oats with Real Strawberries (1 cup)

160 calories
2 g fat
(0 g saturated)
3 g fiber
11 g sugars

Heavy on the carbs and calories with little fiber payoff.

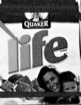

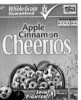

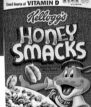
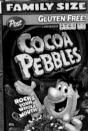
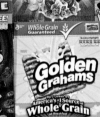
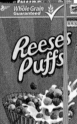
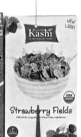

Kellogg's Honey Smacks (1 cup)

133 calories
0.5 g fat
(0 g saturated)
1 g fiber
20 g sugars

This is among the most sugar-loaded boxes in the cereal aisle.

Post Cocoa Pebbles (1 cup)

160 calories
1 g fat
(1 g saturated)
0 g fiber
15 g sugars

Not just devoid of fiber, but also soaked with hydrogenated oils.

General Mills Golden Grahams (1 cup)

160 calories
1 g fat
(0 g saturated)
1 g fiber
15 g sugars

Loaded with sugar, lacking in fiber, and saturated with sodium.

General Mills Reese's Puffs (1 cup)

160 calories
4 g fat
(0.5 g saturated)
1 g fiber
13 g sugars

Oxford researchers rated this the unhealthiest cereal in the supermarket.

General Mills Apple Cinnamon Cheerios (1 cup)

160 calories
2 g fat
(0 g saturated)
3 g fiber
13 g sugars

Worse than most junk cereal.

Kashi Strawberry Fields (1 cup)

120 calories
0 g fat
1 g fiber
9 g sugars

Wholesome Cereals

Eat This

Cinnamon is a worthwhile addition to any cereal. Studies show that it helps your body manage blood sugar.

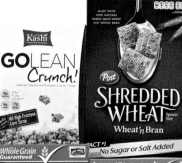

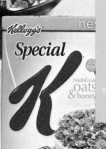

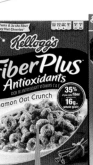

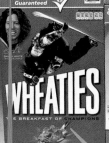

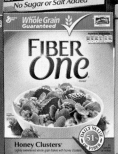

Post Shredded Wheat Spoon Size Wheat 'n Bran
(1 cup)
160 calories
1 g fat
(0 g saturated)
6 g fiber
<1 g sugars
Just add blueberries or sliced banana.

General Mills Total Raisin Bran
(1 cup)
160 calories
1 g fat
(0 g saturated)
5 g fiber
17 g sugars
You'll find an entire day's worth of calcium and vitamin E in each serving.

Kellogg's FiberPlus Cinnamon Oat Crunch
(1 cup)
147 calories
2 g fat
(0 g saturated)
12 g fiber
9 g sugars

Kashi GoLean Crunch!
(1 cup)
190 calories
3 g fat
(0 g saturated)
8 g fiber
13 g sugars
More than a third of these calories come from fiber and protein—an incredible feat for a cereal.

General Mills Wheaties
(1 cup)
133 calories
1 g fat
(0 g saturated)
4 g fiber
5 g sugars
"Eat your Wheaties" might have been a clever marketing campaign, but we can't say we disagree with the advice.

General Mills Fiber One Honey Clusters
(1 cup)
160 calories
1.5 g fat
(0 g saturated)
13 g fiber
6 g sugars
An impressive two-to-one fiber-to-sugar ratio.

Kellogg's Special K Multigrain Oats & Honey
(1 cup)
150 calories
1 g fat
(0 g saturated)
4.5 g fiber
12 g sugars
The sugar count could be lower, but at least it has the fiber to back it up.

Not That!

Quaker Cinnamon Oatmeal Squares
(1 cup)

210 calories
2.5 g fat
(0.5 g saturated)
5 g fiber
9 g sugars

Packs some nice fiber, but the sugar and cheap, refined carbs like maltodextrin drive the calorie count too high.

General Mills Oatmeal Crisp Hearty Raisin
(1 cup)

240 calories
2.5 g fat
(0.5 g saturated)
5 g fiber
20 g sugars

Before adding milk, each bowl has just 10 calories fewer than a McDonald's hamburger.

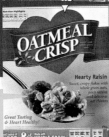
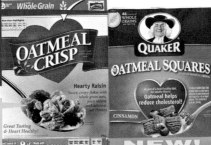
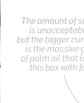

The amount of sugar is unacceptable, but the bigger curiosity is the massive glut of palm oil that loads this box with fat.

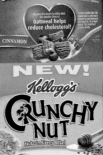
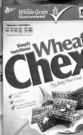
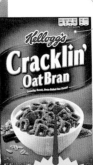

Kellogg's Smart Start Strong Heart Original Antioxidants
(1 cup)

190 calories
0.5 g fat
(0 g saturated)
3 g fiber
14 g sugars

What's so smart about this cereal?

Kellogg's Crunchy Nut Golden Honey Nut
(1 cup)

160 calories
1.5 g fat
(0 g saturated)
<1 g fiber
15 g sugars

Fiber-free cereal is like eating ice cream for breakfast.

General Mills Wheat Chex
(1 cup)

213 calories
1 g fat
(0 g saturated)
7 g fiber
7 g sugars

This fiber-to-sugar ratio is acceptable, but 400 milligrams of sodium and these calorie counts are not.

Quaker Natural Granola Oats & Honey
(1 cup)

400 calories
12 g fat
(1 g saturated)
10 g fiber
20 g sugars

Rumors of granola's healthfulness have been greatly exaggerated.

Kellogg's Cracklin' Oat Bran
(1 cup)

267 calories
9 g fat
(4 g saturated)
8 g fiber
20 g sugars

163

Hot Cereals

Eat This

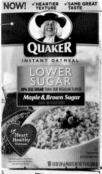
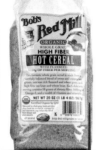
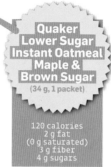

**Quaker
Lower Sugar
Instant Oatmeal
Maple &
Brown Sugar**
(34 g, 1 packet)

120 calories
2 g fat
(0 g saturated)
3 g fiber
4 g sugars

Oat fiber has been shown to lower your LDL cholesterol, but unfortunately the excessive sugar load in most quick-cook oat mixes also lowers your chances of a flat belly. Choose this one and you'll earn the perk without the pitfall.

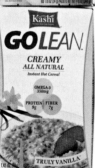
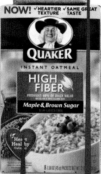
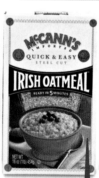
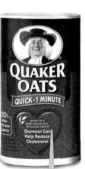

Kashi GoLean Creamy All Natural Instant Hot Cereal Truly Vanilla (40 g, 1 packet)	**Quaker High Fiber Instant Oatmeal Maple & Brown Sugar** (45 g, 1 packet)	**Bob's Red Mill Organic High Fiber Hot Cereal** (45 g, ⅓ cup dry)	**McCann's Quick & Easy Steel Cut Irish Oatmeal** (40 g, ¼ cup dry)	**Quaker Oats Quick Oats** (40 g, ½ cup dry)
150 calories 2 g fat (0 g saturated) 7 g fiber 6 g sugars	160 calories 2 g fat (0 g saturated) 10 g fiber 7 g sugars	150 calories 5 g fat (0 g saturated) 10 g fiber 0 g sugars	150 calories 2.5 g fat (0.5 g saturated) 3 g fiber <1 g sugars	150 calories 3 g fat (0.5 g saturated) 4 g fiber 1 g sugars
Kashi makes some of the best cereals—hot and cold—in the aisles.	Extra oat flour is behind one of the highest-fiber cereals on the shelf.	You should aim for 30 grams of fiber every day. This is a great start.	Steel-cut oats digest slower than the rolled variety, for a gentler effect on blood sugar.	It's worth the extra 30 calories to gain protein, healthy fat, and four times the fiber—all three of which help promote satiety.

Not That!

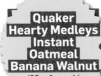

Quaker Hearty Medleys Instant Oatmeal Banana Walnut
(36 g, 1 pouch)

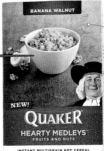

140 calories
2.5 g fat
(0 g saturated)
3 g fiber
12 g sugars

"Hearty" or not, this oatmeal has more sugar than a bowl of Post's Fruity Pebbles.

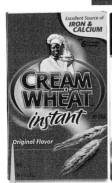

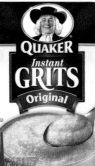

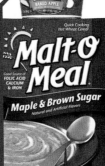

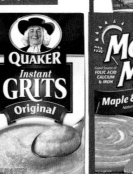

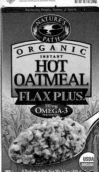

Cream of Wheat
(33 g, 3 Tbsp dry)

120 calories
0 g fat
1 g fiber
0 g sugars

We like the simplicity of Cream of Wheat, we just don't like the fact that it contains only a trace amount of fiber and little else to keep your hunger at bay throughout the morning.

Quaker Instant Grits Original
(56 g, 2 packets)

200 calories
0 g fat
2 g fiber
0 g sugars

This Southern staple is heavy in starch but low in fiber.

Quaker Oatmeal Express Baked Apple
(54 g, 1 cup)

200 calories
2.5 g fat
(0.5 g saturated)
4 g fiber
17 g sugars

A sugar load like this is appropriate for dessert, but not for breakfast.

Malt-O-Meal Maple & Brown Sugar Hot Cereal
(45 g, ¼ cup dry)

170 calories
0 g fat
1 g fiber
13 g sugars

Farina, the cereal Malt-O-Meal is made with, is wheat with the bran and most of the germ removed. As such, it contains almost zero fiber.

Nature's Path Organic Instant Hot Oatmeal Flax Plus
(50 g, 1 packet)

210 calories
3 g fat
(0.5 g saturated)
5 g fiber
10 g sugars

Too many calories and grams of sugar to compete with the best oatmeals in the supermarket.

Breads
Eat This

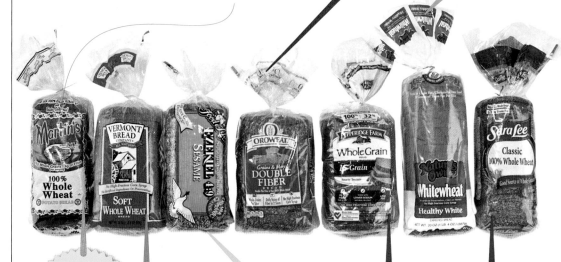

You won't find a softer, tastier bread with more fiber or fewer calories. Plus, two slices have an impressive 12 grams of protein.

Oroweat Double Fiber Bread
(76 g, 2 slices)

160 calories
3 g fat
(0 g saturated)
10 g fiber

This loaf is stacked with a surplus of fiber, which is a proven weapon against high cholesterol. One of the best slices in the supermarket.

Nature's Own Whitewheat
(52 g, 2 slices)

110 calories
1 g fat
(0 g saturated)
4 g fiber

With both soluble and insoluble fibers from soy, this just might be the best white loaf in the supermarket.

Martin's Famous Whole Wheat Potato Bread
(70 g, 2 slices)

140 calories
2 g fat
(0 g saturated)
8 g fiber

Vermont Bread Company Soft Whole Wheat
(76 g, 2 slices)

140 calories
2 g saturated
(0 g saturated)
6 g fiber

Vermont Bread Company doesn't use preservatives, artificial flavors, or high-fructose corn syrup in any of its breads.

Food for Life Ezekiel 4:9 Sprouted Grain Bread Sesame
(70 g, 2 slices)

160 calories
1 g fat
(0 g saturated)
6 g fiber

Sprouted grains are packed with more B vitamins and boast a broader spectrum of amino acids.

Pepperidge Farm Whole Grain 15 Grain
(86 g, 2 slices)

200 calories
4 g fat
(1 g saturated)
8 g fiber

Two slices of almost all of the Farm's Whole Grain Breads line provide a third of your daily recommended fiber intake.

Sara Lee Classic 100% Whole Wheat
(56 g, 2 slices)

140 calories
2 g fat
(0 g saturated)
4 g fiber

"Whole wheat" means you're consuming the fibrous bran and germ layers of the grain. That's exactly what you want.

Not That!

Wonder Made with Whole Grain White
(57 g, 2 slices)

140 calories
2 g fat
(0.5 g saturated)
3 g fiber

Compared to the same variety of bread made by Nature's Own, this loaf has more sugar, more sodium, and less fiber.

Sara Lee Hearty & Delicious 100% Whole Wheat
(86 g, 2 slices)

240 calories
3 g fat
(1 g saturated)
6 g fiber

The fiber's commendable, but these slices are way too calorie dense to qualify as pantry staples.

This "wheat" bread is an imposter. The first ingredient is enriched flour, which is a euphemism for wheat flour stripped of most of its nutrients.

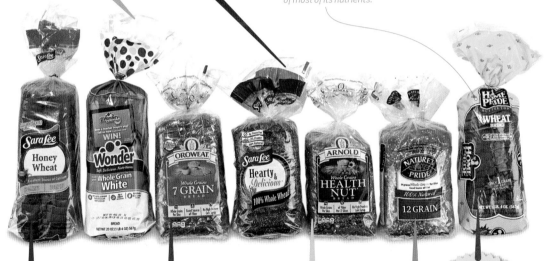

Sara Lee Honey Wheat
(57 g, 2 slices)

150 calories
1.5 g fat
(0.5 g saturated)
2 g fiber

Most breads are made from a form of wheat, but unless it says "whole," you're paying for stripped-down grains with little fiber and miniscule amounts of micronutrients.

Oroweat Whole Grains 7 Grain
(76 g, 2 slices)

180 calories
2 g fat
(0 g saturated)
4 g fiber

Sure this bread contains seven grains, but refined flour is still one of its major constituents.

Arnold Whole Grains Health Nut
(86 g, 2 slices)

240 calories
4 g fat
(0 g saturated)
4 g fiber

The second ingredient is the same white flour you'd find in a slice of Wonder Classic White bread.

Nature's Pride 12 Grain
(86 g, 2 slices)

220 calories
4 g fat
(0 g saturated)
4 g fiber

The wheat is whole grain, sure. Too bad the other 11 grains aren't. You'd need twice as much fiber to justify these calories.

Home Pride Butter Top Wheat
(56 g, 2 slices)

140 calories
2 g fat
(0 g saturated)
2 g fiber

167

Tortillas, Pitas & Wr

Eat This

Ezekiel 4:9 Pocket Bread
(47 g, 1 pita)

100 calories
0.5 g fat
(0 g saturated)
4 g fiber

Stuff with tomatoes and smear with hummus for an incredible midday snack.

The addition of corn bran boosts the fiber count and makes this the ideal shell for taco night.

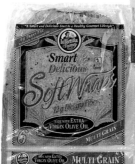
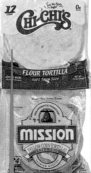
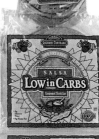
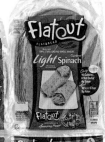

Ortega Whole Grain Corn Taco Shells
(28 g, 2 shells)

110 calories
6 g fat
(1 g saturated)
6 g fiber

La Tortilla Factory Smart & Delicious SoftWraps MultiGrain
(62 g, 1 wrap)

100 calories
3.5 g fat
(0.5 g saturated)
12 g fiber

You won't find a better tortilla.

Chi-Chi's Flour Tortillas Soft Taco Size
(28 g, 1 tortilla)

80 calories
2 g fat
(1 g saturated)
1 g fiber

Cut calories by using smaller tortillas and stuffing them extra full.

Mission Yellow Corn Tortillas Extra Thin
(37 g, 2 tortillas)

80 calories
1 g fat
(0 g saturated)
2 g fiber

Corn trumps flour every time. It's both higher in fiber and lower in calories.

Tumaro's Low in Carbs Tortillas Salsa
(39 g, 1 tortilla)

50 calories
1.5 g fat
(0 g saturated)
6 g fiber

This wrap earns its fiber from two healthy sources: oats and wheat.

Flatout Light Garden Spinach
(53 g, 1 flatbread)

90 calories
2.5 g fat
(0 g saturated)
9 g fiber

Flatout produces America's most impressive line of flatbreads.

168

aps

Not That!

The palm oil in these shells adds saturated fat, but it doesn't add fiber.

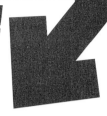
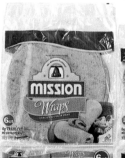
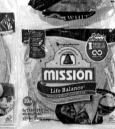
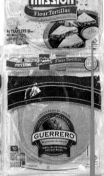
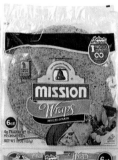
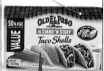

Mission Garden Spinach Herb Wraps
(70 g, 1 tortilla)

210 calories
4.5 g fat
(2 g saturated)
1 g fiber

Contains fats that may cause the same cholesterol-spiking properties as trans fats.

Mission Life Balance Medium/ Soft Taco Whole Wheat Tortillas Plus!
(41 g, 1 tortilla)

120 calories
3.5 g fat
(1.5 g saturated)
3 g fiber

The recipe is 31 ingredients long.

Guerrero Soft Taco Tortillas
(42 g. 1 tortilla)

140 calories
6 g fat
(3 g saturated)
1 g fiber

This tortilla contains seven ingredients and six times the fat of its corn counterpart.

Mission Flour Tortillas Medium/ Soft Taco Size
(49 g, 1 tortilla)

150 calories
3.5 g fat
(1.5 g saturated)
1 g fiber

Each shell delivers about 20 percent of your day's sodium.

Mission Wraps Plus! Multi-Grain
(70 g, 1 wrap)

210 calories
6 g fat
(2.5 g saturated)
7 g fiber

Blame a big dose of vegetable shortening for Mission's high-calorie wraps.

Old El Paso Stand'n Stuff Taco Shells
(27 g, 2 shells)

130 calories
6 g fat
(2.5 g saturated)
1 g fiber

Breakfast Breads
Eat This

Outside of green vegetables, you'll find very few foods that manage to pack 8 grams of fiber into 100 calories. That makes this an unbeatable foundation for breakfast sandwiches.

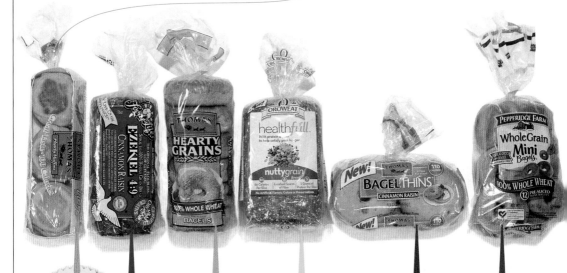

Thomas' Light Multi-Grain English Muffins
(57 g, 1 muffin)

100 calories
1 g fat
(0 g saturated)
26 g carbs
8 g fiber

Food for Life Ezekiel 4:9 Cinnamon Raisin Sprouted 100% Whole Grain Bread
(34 g, 1 slice)

80 calories
0 g fat
(0 g saturated)
18 g carbs
2 g fiber

Thomas' Hearty Grains 100% Whole Wheat Bagels
(95 g, 1 bagel)

240 calories
2 g fat
(0.5 g saturated)
49 g carbs
7 g fiber

Just as impressive as the fiber is the 10 grams of protein in each serving.

Oroweat Health-full Nutty Grain Bread
(38 g, 1 slice)

80 calories
1 g fat
(0 g saturated)
17 g carbs
5 g fiber

An excellent fiber load for an 80-calorie slice.

Thomas' Bagel Thins Cinnamon Raisin
(46 g, 1 bagel)

110 calories
1 g fat
(0 g saturated)
25 g carbs
5 g fiber

Swipe with peanut butter for a near-perfect snack.

Pepperidge Farm 100% Whole Wheat Mini Bagels
(40 g, 1 bagel)

100 calories
0.5 g fat
(0 g saturated)
20 g carbs
4 g fiber

Add a fried egg and 2 slices of ham for a hunger-squashing sandwich.

Not That!

The more fiber you work into your breakfast, the more likely you'll be to make it to lunch without experiencing hunger pangs. That means this muffin is a recipe for midmorning cravings.

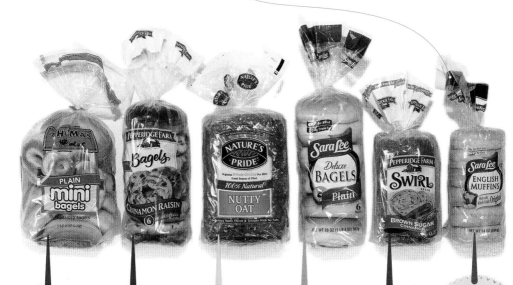

Thomas' Plain Mini Bagels
(43 g, 1 bagel)

120 calories
1 g fat
(0 g saturated)
24 g carbs
<1 g fiber

Just because it's small doesn't excuse it from delivering essentially zero fiber.

Pepperidge Farm Bagels Cinnamon Raisin
(57 g, 1 bagel)

270 calories
1 g fat
(0 g saturated)
57 g carbs
3 g fiber

This bagel packs as many carbs as five slices of toast.

Nature's Pride 100% Natural Nutty Oat Bread
(43 g, 1 slice)

120 calories
2 g fat
(0 g saturated)
20 g carbs
3 g fiber

A 120-calorie slice of bread needs more fiber.

Sara Lee Deluxe Bagels Plain
(95 g, 1 bagel)

260 calories
1 g fat
(0 g saturated)
50 g carbs
2 g fiber

This is a wedge of refined carbs, an invitation for a blood sugar roller coaster.

Pepperidge Farm Brown Sugar Cinnamon Swirl Bread
(38 g, 1 slice)

110 calories
2 g fat
(0 g saturated)
21 g carbs
<1 g fiber

Packs five different forms of sugar.

Sara Lee Original English Muffins
(66 g, 1 muffin)

140 calories
1 g fat
(0 g saturated)
27 g carbs
2 g fiber

171

Breakfast Pastries

Eat This

Hostess SmartBakes Muffins Bananas & Nuts
(50 g, 1 muffin)

150 calories
3 g fat
(0.5 g saturated)
3 g fiber
14 g sugars

This muffin is made with real bananas and whole wheat.

Pepperidge Farms Mini Bagels
(43 g, 1 bagel)

120 calories
0.5 g fat
(0 g saturated)
2 g fiber
6 g sugars

A modestly-sized bagel with a lashing of cinnamon, which has been shown to temper the types of blood sugar spikes routinely caused by carb-heavy breakfasts.

Despite their nasty reputation, doughnuts are no worse than any other carb-heavy pastry. Stick to a single modestly portioned Krispy Kreme and you'll fare pretty well in the battle against the bulge.

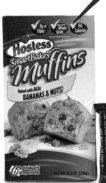
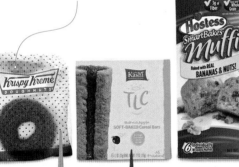

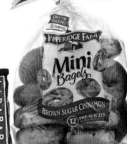
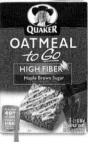

Krispy Kreme Doughnuts Original Glazed
(49 g, 1 doughnut)

190 calories
11 g fat
(4.5 g saturated)
10 g sugars

Kashi TLC Soft-Baked Cereal Bars Baked Apple
(35 g, 1 bar)

110 calories
3 g fat (0 g saturated)
3 g fiber
9 g sugars

The more fiber you get at breakfast, the less likely you are to overeat at lunchtime.

Lärabar Blueberry Muffin
(45 g, 1 bar)

190 calories
8 g fat
(1.5 g saturated)
3 g fiber
17 g sugars

We love Lärabar for its unmatched simplicity. This tasty bar contains just four ingredients: cashews, raisins, blueberries, and blueberry juice.

Quaker Oatmeal to Go High Fiber Maple Brown Sugar
(60 g, 1 bar)

210 calories
4 g fat
(1 g saturated)
10 g fiber
13 g sugars

This bar contains as much fiber as 3 servings of instant oatmeal.

Not That!

Little Debbie Honey Buns
(50 g, 1 pastry)

230 calories
13 g fat
(6 g saturated)
<1 g fiber
13 g sugars

Of the 31 ingredients in this bun, partially hydrogenated oils show up twice.

Ne-Mo's Fine Bakery Products Banana Bread
(113 g, 1 piece)

460 calories
23 g fat
(4 g saturated)
1 g fiber
34 g sugars

You could eat nearly three of the Hostess SmartBakes Muffins and still consume fewer calories.

Little Debbie's Donut Sticks have three strikes against them: more calories, more fat, and more sugar than the Krispy Kreme alternative.

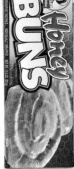
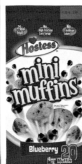
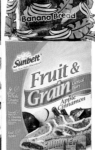
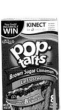
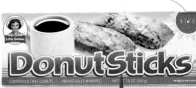

Kellogg's Pop-Tarts Brown Sugar Cinnamon Unfrosted
(50 g, 1 pastry)

210 calories
8 g fat
(2.5 g saturated)
<1 g fiber
12 g sugars

Opting for the unfrosted version does little to boost the nutritional merit of this pathetic pastry.

Hostess Mini Muffins Blueberry
(57 g, 1 pouch)

210 calories
8 g fat
(1.5 g saturated)
<1 g fiber
19 g sugars

Hostess's heavy hand with the soybean oil and added sugar turns these muffins into something more akin to dessert than breakfast.

Sunbelt Fruit & Grain Cereal Bars Apple Cinnamon
(39 g, 1 bar)

140 calories
3 g fat (1 g saturated)
1 g fiber
16 g sugars

Packages can boast all they want about a product being made with whole grains, but if it only contains a single gram of fiber, something has been lost during production.

Little Debbie Donut Sticks
(47 g, 1 doughnut)

230 calories
14 g fat
(7 g saturated)
15 g sugars

Breakfast Condimen

Eat This

One ounce of maple syrup packs more than 50 percent of your daily manganese, a mineral that boosts energy, stabilizes blood sugar, and helps defend against free-radical damage.

Justin's Chocolate Hazelnut Butter
(32 g, 2 Tbsp)
190 calories
16 g fat
(2.5 g saturated)
7 g sugars

This spread is made primarily of hazelnuts, which earn you a load of heart-healthy fats.

Smucker's Sugar Free Breakfast Syrup
(60 ml, ¼ cup)
20 calories
0 g fat
0 g sugars

This is one of the few sugar-free syrups made with sucralose, one of the best noncaloric sweeteners.

Polaner All Fruit with Fiber Blueberry
(64 g, ¼ cup)
120 calories
0 g fat
24 g sugars

The first ingredient is blueberries, which makes this an excellent upgrade from blueberry syrup.

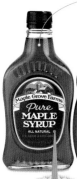
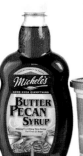

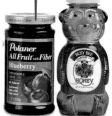

Maple Grove Farms 100% Pure Maple Syrup Dark Amber
(¼ cup)
200 calories
0 g fat
53 g sugars

Michele's Butter Pecan Syrup
(¼ cup)
167 calories
0 g fat
18 g sugars

Contains a mere fraction of the sugar in the typical pancake syrup.

Kraft Philadelphia Whipped Cream Cheese Spread
(21 g, 2 Tbsp)
60 calories
6 g fat
(3.5 g saturated)
<1 g sugars

Fewer calories, easier to spread.

Breakstone's Salted Whipped Butter
(1 Tbsp)
60 calories
7 g fat
(4.5 g saturated)
55 mg sodium

We'll take real butter over margarine any day.

Smart Balance Buttery Spread Made with Extra Virgin Olive Oil
(11 g, 1 Tbsp)
60 calories
7 g fat
(2 g saturated)
70 mg sodium

Laced with potent omega-3 fatty acids.

Honey
(any brand, 42 g, 2 Tbsp)
128 calories
0 g fat
35 g sugars

Honey exhibits antiviral, antibacterial, and antifungal properties. No common syrup can make that claim.

Not That!

Smucker's Blueberry Syrup
(60 ml, ¼ cup)

200 calories
0 g fat
44 g sugars

You'd think a fruit-based topping would be healthy, but regardless of the flavor, syrup is mostly sugar.

Aunt Jemima Lite Syrup
(60 ml, ¼ cup)

100 calories
0 g fat
25 g sugars

High-fructose corn syrup is still the first ingredient in this subpar "lite" product.

Nutella
(37 g, 2 Tbsp)

200 calories
11 g fat
(3.5 g saturated)
21 g sugars

The first two ingredients are sugar and palm oil. Maybe that's why Ferrero USA, the maker of Nutella, was sued last year for misleading marketing.

The majority of pancake syrups are entirely comprised of refined sugar with a touch of artificial maple flavoring. If you want real syrup, make sure it says "maple" on the label.

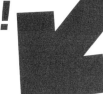

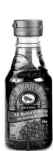
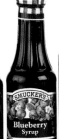
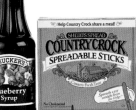
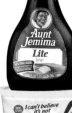

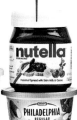
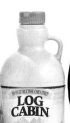
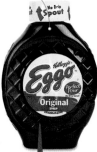

Lyle's Golden Syrup Original
(2 Tbsp)

130 calories
0 g fat
34 g sugars

Don't be fooled by the fancy label. This jar contains nothing more than cane sugar syrup, also known as liquefied sugar.

Shedd's Spread Country Crock Spreadable Sticks
(14 g, 1 Tbsp)

80 calories
8 g fat
(1.5 g saturated, 2 g trans)
90 mg sodium

Banish trans fats from your kitchen.

I Can't Believe It's Not Butter! Olive Oil Soft Spread
(14 g, 1 Tbsp)

70 calories
8 g fat
(2 g saturated)
90 mg sodium

If only they'd ditch the partially hydrogenated oils.

Kraft Philadelphia Garden Vegetable Soft Cream Cheese
(31 g, 2 Tbsp)

80 calories
7 g fat
(4.5 g saturated)
1 g sugars

Not worth the extra calories.

Log Cabin All Natural Table Syrup
(¼ cup)

210 calories
0 g fat
35 g sugars

"All natural" doesn't mean what you think it does. Real maple makes up only 4 percent of this bottle.

Kellogg's Eggo Original Syrup
(¼ cup)

240 calories
0 g fat
40 g sugars

Nut & Seed Butters

Eat This

Unlike other peanut butter powerhouses like Skippy and Peter Pan, Jif doesn't use partially hydrogenated oils. A long-term Harvard study found that people who ate nuts and nut butters lost the most weight.

Peanut Butter & Co. The Bee's Knees
(32 g, 2 Tbsp)

180 calories
14 g fat
(2.5 g saturated)
60 mg sodium

Sweetened with a touch of real honey and delicious on toasted wheat with sliced bananas.

Kettle Creamy Unsalted Cashew Butter
(28 g, 1 oz)

165 calories
14 g fat
(3 g saturated)
4 mg sodium

The chip makers churn out a butter rich in copper that helps protect against joint and bone-loss problems.

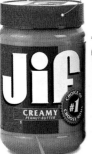
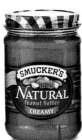
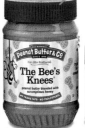
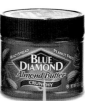
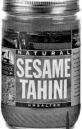

Jif Creamy Peanut Butter
(32 g, 2 Tbsp)

190 calories
16 g fat
(3 g saturated)
150 mg sodium

Smucker's Natural Peanut Butter Creamy
(32 g, 2 Tbsp)

200 calories
16 g fat
(2.5 g saturated)
105 mg sodium

This jar contains only two ingredients: peanuts and salt. That's a massive upgrade from the typical list including adjunct oil, sugar, and corn-based thickeners.

Blue Diamond Almond Butter Crunchy
(32 g, 2 Tbsp)

190 calories
17 g fat
(1.5 g saturated)
75 mg sodium

Don't limit yourself to standard peanut butter. Each serving of this antioxidant-rich almond butter contains 40 percent of your daily vitamin E.

Woodstock Farms Natural Sesame Tahini Unsalted
(30 g, 2 Tbsp)

180 calories
17 g fat
(2 g saturated)
0 mg sodium

Sesame seeds are packed with magnesium, which can help lower blood pressure.

Not That!

Contains the same calorie tariff as regular Jif, but it comes packaged with 10 more unnecessary ingredients. With peanut butter, as with most foods, the simpler the better.

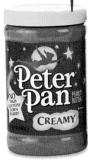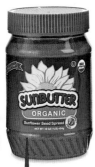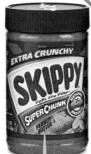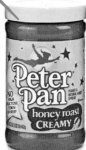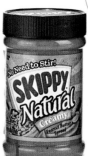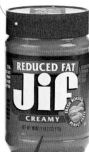

Jellies, Jams & Prese

Eat This

The best jams, jellies, and preserves have one thing in common: They contain more fruit than refined sugar. Polaner's All Fruit line goes one further— it's made with real fruit and sweetened with fruit juice.

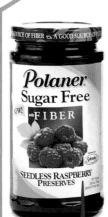

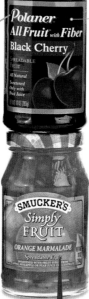

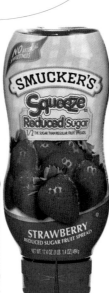

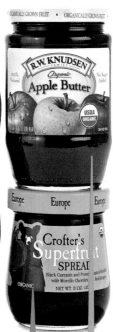

Polaner All Fruit with Fiber Black Cherry
(18 g, 1 Tbsp)

35 calories
0 g fat
7 g sugars

Polaner Sugar Free with Fiber Seedless Raspberry Preserves
(17 g, 1 Tbsp)

10 calories
0 g fat
0 g sugars

Raspberries are a powerful source of antioxidants.

Smucker's Simply Fruit Orange Marmalade Spreadable Fruit
(19 g, 1 Tbsp)

40 calories
0 g fat
8 g sugars

Made with nothing but ingredients derived from fruit.

Smucker's Squeeze Reduced Sugar Strawberry
(17 g, 1 Tbsp)

20 calories
0 g fat
5 g sugars

This version cuts the sugar load in half, reducing overall waistline impact.

Crofter's Superfruit Spread Europe
(18 g, 1 Tbsp)

30 calories
0 g fat
7 g sugars

Made with an antioxidant-rich blend that includes black currants and pomegranates.

R.W. Knudsen Family Organic Apple Butter
(18 g, 1 Tbsp)

35 calories
0 g fat
8 g sugars

This jar contains exactly two ingredients: apples and apple juice concentrate.

178

rves

Not That!

The "gold standard" of spreads, proclaims the label. That's only true if you count multiple sweeteners as the gold standard.

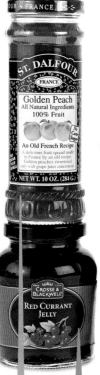
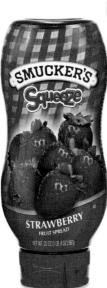
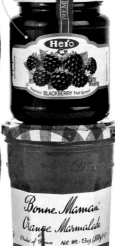
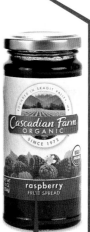

St. Dalfour Golden Peach Preserves
(20 g, 1 Tbsp)

45 calories
0 g fat
11 g sugars

It's nice that St. Dalfour uses only juice to sweeten this jar, but it still has too many calories for regular consumption.

Crosse & Blackwell Red Currant Jelly
(20 g, 1 Tbsp)

50 calories
0 g fat
12 g sugars

A highbrow jar with a lowbrow ingredients roster, including high-fructose corn syrup.

Smucker's Squeeze Strawberry Fruit Spread
(20 g, 1 Tbsp)

50 calories
0 g fat
12 g sugars

It takes Smucker's three forms of sugar to sweeten this squeeze bottle.

Bonne Maman Orange Marmalade
(20 g, 1 Tbsp)

50 calories
0 g fat
13 g sugars

The artisanal-looking jar won't protect you from the 13 grams of sugar in each tablespoon.

Cascadian Farm Organic Raspberry Fruit Spread
(19 g, 1 Tbsp)

40 calories
0 g fat
10 g sugars

Organic or not, the first ingredient here is sugar.

Hero Blackberry Fruit Spread
(20 g, 1 Tbsp)

50 calories
0 g fat
11 g sugars

Grains
Eat This

Quinoa ranks high in the running for World's Healthiest Food. It functions like any other grain in your cupboard, but genetically it's closer to spinach or chard. And the best part: It cooks in just 12 to 15 minutes.

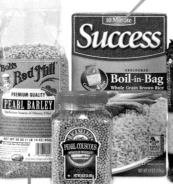
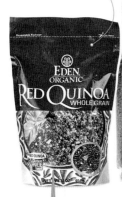
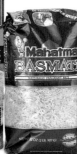
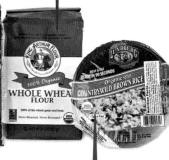

Success Boil-in-Bag Whole Grain Brown Rice
(43 g, ½ cup dry, 1 cup cooked)
150 calories
1 g fat
(0 g saturated)
2 g fiber

Whole grains don't have to be difficult. Just plunk one of these bags in boiling water or toss it in the microwave.

King Arthur Flour Premium 100% Whole Wheat Flour
(30 g, ¼ cup)
110 calories
0.5 g fat
(0 g saturated)
4 g fiber

The red wheat in this bag is more nutrient dense and protein packed than regular white wheat.

Eden Organic Red Quinoa
(45 g, ¼ cup)
170 calories
2 g fat
(0 g saturated)
5 g fiber

Bob's Red Mill Pearl Barley
(50 g, ¼ cup dry)
180 calories
1 g fat
(0 g saturated)
8 g fiber

Use this fiber-loaded grain as a replacement for noodles or rice in soups like minestrone and chicken.

RiceSelect Whole Wheat Pearl Couscous
(50 g, ½ cup dry)
190 calories
1 g fat
(0 g saturated)
6 g fiber

Couscous is rolled spheres of wheat, so when purchasing it, you should adhere to the same principle as for bread and pasta: Whole wheat is king.

Mahatma Basmati Rice
(45 g, ¼ cup dry)
160 calories
0.5 g fat
(0 g saturated)
<1 g fiber

Basmati rice is easier on your blood sugar than jasmine. Improve matters even more by picking up brown basmati, which packs more fiber than the normal white variety.

Lundberg Heat & Eat Organic Countrywild Brown Rice
(210 g, 1 bowl)
280 calories
3 g fat
(0 g saturated)
6 g fiber

Three strains of whole-grain rice means more texture and flavor than typical brown rice.

Not That!

Gold Medal Organic All-Purpose Flour
(30 g, ¼ cup)

100 calories
0 g fat
1 g fiber

We applaud the organic effort, but it doesn't mean much once Gold Medal strips most of the fiber from the grain.

Minute Ready to Serve Brown Rice
(125 g, 1 container, 1 cup)

230 calories
3.5 g fat
(0 g saturated)
2 g fiber

Many quick-serve rice packages contain unnecessary oil. You can do better.

Wild rice has more protein than brown rice, but it still comes up short when stacked against more-robust whole grains and seeds.

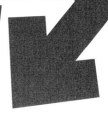

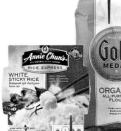
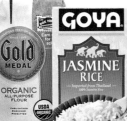
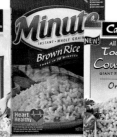
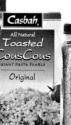
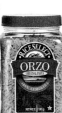
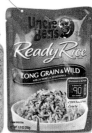

Annie Chun's Rice Express White Sticky Rice
(210 g, 1 bowl)

300 calories
0 g fat
0 g fiber

Choose this over Lundberg's and you'll sacrifice about a quarter of your day's recommended fiber intake.

Goya Thai Jasmine Rice
(45 g, ¼ cup dry)

170 calories
0 g fat
0 g fiber

Refined grains like this tend to prime your body for belly fat storage.

Casbah Toasted CousCous Original
(45 g, ⅓ cup dry)

170 calories
0 g fat
2 g fiber

The 20 calories you save by opting for toasted over whole wheat comes at a two-thirds reduction in fiber. It's not worth it.

RiceSelect Orzo
(56 g, ½ cup dry)

210 calories
1 g fat
(0 g saturated)
2 g fiber

Orzo looks like a grain, but it's actually a tiny form of pasta. As such, it delivers a mere fraction of the fiber of a true grain like barley.

Uncle Ben's Ready Rice Long Grain & Wild
(1 cup prepared)

220 calories
3 g fat
(0 g saturated)
2 g fiber

Rice Sides
Eat This

The chickpeas in this mix are loaded with cancer-fighting folate and help boost the dish's fiber to a level typically associated with more robust grains like barley and quinoa.

Near East Rice Pilaf Mix Lentil
(1 cup prepared)

200 calories
3.5 g fat
(2 g saturated)
680 mg sodium
8 g fiber

Lentils provide a healthy mixture of soluble and insoluble fiber and are loaded with protein, making this one of the healthiest side dishes in the supermarket.

Uncle Ben's Ready Rice Spanish Style
(1 cup prepared)

200 calories
2.5 g fat
(0 g saturated)
620 mg sodium
2 g fiber

Tomatoes and poblano peppers are listed right after rice, making this Uncle Ben's most nutritious variety of Ready Rice.

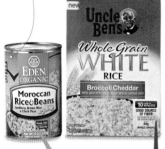 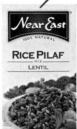 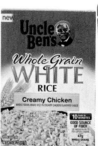 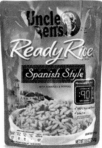 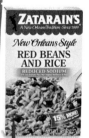

Eden Organic Moroccan Rice & Beans
(1 cup prepared)

220 calories
2 g fat (0 g saturated)
460 mg sodium
6 g fiber

Uncle Ben's Whole Grain White Rice Broccoli Cheddar
(1 cup prepared)

200 calories
2 g fat
(0.5 g saturated)
600 mg sodium
4 g fiber

Typically, white rice is devoid of the grain's bran and germ, but Ben's new line keeps some in place and fortifies it with extra fiber from chicory root.

Uncle Ben's Whole Grain White Rice Creamy Chicken
(1 cup prepared)

200 calories
2 g fat (0 g saturated)
590 mg sodium
5 g fiber

If you can't stomach brown rice, make Ben's Whole Grain White Rice your new go-to option for white.

Zatarain's New Orleans Style Reduced Sodium Red Beans and Rice
(⅓ cup dry, 1 cup prepared)

190 calories
0 g fat
720 mg sodium
5 g fiber

After rice, red beans are the first ingredient. If only all supermarket products were this straightforward.

**Knorr
Cajun Sides
Dirty Rice**
(1 cup prepared)

270 calories
5.5 g fat
(1 g saturated)
830 mg sodium
2 g fiber

More calories, fat, sodium,
and ingredients
than Uncle Ben's version.

**Goya
Fiesta Rice
with Wild Rice
& Vegetables**
(1 cup prepared)

320 calories
0 g fat
1,000 mg sodium
4 g fiber

The "broth-type flavor"
in this box consists of
monosodium glutamate
(aka MSG), maltodextrin,
partially hydrogenated oil,
and sugar.

Not That!

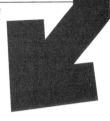

*Not one of Rice-A-Roni's
Whole Grain Blends has fewer than
250 calories—not to mention the fact that
a single serving chews through
about a third of your day's sodium allotment.*

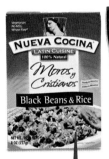
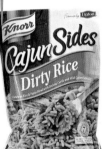
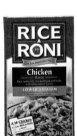
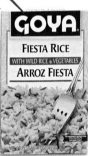
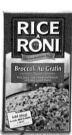
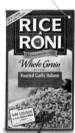

**Nueva Cocina
Black Beans
& Rice**
(⅓ cup dry)

220 calories
0 g fat
760 mg sodium
3 g fiber

A few more black beans
would earn this dish
a stronger hit of fiber.
Three grams isn't
enough to justify
this caloric price tag.

**Rice-A-Roni
Chicken Flavor
Lower Sodium**
(1 cup prepared)

270 calories
5 g fat (1 g saturated,
0.5 g trans)
670 mg sodium
2 g fiber

Lower sodium? Lower
than what, a salt shaker?

**Rice-A-Roni
Broccoli
Au Gratin**
(1 cup prepared)

350 calories
16 g fat
(5 g saturated,
2 g trans)
910 mg sodium
2 g fiber

Neither cheese nor
broccoli places higher
than partially
hydrogenated oil in this
box's ingredient list.

**Rice-A-Roni
Whole Grain
Blends
Roasted Garlic
Italiano**
(1 cup prepared)

270 calories
9 g fat
(1.5 g saturated)
760 mg sodium
3 g fiber

183

Dry Noodles
Eat This

Diets rich in fiber have been shown to decrease the risks of diabetes and heart disease. Each serving of this pasta has more than 20 percent of your daily requirement.

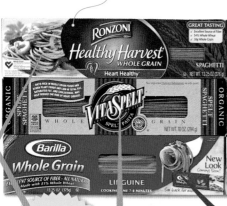

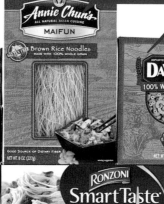

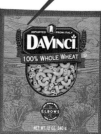

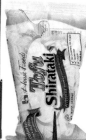

Annie Chun's Maifun Brown Rice Noodles
(56 g dry)

200 calories
1 g fat
(0.5 g saturated)
4 g fiber

These noodles are made with a refreshingly simple recipe of just brown rice flour and water.

DaVinci 100% Whole Wheat Elbows
(59 g dry)

180 calories
1.5 g fat
(0 g saturated)
5 g fiber

For your next batch of mac and cheese, swap out the cream for milk and toss with these noodles. You'll cut hundreds of calories and triple up on fiber.

Ronzoni Healthy Harvest Whole Grain Spaghetti
(56 g dry)

180 calories
1 g fat
(0 g saturated)
6 g fiber

Vita-Spelt Whole Grain Spelt Spaghetti
(57 g, 2 oz dry)

190 calories
1.5 g fat
(0 g saturated)
5 g fiber

Spelt is a nutrient-dense grain related to wheat, but many people with wheat sensitivity find it more tolerable.

Barilla Whole Grain Linguine
(56 g dry)

200 calories
1.5 g fat
(0 g saturated)
6 g fiber

Nearly all dried pasta varieties pack similar amounts of calories and fat, which is why the fiber count is the single most important number on the nutrition label.

Ronzoni Smart Taste Angel Hair
(57 g dry)

170 calories
0.5 g fat
(0 g saturated)
5 g fiber

For those who just can't do wheat pasta, Ronzoni combines the taste and texture of white noodles with the fiber of whole wheat.

House Foods Tofu Shirataki Fettuccine Shaped Noodle Substitute
(113 g)

20 calories
0.5 g fat
(0 g saturated)
2 g fiber

Find these tofu-based noodles in specialty stores or online at www.house-foods.com.

Not That!

American Beauty Quick Cook Elbows
(56 g dry)

210 calories
1 g fat
(0 g saturated)
2 g fiber

If you're going to make a cheesy pasta dish, the least you can do is start with a more wholesome noodle.

Roland Organic Buckwheat Soba Noodles
(56 g dry)

200 calories
1 g fat
(0 g saturated)
1 g fiber

These noodles would be commendable if they were made with whole-grain buckwheat.

When it comes to noodles and grains, organic is far less important nutritionally than high fiber.

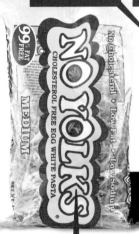
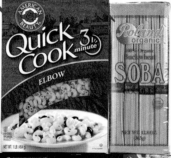
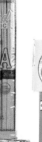
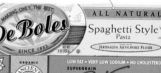
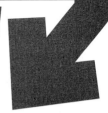

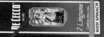
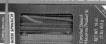

No Yolks Egg White Pasta
(56 g dry)

210 calories
0.5 g fat
(0 g saturated)
3 g fiber

Yolks or not, this pasta is still made with regular, nutrient-hollow refined flour.

Barilla Angel Hair
(56 g dry)

200 calories
1 g fat
(0 g saturated)
2 g fiber

These numbers are pretty standard for run-of-the-mill white pasta. Aim for better.

De Cecco 7. Linguine with Spinach
(56 g dry)

200 calories
1 g fat
(0 g saturated)
2 g fiber

Not even spinach can save this linguine. The green leaf is the second ingredient, yet it brings more color than it does nutrients to these noodles.

Ancient Harvest Quinoa Spaghetti Wheat Free
(57 g, 2 oz dry)

205 calories
1 g fat
(0 g saturated)
4 g fiber

You may think these noodles are made strictly from healthy quinoa, yet the primary ingredient is corn flour, which contains less protein and fiber.

DeBoles Organic Spaghetti Style Pasta
(56 g dry)

210 calories
1 g fat
(0 g saturated)
1 g fiber

185

Packaged & Seasoned
Eat This

Kraft's Deluxe mac line is a huge step up from the standard blue box. Not only is it low in calories, it also packs 13 grams of protein and 2 grams of fiber.

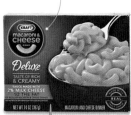
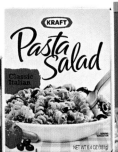
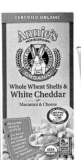
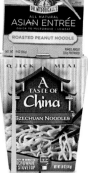
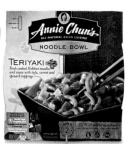

Kraft Deluxe Macaroni and Cheese Original ½ the Fat
(1 cup prepared)

290 calories
4.5 g fat
(2 g saturated)
850 mg sodium

Kraft Pasta Salad Italian
(1 cup prepared)

220 calories
7 g fat
(1 g saturated)
630 mg sodium

Kraft replaces standard oil with water in this pasta salad. The result is a dish with superior numbers across the board.

Annie's Whole Wheat Shells & White Cheddar
(1 cup prepared)

260 calories
5 g fat
(2.5 g saturated)
580 mg sodium

This box delivers 5 grams of fiber, which is a feat unmatched in the world of macs.

Dr. McDougall's Roasted Peanut Noodle
(1 cup, 60 g)

220 calories
3 g fat
(0 g saturated)
580 mg sodium

Ramen doesn't get lower in sodium.

A Taste of China Szechuan Noodles
(141 g, 1 package)

375 calories
7.5 g fat
(1.5 g saturated)
1,125 mg sodium

High in sodium, but built with an impressive list of high-quality ingredients.

Annie Chun's Teriyaki Noodle Bowl
(232 g, 1 bowl)

400 calories
5 g fat
(0 g saturated)
880 mg sodium

This is a substantially sized bowl for only 400 calories.

Noodles

Not That!

This iconic box is a nutritional disaster, complete with more than 2 days' worth of trans fats per serving.

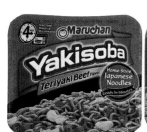

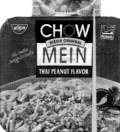

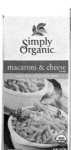

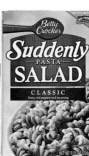

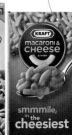

Maruchan Yakisoba Teriyaki Beef
(113 g, 1 package)

520 calories
20 g fat
(10 g saturated)
1,320 mg sodium

Half the size, four times the fat.

Nissin Chow Mein Thai Peanut
(114 g, 1 container)

560 calories
28 g fat
(10 g saturated)
1,280 mg sodium

This bowl is filled with half your day's saturated fat and sodium, plus a pool of partially hydrogenated oil.

Nissin Cup Noodles Chicken
(64 g, 1 container)

300 calories
13 g fat
(7 g saturated)
1,060 mg sodium

Loaded with 45 percent of your daily sodium and 35 percent of your day's saturated fat.

Simply Organic Macaroni & Cheese
(1 cup prepared)

360 calories
14 g fat
(11 g saturated)
859 mg sodium

Organic it may be, but that does not forgive the sin of excess sodium and saturated fat.

Betty Crocker Suddenly Pasta Salad Classic
(1 cup prepared)

330 calories
10 g fat
(1.5 g saturated)
1,040 mg sodium

This side dish packs a staggering 40 percent of your daily sodium.

Kraft Macaroni & Cheese Dinner Original
(1 cup prepared)

400 calories
19 g fat
(4.5 g saturated,
4 g trans)
710 mg sodium

187

Pasta Sauces
Eat This

We love traditional pesto as a sauce and as a condiment, but choose the wrong one and calorie counts climb to stratospheric levels. Classico solves the problem by bolstering this pesto with sweet, dried tomatoes, reducing the need for an oily deluge.

DeLallo Red Clam Sauce
(½ cup)

40 calories
1.5 g fat
(0 g saturated)
490 mg sodium

Tomatoes, clams, water, and red peppers are the first four ingredients —a recipe for a healthy sauce.

Muir Glen Cabernet Marinara
(125 g, ½ cup)

60 calories
1 g fat
(0 g saturated)
360 mg sodium

Cabernet is king of the alcohol-imbued pasta sauces. It brings a layer of complexity without a heavy calorie tax.

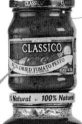
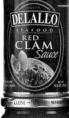
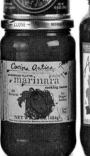
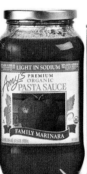
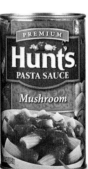
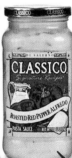
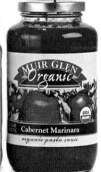

Classico Sun-Dried Tomato Pesto
(62 g, ¼ cup)

90 calories
5 g fat
(1 g saturated)
630 mg sodium

Ragú Light No Sugar Added Tomato & Basil
(125 g, ½ cup)

60 calories
1 g fat
(0 g saturated)
320 mg sodium

Why add sugar when tomatoes are packed with natural sweetness?

Cucina Antica Garlic Marinara
(118 g, ½ cup)

36 calories
2 g fat
(0 g saturated)
246 mg sodium

This lean sauce earns its naturally sweet flavor from San Marzano tomatoes instead of fats or added sugars.

Amy's Light in Sodium Organic Family Marinara
(125 g, ½ cup)

80 calories
4.5 g fat
(0.5 g saturated)
290 mg sodium

Amy's regular marinara has twice the sodium.

Hunt's Pasta Sauce Mushroom
(126 g, ½ cup)

50 calories
0.5 g fat
(0 g saturated)
590 mg sodium

Amidst a wall of bottled artisan sauces, the low-cal leader lives in a humble can.

Classico Roasted Red Pepper Alfredo
(¼ cup)

60 calories
5 g fat
(3 g saturated)
310 mg sodium

Brilliant: The red peppers in this jar displace calories from heavy cream.

188

Not That!

Bertolli Vodka Sauce
(125 g, ½ cup)

150 calories
9 g fat
(4.5 g saturated)
700 mg sodium

It's not the vodka you have to worry about, it's the belt-buckling triad of cream, oil, and sugar.

DeLallo White Clam Sauce
(½ cup)

160 calories
15 g fat
(2 g saturated)
540 mg sodium

"White sauce" typically denotes an ample dose of oil or cream. As such, this sauce is 10 times as fatty as its tomato-based cousin.

Thanks mostly to the heavy use of oil and cheese, nearly every calorie in this sauce comes from fat.

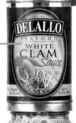

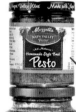

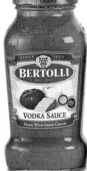

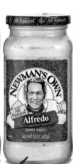

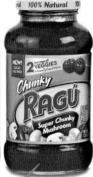

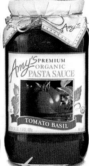

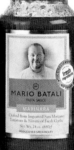

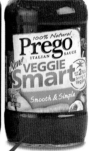

Newman's Own Alfredo Pasta Sauce
(¼ cup)

90 calories
8 g fat
(4.5 g saturated)
410 mg sodium

Worse Alfredo sauces exist, but that doesn't make Newman's a winner.

Chunky Ragú Super Chunky Mushroom
(128 g, ½ cup)

80 calories
2.5 g fat
(0 g saturated)
470 mg sodium

Like sugar with your mushrooms? Ragu dusts them 10 grams of sugar per serving.

Amy's Organic Tomato Basil
(125 g, ½ cup)

110 calories
6 g fat
(1 g saturated)
580 mg sodium

We applaud Amy's use of organic tomatoes, but 110 calories is just far too much for a tomato-based pasta sauce.

Mario's Original Marinara
(122 g, ½ cup)

130 calories
10 g fat
(1.5 g saturated)
580 mg sodium

Chef Mario Batali isn't known for his light cuisine.

Prego Veggie Smart Smooth & Simple
(120 ml, ½ cup)

90 calories
1.5 g fat
(0 g saturated)
410 mg sodium

A full 14 grams of sugar means this sauce packs more of the sweet stuff than a serving of Frosted Flakes.

Mezzetta Homemade Style Basil Pesto
(60 ml, ¼ cup)

300 calories
32 g fat
(2.5 g saturated)
640 mg sodium

Condiments
Eat This

This swap makes the Eat This, Not That! hall of fame. Not only do you cut calories in half, but you also boost your healthy fat intake.

Annie's Naturals Organic Ketchup
(17 g, 1 Tbsp)

15 calories
0 g fat
170 mg sodium
4 g sugars

Go ahead and spring for organic. Research shows that organically raised tomatoes produce nearly twice as much cancer-fighting lycopene.

McCormick Fat Free Tartar Sauce
(32 g, 2 Tbsp)

30 calories
0 g fat
250 mg sodium
5 g sugars

Although by no means a nutritious condiment, this light take on tartar does eliminate more than 100 calories per serving.

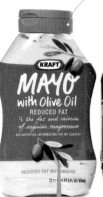
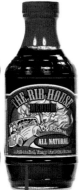
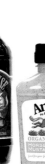
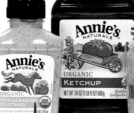
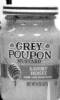
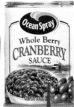
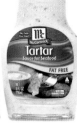

Kraft Mayo with Olive Oil
(15 g, 1 Tbsp)

45 calories
4 g fat
(0 g saturated)
95 mg sodium
<1 g sugars

The Rib House Medium BBQ Sauce
(31 g, 2 Tbsp)

25 calories
0 g fat
240 mg sodium
6 g sugars

The Rib House's sauce earns a touch of sweetness from brown sugar, but its primary ingredients are tomato paste and vinegar.

Annie's Naturals Organic Horseradish Mustard
(10 g, 2 tsp)

10 calories
0 g fat
120 mg sodium
0 g sugars

This bottle contains no ingredients that you wouldn't have on hand at home.

Grey Poupon Savory Honey Mustard
(15 g, 1 Tbsp)

30 calories
0 g fat
15 mg sodium
3 g sugars

Made mostly from mustard seeds, which are loaded with omega-3 fatty acids.

Ocean Spray Whole Berry Cranberry Sauce
(35 g, 2 Tbsp)

55 calories
0 g fat
5 g carbohydrates
5 mg sodium
11 g sugars

Not just for Thanksgiving anymore. Turn to cranberry sauce for a low-calorie, high-antioxidant sandwich companion.

Not That!

Aside from pure oil, mayonnaise is the most calorie-dense thing you can put on a sandwich. Every one of its 90 calories comes from fat.

Kraft Tartar Sauce Natural Lemon Flavor & Herb (28 g, 2 Tbsp)

150 calories
16 g fat
(2.5 g saturated)
180 mg sodium
<1 g sugars

Tartar sauce is little more than mayonnaise with relish stirred in. Go with a light version or switch to cocktail sauce.

Heinz Tomato Ketchup (17 g, 1 Tbsp)

20 calories
0 g fat
160 mg sodium
4 g sugars

Placed last in our ketchup taste test on page 46. Switch to Annie's and you earn the benefits of organic tomatoes and eliminate the high-fructose corn syrup in Heinz's.

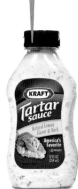

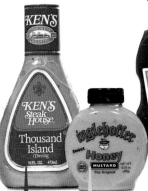

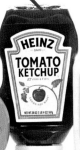

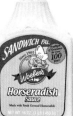

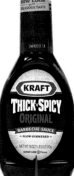

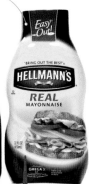

Ken's Steak House Thousand Island Dressing (30 g, 2 Tbsp)

140 calories
13 g fat
(2 g saturated)
300 mg sodium
3 g sugars

There's no secret with this sauce: Thousand Island is big on calories and low on nutrients.

Inglehoffer Sweet Honey Mustard (15 g, 1 Tbsp)

45 calories
0 g fat
105 mg sodium
6 g sugars

The first two ingredients are water and sugar, and corn syrup trails close behind.

Woeber's Sandwich Pal Horseradish Sauce (10 g, 2 tsp)

40 calories
3 g fat
(0 g saturated)
60 mg sodium
0 g sugars

"Sauce" is a euphemism; what they meant to say is soybean oil and corn syrup.

Kraft Thick 'n Spicy Original Barbecue Sauce (37 g, 2 Tbsp)

70 calories
0 g fat
340 mg sodium
13 g sugars

High-fructose corn syrup is the primary ingredient, which is why this bottle delivers twice as much sugar as the more modest option on the opposite page.

Hellmann's Real Mayonnaise (13 g, 1 Tbsp)

90 calories
10 g fat
(1.5 g saturated)
90 mg sodium
0 g sugars

Dressings
Eat This

Bolthouse Farms casts yogurt as the star in classic flavors such as ranch, honey mustard, Thousand Island, and blue cheese, allowing you to swap out vegetable oil for worthwhile hits of calcium and probiotic bacteria.

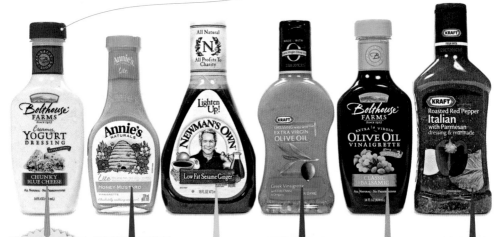

Bolthouse Farms Creamy Yogurt Dressing Chunky Blue Cheese
(30 g, 2 Tbsp)

50 calories
4.5 g fat
(1.5 g saturated)
140 mg sodium

Annie's Naturals Lite Honey Mustard Vinaigrette
(31 g, 2 Tbsp)

40 calories
3 g fat
(0 g saturated)
125 mg sodium

Finally, a honest mustard dressing not spoiled with oil.

Newman's Own Lighten Up! Low Fat Sesame Ginger
(30 g, 2 Tbsp)

35 calories
1.5 g fat
(0 g saturated)
330 mg sodium

Vinegar, soy sauce, and ginger can drive the flavor.

Kraft Greek Vinaigrette with Feta Cheese and Oregano
(31 g, 2 Tbsp)

60 calories
5 g fat
(1 g saturated)
360 mg sodium

This bottle keeps it real with a healthy dose of olive oil.

Bolthouse Farms Classic Balsamic Olive Oil Vinaigrette
(30 g, 2 Tbsp)

30 calories
0 g fat
150 mg sodium

The lightest vinaigrette we've ever come across.

Kraft Roasted Red Pepper Italian with Parmesan
(32 g, 2 Tbsp)

40 calories
2 g fat
(0 g saturated)
340 mg sodium

The bulk of this bottle is filled with vinegar and tomato puree, a perfect low-cal formula.

Not That!

Virtually every calorie in this bottle comes from soybean oil, which is a common theme in the dressing aisle. Consider them wasted calories; soybean oil doesn't have the same heart-healthy cachet as olive or canola oil.

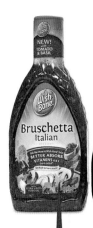
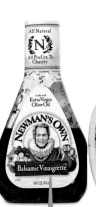
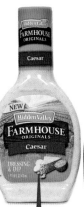
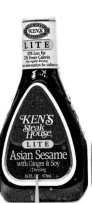
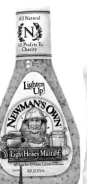
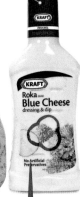

Wish-Bone Bruschetta Italian
(2 Tbsp, 30 mL)

60 calories
5 g fat
(1 g saturated)
340 mg sodium

The front label boasts about olive oil, but it accounts for less than 2 percent of the recipe.

Newman's Own Balsamic Vinaigrette
(30 g, 2 Tbsp)

90 calories
9 g fat
(1 g saturated)
290 mg sodium

A totally standard vinaigrette. You can do much better.

Hidden Valley Farmhouse Originals Caesar
(30 g, 2 Tbsp)

120 calories
11 g fat
(1.5 g saturated)
220 mg sodium

You're committing yourself to nearly 3,000 calories with this bottle.

Ken's Steak House Lite Asian Sesame
(30 g, 2 Tbsp)

70 calories
4 g fat
(0.5 g saturated)
440 mg sodium

After water, sugar is the first ingredient in this bottle.

Newman's Own Lighten Up! Light Honey Mustard Dressing
(30 g, 2 Tbsp)

70 calories
4 g fat
(0.5 g saturated)
280 mg sodium

"Light" is a relative term.

Kraft Roka Brand Blue Cheese
(29 g, 2 Tbsp)

120 calories
13 g fat
(2 g saturated)
380 mg sodium

193

Asian Sauces
Eat This

A scoop of curry paste can bring a world of flavor to a common stir-fry, and this one is among the best. It's made primarily from red chili peppers, garlic, and lemongrass.

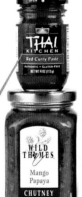
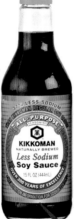
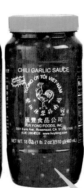
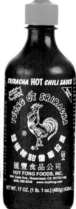
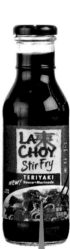
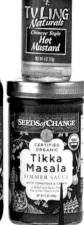

Thai Kitchen Red Curry Paste
(30 g, 2 Tbsp)

30 calories
0 g fat
780 mg sodium
2 g sugars

Wild Thymes Mango Papaya Chutney
(1 Tbsp)

15 calories
0 g fat
0 mg sodium
3 g sugars

This jar contains an antioxidant-rich blend of mango, apples, pineapple, and papaya.

Kikkoman Less Sodium Soy Sauce
(15 ml, 1 Tbsp)

10 calories
0 g fat
575 mg sodium
0 g sugars

All soy sauces are low in calories, so it's the sodium count that matters most. Kikkoman keeps it in check.

Huy Fong Chili Garlic Sauce
(1 tsp)

0 calories
0 g fat
115 mg sodium
<1 g sugars

The ground chili peppers found in here help break up blood clots and speed up metabolism.

La Choy Stir-Fry Teriyaki Sauce & Marinade
(1 Tbsp)

10 calories
0 g fat
105 mg sodium
1 g sugars

By cutting sugar and soy, La Choy has created the best teriyaki sauce in the supermarket.

Seeds of Change Tikka Masala
(⅓ cup)

90 calories
7 g fat
(2.5 g saturated)
280 mg sodium

Each serving also boasts 2 grams of fiber from the tomato puree.

Not That!

True curries are flavorful pastes made largely of nutrient-packed spices and herbs, but two of the first few ingredients in this jar are oil and salt.

SunLuck Duck Sauce
(1 Tbsp)
35 calories
0 g fat
170 mg sodium
8 g sugars
Duck sauce is essentially flavored sugar.

Mae Ploy Sweet Chilli Sauce
(15 g, 1 Tbsp)
35 calories
0 g fat
200 mg sodium
7 g sugars
Avoid sauces that feature sugar as the first ingredient.

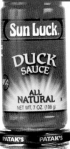
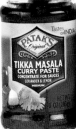
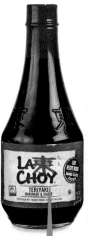
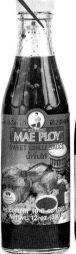
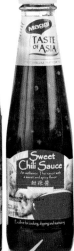
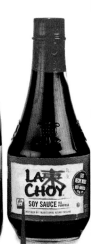
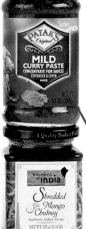
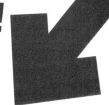

Patak's Tikka Masala
(46 g, ⅓ cup)
133 calories
9 g fat
(1 g saturated)
585 mg sodium
A heavy-handed application of canola oil fattens up this sauce.

La Choy Teriyaki Marinade & Sauce
(1 Tbsp)
40 calories
0 g fat
570 mg sodium
8 g sugars
Eight times the sugar and five times the sodium of La Choy's other teriyaki sauce.

Maggi Sweet Chili Sauce
(15 ml)
35 calories
0 g fat
250 mg sodium
8 g sugars
Nearly every calorie in this bottle comes from pure sugar, the first ingredient on the list.

La Choy Soy Sauce
(15 ml, 1 Tbsp)
10 calories
0 g fat
1,160 mg sodium
<1 g sugars
One tablespoon has half your day's sodium intake.

Kitchens of India Shredded Mango Chutney
(1 Tbsp)
80 calories
0 g fat
150 mg sodium
17 g sugars
The first ingredient is sugar.

Patak's Mild Curry Paste
(35 g, 2 Tbsp)
110 calories
9 g fat
(0.5 g saturated)
480 mg sodium
1 g sugars

195

Barbecue Sauces &

Eat This

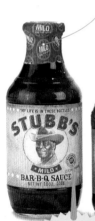

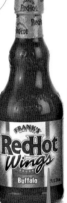

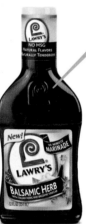

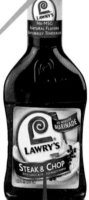

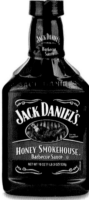

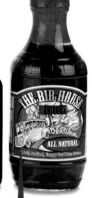

Lawry's 30-Minute Marinade Balsamic Herb
(30 ml, 2 Tbsp)

20 calories
720 mg sodium

Every one of the Lawry's marinades beats every one of KC Masterpiece's.

Jack Daniel's Honey Smokehouse Barbecue Sauce
(34 g, 2 Tbsp)

45 calories
0 g fat
280 mg sodium

Most sauce purveyors use the word "honey" as an excuse to turn their products into dessert. We love that the guys at Jack Daniel's resisted the urge.

Stubb's Bar-B-Q Sauce Mild
(32 g, 2 Tbsp)

25 calories
0 g fat
230 mg sodium

Frank's Red Hot Wings Buffalo Sauce
(30 ml, 2 Tbsp)

0 calories
0 g fat
920 mg sodium

The sodium is a bit high, but Frank's is potent enough that a few shakes will do.

Lawry's 30-Minute Marinade Steak & Chop
(30 ml, 2 Tbsp)

10 calories
0 g fat
780 mg sodium

Unlike many sugar-heavy marinades, Lawry's uses mostly lemon juice and vinegar, which serve to both flavor and tenderize poultry and red meat.

The Rib House Medium BBQ Sauce
(31 g, 2 Tbsp)

25 calories
0 g fat
240 mg sodium

Barbecue sauce is a condiment often abused by manufacturers eager to cut costs with low-quality sugars. The Rib House uses mainly tomato paste, vinegar, and brown sugar.

Marinades

Not That!

Famous Dave's BBQ Sauce Sweet & Zesty
(38 g, 2 Tbsp)

70 calories
0 g fat
320 mg sodium

With 15 grams of sugar in every serving, Famous Dave is a dead ringer for Willy Wonka.

KC Masterpiece Marinade Honey Teriyaki
(30 ml, 2 Tbsp)

70 calories
0 g fat
740 mg sodium

High-fructose corn syrup is the first ingredient. Grill masters don't reach for HFCS when they fire up the grill, so you shouldn't either.

The first ingredient in this bottle is high-fructose corn syrup. That provides an excessive sugar load that turns into bitter-tasting carbon once it meets the heat of the grill.

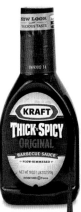
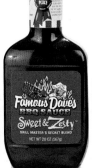
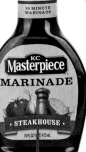
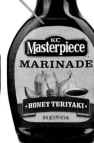
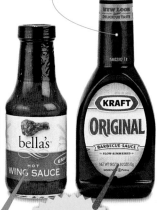

Kraft Thick'n Spicy Barbecue Sauce Original
(37 g, 2 Tbsp)

70 calories
0 g fat
340 mg sodium

Every tablespoon of this sauce contains more sugar than a Chewy Chips Ahoy! cookie.

KC Masterpiece Marinade Steakhouse
(30 ml, 2 Tbsp)

60 calories
2 g fat (0 g saturated)
660 mg sodium

KC Masterpiece always falls back on excessive sweeteners to flavor its sauces, in this case producing a marinade with six times the sugar count of its Lawry's counterpart.

Bella's Hot Wing Sauce
(30 g, 2 Tbsp)

70 calories
5 g fat (0 g saturated)
760 mg sodium

Wings have plenty of fat as it is, so you don't need more from your sauce.

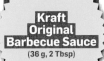

Kraft Original Barbecue Sauce
(36 g, 2 Tbsp)

60 calories
0 g fat
450 mg sodium

Soups
Eat This

Carrots and red peppers are among the primary ingredients in this carton. That's how each serving earns you nearly half of your daily vitamin A requirement.

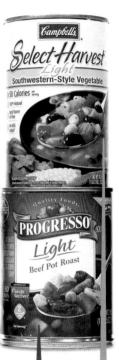

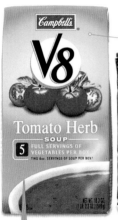

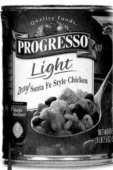

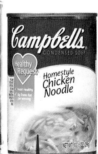

V8 Tomato Herb
(1 cup)

90 calories
0 g fat
480 mg sodium
3 g fiber

Progresso Light Zesty Santa Fe Style Chicken
(1 cup)

80 calories
1 g fat
(0 g saturated)
460 mg sodium
2 g fiber

The black beans in this soup bolster the fiber content, plus add a shot of brain-boosting antioxidants.

Campbell's Healthy Request Condensed Chicken Noodle
(1 cup prepared)

60 calories
1.5 g fat
(0.5 g saturated)
440 mg sodium
1 g fiber

Has less than half the sodium of Campbell's regular chicken noodle.

Progresso Light Beef Pot Roast
(1 cup)

80 calories
2 g fat
(1 g saturated)
470 mg sodium
2 g fiber

There's a bounty of vegetation in this can, and it includes carrots, green beans, potatoes, tomatoes, celery, and peas.

Campbell's Select Harvest Light Southwestern-Style Vegetable
(1 cup)

50 calories
0 g fat
480 mg sodium
4 g fiber

The heavy vegetable load packs 4 grams of fiber into a 50-calorie serving.

Not That!

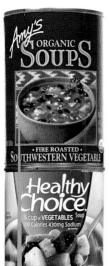

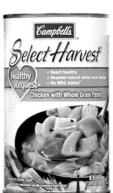

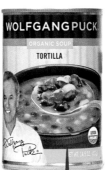

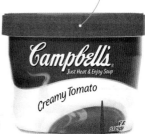

Call it junk stew: The third ingredient is high-fructose corn syrup, and the "dairy base" is made with oil.

Amy's Organic Fire Roasted Southwestern Vegetable (1 cup)

140 calories
4 g fat
(0.5 g saturated)
680 mg sodium
4 g fiber

We love all of the vegetables, but Campbell's does it with a fraction of the calories.

Healthy Choice Beef Pot Roast (1 cup)

110 calories
0.5 g fat
(0 g saturated)
430 mg sodium
3 g fiber

Switch to Progresso's version and save 30 calories per serving.

Campbell's Select Harvest Healthy Request Chicken with Whole Grain Pasta (1 cup)

100 calories
2 g fat
(0.5 g saturated)
410 mg sodium
1 g fiber

The "whole grain" pasta provides 1 gram of fiber.

Wolfgang Puck Organic Signature Tortilla Soup (1 cup)

160 calories
3.5 g fat
(1 g saturated)
670 mg sodium
6 g fiber

We'd expect Chef Puck to be above the excessive sugar and sodium that other soup makers fall back on.

Campbell's Microwavable Bowls Creamy Tomato (1 cup)

160 calories
5 g fat
(1 g saturated)
480 mg sodium
3 g fiber

Beans and Chili

Eat This

When properly prepared, chili is a potent mix of muscle-building protein and gut-scrubbing fiber. This one achieves those objectives while also reining in fat.

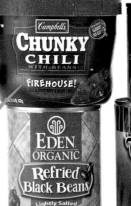
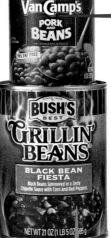
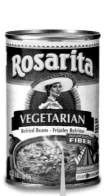
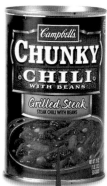

Campbell's Chunky Chili Firehouse Beef & Bean Chili
(1 cup)

230 calories
8 g fat
(3.5 g saturated, 0.5 g trans)
870 mg sodium
8 g fiber

Eden Organic Refried Black Beans
(½ cup)

110 calories
1.5 g fat
(0 g saturated)
180 mg sodium
7 g fiber

Black beans contain the same dark-hued antioxidants that give blueberries the ability to boost brainpower.

Bush's Grillin' Beans Black Bean Fiesta
(½ cup)

110 calories
1 g fat
(0 g saturated)
570 mg sodium
5 g fiber

Bush's skips the normal spoonful of sugar and instead sweetens this can with corn and peppers.

Rosarita Vegetarian Refried Beans
(½ cup)

120 calories
2 g fat
(0 g saturated)
540 mg sodium
6 g fiber

"Vegetarian" means Rosarita omits the lard found in Ortega's version.

Campbell's Chunky Grilled Steak Chili with Beans
(1 cup)

200 calories
3 g fat
(1 g saturated)
870 mg sodium
7 g fiber

Impressively lean for a beefed-up can of chili. When choosing chili, Campbell's is a good bet.

Not That!

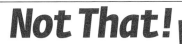

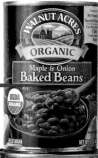

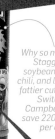

Why so much fat? Stagg adds soybean oil to its chili, and likely uses fattier cuts of beef. Switch to Campbell's and save 220 calories per can.

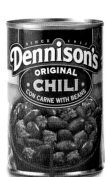

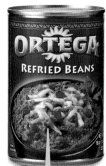

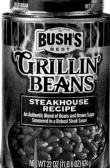

Dennison's Original Chili with Beans
(1 cup)

360 calories
14 g fat
(6 g saturated, 1 g trans)
1,030 mg sodium
11 g fiber

Each can has more than half your day's saturated fat and more than a full day's sodium.

Ortega Refried Beans
(½ cup)

150 calories
2.5 g fat
(1 g saturated)
570 mg sodium
9 g fiber

Ortega's beans tend to be the most calorically dense in the supermarket.

Bush's Grillin' Beans Steakhouse Recipe
(½ cup)

180 calories
0.5 g fat
(0 g saturated)
510 mg sodium
5 g fiber

Contains 21 grams of sugar, 10 times that of Bush's black bean version.

Ortega Refried Beans Fat Free
(½ cup)

130 calories
0 g fat
570 mg sodium
9 g fiber

By the time you finish this can, you'll have taken in nearly 2,000 milligrams of sodium.

Stagg Chili Dynamite Hot Chili with Beans
(1 cup)

340 calories
17 g fat
(7 g saturated, 1 g trans)
800 mg sodium
8 g fiber

Canned & Cupped Fru

Eat This

To get the most from a piece of fruit, eat it raw.
In lieu of that, fruits canned
in their own juices are far easier on
your blood sugar than those sopped in syrup.

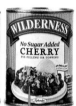

**Del Monte
No Sugar
Added
Diced
Peaches**
(106 g, 1 cup)

25 calories
0 g fat
5 g sugars

Peaches are
plenty sweet enough
on their own.

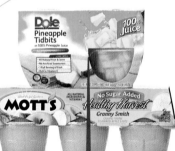

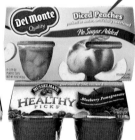

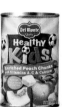

**Dole
Tropical Fruit
in 100%
Fruit Juice**
(122 g, ½ cup)

70 calories
0 g fat
15 g sugars

**Dole
Pineapple
Tidbits in
100%
Pineapple
Juice**
(113 g, 1 container)

60 calories
0 g fat
14 g sugars

Pineapple packs
loads of powerful
antioxidants.

**Mott's Healthy
Harvest No
Sugar Added
Granny Smith**
(111 g, 1 container)

50 calories
0 g fat
11 g sugars

The lack of added
sugars makes
this as close to
real fruit as
applesauce comes.

**Musselman's
Healthy Picks
Blueberry
Pomegranate**
(113 g, 1 unit)

70 calories
0 g fat
10 g sugars

This has added
dextrin, a natural
fiber that will help
keep your blood
sugar from spiking.

**Del Monte
Healthy Kids
Peach
Chunks**
(124 g, ½ cup)

60 calories
0 g fat
14 g sugars

You don't have to
be a kid to benefit
from the day's
worth of vitamin C
that's in this can.

**Wilderness
No Sugar
Added Cherry
Pie Filling**
(85 g, ⅓ cup)

35 calories
0 g fat
4 g sugars

Stuff it into
a crepe and drizzle
with dark
chocolate for an
insanely decadent,
low-calorie dessert.

its

Not That!

Del Monte Fruit Cocktail in Heavy Syrup
(127 g, ½ cup)

100 calories
0 g fat
23 g sugars

"Heavy syrup" amounts to little more than viscous, sugary goo. In other words, it's liquid candy.

As used on this can, "lightly sweetened" means that Dole used sugar instead of corn syrup to coat its fruit. The result is the same—spiked insulin and a dose of unneeded sugars.

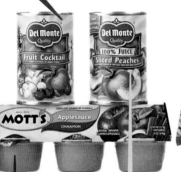
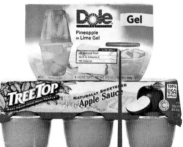

Wilderness Original Country Cherry Pie Filling
(89 g, ⅓ cup)

90 calories
0 g fat
19 g sugars

This can packs five times the sugar of the alternative.

Mott's Cinnamon Apple Sauce
(113 g, 1 container)

100 calories
0 g fat
24 g sugars

The extra calories come from high-fructose corn syrup.

Del Monte 100% Juice Sliced Peaches
(124 g, ½ cup)

60 calories
0 g fat
14 g sugars

Fruit juice trumps syrup, but it still doesn't compete with unadulterated natural fruit.

Tree Top Naturally Sweetened Apple Sauce
(113 g, 1 unit)

70 calories
0 g fat
15 g sugars

Not a bad product, but when there is a pure applesauce alternative, you should take it.

Dole Pineapple in Lime Gel
(123 g, 1 container)

90 calories
0 g fat
22 g sugars

Dole encases perfectly sweet chunks of pineapple in a neon shell of processed sugar.

Dole Tropical Fruit in Lightly Sweetened Passion Fruit Juice
(122 g, ½ cup)

90 calories
0 g fat
20 g sugars

Canned & Jarred Vege

Eat This

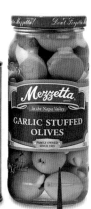

Green Giant Southwestern Style Corn
(94 g, ½ cup)

60 calories
0.5 g fat
(0 g saturated)
240 mg sodium

The black beans help push the fiber count up to 3 grams per serving. Serve next to a grilled sirloin.

Pickles make for a great snack just before a sweaty cardio workout. The sodium helps your body retain water.

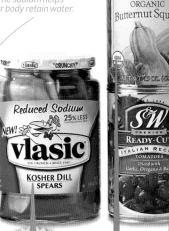

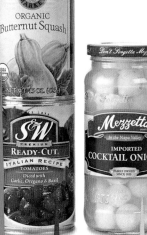

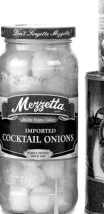

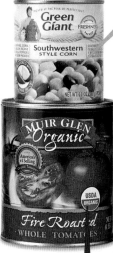

Vlasic Reduced Sodium Kosher Dill Spears
(84 g, 2 spears)

0 calories
0 g fat
450 mg sodium

Farmer's Market Organic Butternut Squash
(100 g, ½ cup)

50 calories
0 g fat
5 mg sodium

A cup of this contains nearly a full day's vitamin A.

S&W Ready-Cut Tomatoes Diced with Garlic, Oregano & Basil
(121 g, ½ cup)

25 calories
0 g fat
190 mg sodium

Nothing but tomatoes and spices.

Mezzetta Imported Cocktail Onions
(2 Tbsp)

5 calories
0 g fat
300 mg sodium

Cocktail onions add a vinegar kick to everything they touch—salads, side dishes, cocktails.

Muir Glen Organic Fire Roasted Whole Tomatoes
(122 g, ½ cup)

25 calories
0 g fat
290 mg sodium

Exposing tomatoes to heat brings out more of the fruit's lycopene.

Mezzetta Garlic Stuffed Olives
(19 g, 2 olives)

20 calories
2 g fat
(0 g saturated)
280 mg sodium

Stuffing olives with garlic heightens the heart-healthy effects while minimizing the caloric impact.

tables

Not That!

Green Giant Chipotle White Corn
(95 g, ⅔ cup)

90 calories
0.5 g fat
(0 g saturated)
250 mg sodium

Beware of spicy products; manufacturers usually add plenty of sugar to balance out the heat.

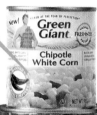

High-fructose corn syrup pollutes these pickles with as much sugar as a handful of M&M's.

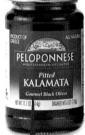
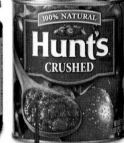
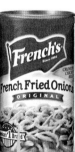
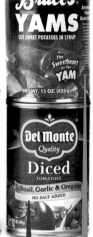
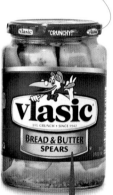
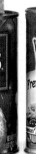

Peloponnese Pitted Kalamata Olives
(18 g, 6 olives)

54 calories
5.5 g fat
(0.5 g saturated)
252 mg sodium

Stuffed olives make for better snacking; save these for cooking.

Hunt's Crushed Tomatoes
(121 g, ¼ cup)

45 calories
0 g fat
230 mg sodium

Compared to Muir Glen's, Hunt's tomatoes have more calories and sodium and less vitamin E and iron.

French's French Fried Onions
(2 Tbsp)

45 calories
3.5 g fat
(1.5 g saturated)
60 mg sodium

These are far closer to onion rings than they are to onions. Which is to say, lots of fat, few nutrients.

Del Monte Diced Tomatoes with Basil, Garlic & Oregano No Salt Added
(126 g, ½ cup)

50 calories
0 g fat
50 mg sodium

Like high-fructose corn syrup with your tomatoes?

Bruce's Yams Cut Sweet Potatoes
(124 g, ½ cup)

143 calories
0 g fat
41 mg sodium
16 g sugars

Yams are one of the food world's most abused vegetables. Next time you eat them, try them without sugar.

Vlasic Bread & Butter Spears
(84 g, 2 spears)

75 calories
0 g fat
510 mg sodium

Canned & Packaged
Eat This

206

Bumble Bee Premium Light Tuna in Water
(71 g, 1 pouch)

70 calories
1 g fat
(0 g saturated)
240 mg sodium

The cans typically used to package tuna are lined with the hormone-disrupting chemical BPA (bisphenol A). Switch to pouches and eliminate the risk.

Lean roast beef—the kind found here—is one of the best sources of heme iron, the type most easily absorbed by the body.

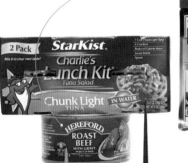
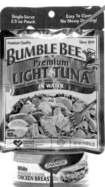
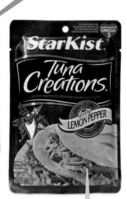
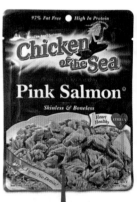

Hereford Roast Beef with Gravy
(152 g, ⅔ cup)

140 calories
3 g fat
(1.5 g saturated)
800 mg sodium

StarKist Charlie's Lunch Kit Tuna Salad Chunk Light Tuna
(123 g, 1 kit)

210 calories
8 g fat
(1 g saturated)
580 mg sodium

StarKist scores points by swapping out a fattier spread for reduced-calorie mayo.

Swanson White Premium Chunk Chicken Breast in Water
(2 oz, 56 g)

60 calories
1 g fat
(0 g saturated)
260 mg sodium

Choosing canned chicken over canned ham will save you calories, fat and 360 milligrams of sodium.

StarKist Tuna Creations Zesty Lemon Pepper
(140 g, 1 pouch)

150 calories
1 g fat
(0 g saturated)
550 mg sodium

Each pouch has 150 percent of your daily selenium, a small but key trace element shown to help reduce the risk of everything from cancer to arthritis.

Chicken of the Sea Pink Salmon
(4 oz)

120 calories
4 g fat
(2 g saturated)
560 mg sodium

Each serving has 1 gram of omega-3 fatty acids. That's half a week's recommended dose for healthy adults.

Protein

Not That!

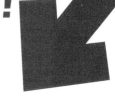

StarKist Albacore White Tuna in Water
(74 g, 1 pouch)

90 calories
2 g fat
(0.5 g saturated)
310 mg sodium

Albacore in a pouch contains just as much mercury as it does in a can. Make chunk light your go-to tuna.

Even Spam's light version contains the fat of 10 pieces of Oscar Mayer Center Cut Bacon and the sodium of a sleeve and a half of saltine crackers.

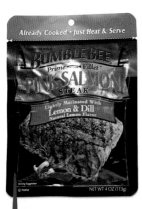

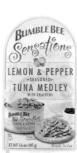

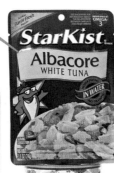

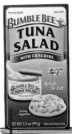

Bumble Bee Prime Fillet Pink Salmon Steak Lightly Marinated with Lemon & Dill
(4 oz, 1 pouch)

150 calories
4.5 g fat
(1 g saturated)
600 mg sodium

The addition of soybean oil undermines the healthful effects of the omega-3 fats.

Bumble Bee Easy Peel Sensations Lemon & Pepper Seasoned Tuna Medley with Crackers
(103 g, 1 can with crackers)

200 calories
7.5 g fat
(3.5 g saturated)
460 mg sodium

Blame the oily marinade.

Hormel Lean Ham with Smoke Flavoring
(2 oz, 56 g)

90 calories
6 g fat
(2 g saturated)
620 mg sodium

Canned ham carries far more sodium than fresh ham. Unless you simply must have it, switch to chicken and save yourself the added cardiovascular strain.

Bumble Bee Tuna Salad with Crackers
(99 g, 1 kit)

300 calories
22 g fat
(3.5 g saturated)
435 mg sodium

If you choose Bumble Bee over StarKist three times per week, you'll take in 4 extra pounds of pure fat in 1 year's time.

Spam Lite
(6 oz, 168 g)

330 calories
24 g fat
(9 g saturated)
1,740 mg sodium

Sugar-Free Foods

Eat This

Hershey's Sugar Free Special Dark
(40 g, 5 pieces)

160 calories
13 g fat
(8 g saturated)
0 g sugars

The darker the chocolate, the more heart-healthy fat it contains. By no means is it a low-calorie food, but eaten in moderation, it can be a decent snack.

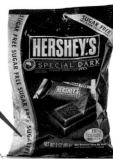

The refined carbohydrates in these Oreos still make them a poor choice for those with diabetes, but with 1.5 grams of fiber and only 45 calories per cookie, they're a nice step toward weaning yourself off sugar.

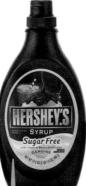
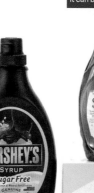
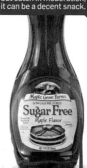
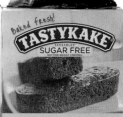

Oreos Sugar Free
(24 g, 2 cookies)

90 calories
5 g fat
(1.5 g saturated)
0 g sugars

Hershey's Chocolate Syrup Sugar Free
(32 g, 2 Tbsp)

15 calories
0 g fat
0 g sugars
4 g sugar alcohols

This syrup is sweetened with erythritol, a sugar alcohol that doesn't exhibit the laxative qualities associated with other sugar alcohols.

Truvia
(3.5 g, 1 packet)

0 calories
0 g fat
0 g sugars
3 g sugar alcohols

There's no perfect noncaloric sweetener, but Truvia is one of our favorites. Unlike other chemical sweeteners, Truvia is derived from the leaves of the stevia plant.

Maple Grove Farms Sugar Free Maple Flavor Syrup
(60 ml, ¼ cup)

35 calories
0 g fat
10 g sugar alcohols

Made with sorbitol, a safer sugar alternative.

Tastykake Sugar Free Sensables Finger Cakes Chocolate Chocolate Chip
(32 g, 1 cake)

100 calories
6 g fat
(2 g saturated)
0 g sugars
9 g sugar alcohols

Sugar is replaced with a solid 4 grams of fiber.

Not That!

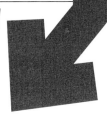

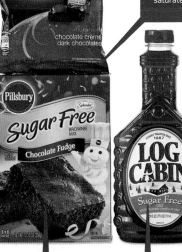

Dove Sugar Free Chocolate Crème Dark Chocolates
(40 g, 5 pieces)

190 calories
15 g fat
(10 g saturated)
0 g sugars

Each small piece contains 10 percent of your day's saturated fat limit.

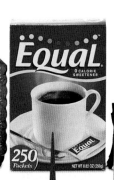

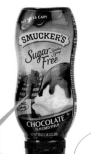

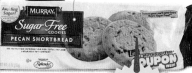

The fat here comes primarily from soybean and palm oils. Remember, even if you remove sugar from the equation, calories still matter.

Pillsbury Sugar Free Brownie Mix Chocolate Fudge
(1/12 package, 29 g baked)

150 calories
8.5 g fat
(1.5 g saturated)
0 g sugars
9 g sugar alcohols

Pillsbury laces its brownie with partially hydrogenated oils. This one's a no-brainer.

Log Cabin Sugar Free Syrup
(60 ml, 1/4 cup)

20 calories
8 g sugar alcohols

No need to use an aspartame-based sweetener when there's an easy-to-find sucralose version on the market.

Equal
(1 g, 1 packet)

0 calories
0 g fat
0 g sugars
0 g sugar alcohols

The FDA deems aspartame safe, but more than a few studies have challenged the artificial sweetener's safety.

Smucker's Sugar Free Chocolate Topping
(38 g, 2 Tbsp)

90 calories
0.5 g fat
(0 g saturated)
0 g sugars
17 g sugar alcohols

In large doses, the maltitol in the Smucker's topping can have a laxative effect.

Murray Sugar Free Pecan Shortbread Cookies
(32 g, 3 cookies)

160 calories
11 g fat
(3 g saturated)
0 g sugars

209

Gluten-Free Foods
Eat This

Gluten is a grain-based protein that some people have trouble digesting. If you're among the unlucky, seek out products like this multigrain bread from Rudi's. Studded with sunflower seeds and flaxseeds, it's nutritionally stacked despite the lack of whole wheat.

Snyder's of Hanover Gluten-Free Pretzel Sticks
(30 g, 30 sticks)

120 calories
1.5 g fat
(0.5 g saturated)
260 mg sodium

Packs more fiber for nearly half the sodium.

Pamela's Products Chocolate Cake Mix
(1/12 package, 50 g mix, 1/12 cake prepared)

260 calories
10 g fat
(2 g saturated)
4 g fiber
22 g sugars

Loaded with fiber.

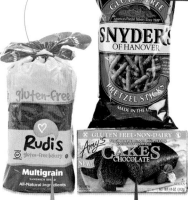
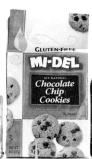
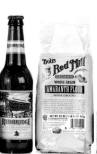
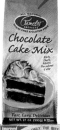
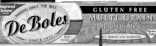

Rudi's Gluten-Free Multigrain Sandwich Bread
(74 g, 2 slices)

180 calories
4 g fat
(0 g saturated)
2 g fiber

Amy's Gluten Free Non-Dairy Organic Cakes Chocolate
(52 g, 1 slice)

180 calories
7 g fat
(1 g saturated)
2 g fiber
17 g sugars

Brown rice flour packs in the fiber.

Mi-Del Gluten-Free Chocolate Chip Cookies
(30 g, 5 cookies)

130 calories
4.5 g fat
(1.5 g saturated)
11 g sugars

Each cookie contains a mere 26 calories.

Anheuser-Busch Redbridge
(12 fl oz)

127 calories
12.3 g carbs
4% ABV

Anheuser uses sorghum to create a flavorful brew with the calories of a light beer.

Bob's Red Mill Organic Whole Grain Amaranth Flour
(30 g, 1/4 cup)

110 calories
2 g fat
(0.5 g saturated)
3 g fiber

Made from one of nature's best grains.

DeBoles Gluten Free Whole Grain Spaghetti Style Pasta
(56 g, 1/4 package)

200 calories
1.5 g fat
(0 g saturated)
3 g fiber

The superstars of the grain world all in one noodle.

Not That!

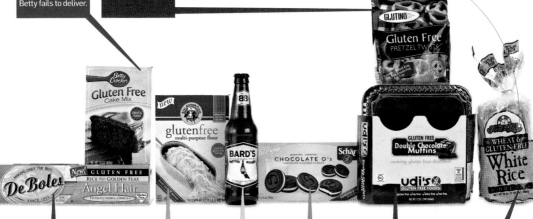

Betty Crocker Gluten Free Cake Mix Devil's Food
(¹⁄₁₀ package, 43 g mix, ¹⁄₁₀ cake prepared)

260 calories
12 g fat
(7 g saturated)
1 g fiber
20 g sugars

Betty fails to deliver.

Glutino Gluten Free Pretzel Twists
(30 g, 24 pretzels)

140 calories
6 g fat
(2.5 g saturated)
420 mg sodium

Glutino packs in the calories thanks to a heavy hand with the palm oil.

Craft your gluten-free-bread sandwich masterpiece with Rudi's and save 40 calories per serving.

DeBoles Gluten Free Rice Plus Golden Flax Angel Hair
(56 g, ¼ package)

210 calories
1.5 g fat
(0 g saturated)
1 g fiber

The omega-3 fats here come at the expense of fiber.

King Arthur Gluten Free Flour
(30 g, 3 Tbsp)

110 calories
0 g fat
0 g fiber

White rice flour is nutritionally bankrupt, just like all white flours.

Bard's Gold
(12 fl oz)

155 calories
14 g carbs
5% ABV

With more and more food and beverage options available to the gluten-free crowd, don't settle for high-calorie alternatives.

Schär Cookies Chocolate O's
(30 g, 3 cookies)

150 calories
7 g fat
(4 g saturated)
9 g sugars

Contains 20 percent of your day's saturated fat intake.

Udi's Gluten Free Double Chocolate Muffins
(85 g, 1 muffin)

270 calories
12 g fat
(4 g saturated)
2 g fiber
25 g sugars

Contains more sugar than a Snickers bar.

Food for Life Wheat & Gluten Free White Rice Bread
(86 g, 2 slices)

220 calories
4 g fat
(0 g saturated)
2 g fiber

Pre- & Postworkout
Eat This

A trio of proteins from soy, whey, and casein help rebuild muscles with both rapid- and slow-digesting proteins.

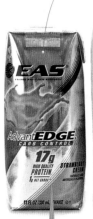
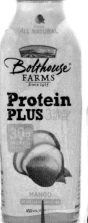
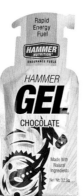
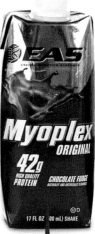
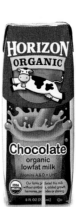
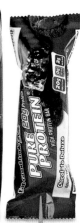

**EAS
AdvantEDGE
Carb Control
Strawberry
Cream**
(11 fl oz, 1 bottle)

110 calories
3 g fat
(0 g saturated)
0 g sugars
17 g protein

**Bolthouse
Farms
Protein Plus
Mango**
(16 oz, 1 bottle)

380 calories
2 g fat
(0 g saturated)
52 g sugars
32 g protein

A full third of these calories come from protein.

**Hammer Gel
Chocolate**
(32.9 g, 1 packet)

90 calories
0 g fat
4 g sugars

This packet is made almost entirely from long-chain complex carbs, which supply a more constant, steady stream of energy.

**Horizon
Organic 1%
Chocolate
Milk**
(240 mL, 1 cup)

160 calories
2.5 g fat
(1.5 g saturated)
26 g sugars
8 g protein

A perfect balance of protein, fat, and carbs.

**EAS Myoplex
Original
Chocolate
Fudge**
(17 fl oz, 1 bottle)

300 calories
7 g fat
(1 g saturated)
2 g sugars
42 g protein

Made with high quality proteins like casein.

**Pure Protein
High Protein
Bar
Chocolate
Deluxe**
(50 g, 1 bar)

180 calories
4.5 g fat
(3 g saturated)
2 g sugars
20 g protein

Almost 50 percent protein.

Foods

Not That!

Special K is marketed as a weight-loss food, yet it contains as much sugar as a Hershey's Take 5 candy bar.

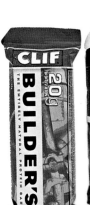
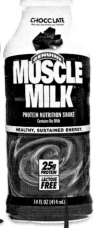
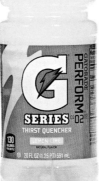
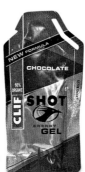
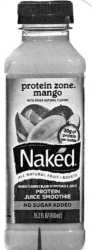
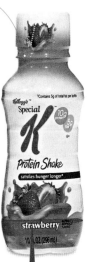

Clif Builder's Cookies 'n Cream
(68 g, 1 bar)

270 calories
8 g fat
(5 g saturated)
20 g sugars
20 g protein

Contains a quarter of your day's saturated fat and enough sugar to qualify as dessert.

CytoSport Muscle Milk Chocolate
(14 fl oz, 1 bottle)

240 calories
9 g fat
(1.5 g saturated)
2 g fiber
3 g sugars
25 g protein

Vegetable oil is the fourth ingredient in this bottle.

Gatorade G Series Lemon Lime
(20 fl oz, 1 bottle)

125 calories
0 g fat
35 g sugars
0 g protein

Milk offers a more complete workout recovery package. If you want a sports drink, switch to lower-calorie G2.

Clif Shot Energy Gel Chocolate
(34 g, 1 pack)

110 calories
1.5 g fat
(1 g saturated)
12 g sugars

This gel derives much of its energy from sugar. Not advisable for casual workouts.

Naked Protein Juice Smoothie Protein Zone Mango
(16 oz, 1 bottle)

440 calories
2 g fat
(0 g saturated)
56 g sugars
32 g protein

Contains a dinner's worth of calories.

Kellogg's Special K Protein Shake Strawberry
(10 fl oz, 1 bottle)

180 calories
5 g fat
(0.5 g saturated)
18 g sugars
10 g protein

EAT
THIS
NOT
THAT!
**SUPERMARKET
SURVIVAL GUIDE**

THE
SNACKS &
SWEETS
AISLES

RODALE
EAT THIS, NOT THAT!
CHAPTER 7

Stay Hungry.
No Pain, No Gain.
Where there's a will, there's a way.

You've heard these inspirational mantras a million times. Anybody who makes money motivating others, from politicians to business leaders to the trainers at the gym to whoever is featured in the latest Nike commercial, is probably spouting some variation of these clichés. But when it comes to controlling your weight, this is just about the worst advice imaginable.

How about this approach: Don't get hungry. Don't feel pain. And for heaven's sake, don't rely on willpower for anything. In fact, if you want to lose weight, do something that every hard-nosed weight-loss guru will tell you not to do:

Snack. A lot.

Now, wait: Before you assume that the *Eat This, Not That* team is on the take from Little Debbie, hear me out. There's a scientifically sound rationale for noshing between meals.

Our bodies are, for the most part, incredibly lazy. While our minds want to roam free and do great things—climb Everest, invent the new iPad, play third base for the Red Sox, and star alongside Ryan Gosling in his new action thriller—our bodies just want to lay down on the couch and keep up with the Kardashians. (In fact, if the show were called Slacking Off with the Kardashians, its ratings would probably be even higher.)

The reason is simple: For most of human existence, food has been scarce. So we're programmed to conserve energy, especially when we get hungry. That means that when we skip meals, or don't snack between meals, our metabolisms slow down and we burn fewer calories throughout the day. Then, like greedy bank CEOs, our bodies demand even more food at mealtime. In fact, studies show that people who don't snack between meals actually eat more calories during the course of the day, because their bodies tell them to load up on energy in case another bout of famine comes. To make matters worse, our bodies then horde all those calories in our butts and bellies instead of loaning them out to needy but qualified applicants like our muscles and brains. The result: A bloated network of fat cells, weakened muscles, and less energy.

The solution: More regulation. Not bank regulation, but energy regulation. Snack regularly so you don't run short of calories during the day, shuttle all your available energy into your love handles, and make up for it by overeating at night.

Oh, but what about willpower? Can't you just muster up your inner General Petraeus and order yourself to resist the extra food at dinnertime? Well, no. Willpower comes, of course, from your brain, and your brain runs on glucose, the blood sugar our bodies create from food. When you're short on food, you're low on glucose—so you literally have less willpower when you're hungry than you do when you're full.

Damn, our bodies are tricky little buggers! No wonder weight loss is so challenging.

But the snacking solution is not only easy (and delicious), it's super-effective too. A study conducted by the National Weight Control Registry looked at more than 5,000 men and women who have lost an average of 70 pounds and kept it off and found that most of them reported eating frequently throughout the day, instead of limiting themselves to three meals. And here's a mind-blowing little chart, taken from a 2010 government study of 5,800 US teenagers who reported their own snack intakes.

NUMBER OF SNACKS PER DAY	% OVERWEIGHT OR OBESE
0	39
2	30
3	28
4	22

That's right—the more you snack, the less likely you are to be overweight!

But in weight management, as in banking strategy, investing wisely is critical to maintaining a healthy bottom line. And Americans don't seem to be very good at making smart investments—with our finances, or with our snacking. While plenty of banks have gotten in trouble by buying into shaky institutions (like Greece, for example), our bodies get in trouble by investing in shaky nutritional choices (like grease, for example). Here's how to make sure you don't get stuck with the food equivalent of junk bonds.

DON'T BE SWEET.

The American Heart Association recommends that men eat no more than 9 teaspoons of sugar a day, and women, no more than 6. Well, that ought to be easy, right? When was the last time you ate 6 or 9 teaspoons of sugar in 1 day? Answer: Probably yesterday. And, if it's after noon, probably today as well. In fact, Americans now eat, on average, 33 teaspoons of sugar a day, according to the most recent National Health and Nutrition Examination Survey. A third of that sugar comes from sweetened beverages (you'll read more about this threat in Chapter 9), but even if you eliminate sodas and sweetened teas altogether, you'll still be way over your allotment: Snacks and sweets provide another 29 percent of our intake, or more than 9.5 teaspoons. The information on the following pages will show you how to dramatically strip sugar calories from your snacking.

ONLY SNACK WHEN YOU'RE HUNGRY.

Just because snacking is good for you doesn't mean you should overdo it. French researchers found that when people who

The Real Calorie Counter

OUR RESEARCH SHOWS YOU COULD BE UNDER-ESTIMATING YOUR CALORIE INTAKE BY 10 PERCENT OR MORE

PRODUCT	Listed calories per serving	Calories based on actual weight of serving size
Back to Nature Granola	200	270
Bear Naked Granola	140	163
Cheerios (without milk)	100	103
Doritos	150	156
Entenmann's Chocolate Glazed Mini Donuts	150	171
Entenmann's Marble Cake	280	301
Kellogg's Nutri-Grain Bars Strawberry	130	137
Hostess Cupcakes	180	186
Oreos	160	162
SunChips Garden Salsa Flavor	140	152
Wonder Classic White Bread	60	65

weren't hungry ate a snack a few hours after lunch, they did not eat fewer calories at dinner.

GO HIGH PROTEIN, LOW SUGAR.

Another study found that high-protein snacks help people feel fuller longer and eat less at the next meal. Study participants ate 200 calories of protein or of carbs or nothing at all. Those who ate high-carb snacks were hungry again just as quickly as those who didn't snack at all.

GO NUTS. LITERALLY.

A study in the journal *Obesity* found that women who eat nuts just twice a week are about 30 percent less likely to gain weight than people who rarely eat nuts.

Snacking 4 times a day can cut your obesity risk nearly in half!

Similar research found that dieters who ate a few ounces of almonds every day lost 6½ inches from their waists in 24 weeks, 50 percent more than dieters who ate the same number of calories, but not as fiber- and protein-rich nuts.

BUT WATCH THE SODIUM.

Salted almonds, on the other hand, could blow your whole strategy. A study published in the American Heart Association journal *Hypertension* found that kids who eat salty snacks get thirstier—duh—but they're also more likely to reach for sugary drinks to tame their thirst. Just 12 percent of all the sodium we take in daily occurs naturally; another 11 percent comes from our salts-hakers. The additional whopping 77 percent comes in the form of salt added by food manufacturers.

LOOK FOR DARK CHOCOLATE.

A study from Denmark found that men who ate dark chocolate consumed 15 percent fewer calories at the next meal and were less interested in fatty, salty, or sugary foods. And research shows that people who eat 30 calories a day of dark chocolate—that's just a small piece, of course—can improve heart health, lower blood pressure, reduce LDL cholesterol, decrease the risk of blood clots, and increase bloodflow to the brain.

MAKE ICE CREAM YOUR REWARD.

British researchers conducted MRI scans and found that a single spoonful of ice cream triggers the pleasure centers in the brain. Plus, just half a cup of vanilla ice cream gives you 17 milligrams of choline, which recent USDA studies show lowers blood levels of homocysteine—an indicator of potential heart trouble—by 8 percent.

The Science of Serving Vessels

FOUR COUNTERMOVES AGAINST THE FORCES OF FAT

1

Downsize your dishes

Unless you're eating off decades-old dishes, you probably have the newer, plus-size plates—the kind that cause your eyes to override your appetite. Give them to Goodwill, and pick up either the 16-piece Santiago set by Dansk (10½-inch dinner plates, 8-inch salad plates, and 7-inch soup bowls, $80) or the 20-piece Platinum Band set by Majestry (10⅝-inch dinner plates, 7¾-inch salad plates, and 7¾-inch soup bowls, $60). Both are sold at bedbathand beyond.com.

2

Be small-minded about snacks

In a recent experiment at the Cornell University food and brand lab, researchers gave study participants either a single bag containing 100 Wheat Thins or four smaller bags holding 25 Thins each, waited for the munching to subside, then did a cracker count. The tally: Those given the jumbo bag ate up to 20 percent more. Outsmart your snack habit by sticking with the tiny 100-calorie packs now being used for everything from Doritos to Goldfish.

3

Raise your glasses

Since even experienced bartenders pour more into short, wide glasses than they do into tall, narrow ones, you'll need to be creative when you play mixmaster at home. Start by using highball glasses to replace the squat tumblers you use for scotch and brandy. Next, put away your pint beer glasses and buy the pilsner kind. Finally, if you own balloon wine glasses, switch them with regular wine glasses. Just watch the red: Cornell researchers found that people inadvertently pour more red wine than white into the same-size glass.

4

Divide and dine

Until all restaurants become BYOP (bring your own plate), you'll need to shrink your serving in a different way: When your entrée arrives, dive in and eat half, then wait at least 10 minutes before coming out for round 2. While you chat and sip water, your stomach will have a chance to digest and decide whether you've had enough—no matter what the plate's saying.

The Ultimate Snack Scorecard

Your hunger is a sleeping beast, and as long as you keep it fed, it will continue sleeping. We created this scorecard to help you identify the perfect snacks for keeping the beast at bay. We analyzed 50 common snacks and snack combinations, and we tallied what percentage of those calories came from protein, fiber, and healthy fats, the sultans of satiety. Then we docked points for sodium and trans fats. Snacks with the highest scores are best at fighting hunger, while snacks with the lowest scores are little more than fast-burning, nutritionally hollow calories. Pack two of the highest-scoring foods on this list into your day—one in the late morning, another in the long hours between lunch and dinner—and you'll fight hunger, energize your body, and watch the body fat melt away.

SNACK FOODS	GRADE	SCORE	CALORIES
Jack Link's Beef Jerky Original (1 oz)	A+	6.50	80
Cottage Cheese 1% (1 cup) + strawberries (1 cup)	A+	5.58	216
Fage Total 2% Greek Yogurt Plain (1 cup)	A+	5.33	150
Avocado (½)	A	4.01	161
String Cheese (1 piece)	A	4.00	80
Orange	A	3.79	62
Pistachios, unshelled raw (1 oz)	A	3.54	159
Triscuits (1 oz) + deli turkey (2 oz)	A	3.51	186
Lärabar Peanut Butter & Jelly	A−	3.29	210
Planters Mixed Nuts (1 oz)	A−	3.12	170
Triscuits (1 oz) + Tribe Hummus (2 Tbsp)	A−	3.09	170
Cheerios (1 cup) + fat-free milk (½ cup)	A−	3.00	140
Apple	B+	2.98	95
Kozy Shack Pudding Chocolate (1 cup)	B+	2.92	110
Jolly Time Better Butter Microwave Popcorn (4cups popped)	B+	2.75	140
Peanut butter (2 Tbsp) + celery (1 large rib)	B+	2.73	196

SNACK FOODS	GRADE	SCORE	CALORIES
Dannon Light & Fit Yogurt Strawberry	B	2.50	80
Baked! Tostitos Scoops! (1 oz) + guacamole (2 Tbsp)	B -	2.25	180
Sunsweet Apricots Mediterranean (6 pieces)	B -	2.20	100
Kellogg's Nutri-Grain Cereal Bars, Apple Cinnamon (1 bar)	B -	2.17	120
Food Should Taste Good Multigrain Chips (1 oz)	B -	2.14	140
Sun Chips Original (1 oz)	C+	1.86	140
Dark chocolate (1 oz)	C+	1.77	164
Ore-Ida Bagel Bites Supreme (4 pieces)	C+	1.72	180
Nature Valley Crunchy Granola Bars, Oats'n Honey (1 pack)	C	1.47	190
Baked! Tostitos Scoops! (1 oz) + salsa (4 Tbsp)	C	1.43	140
Quaker Chewy Granola Bars Peanut Butter Chocolate Chip (1 bar)	C	1.40	100
Carrot sticks (1 cup) + Hidden Valley Ranch Original (2 Tbsp)	C	1.27	190
Smartfood Popcorn White Cheddar (1 oz)	C -	1.25	160
Wheat Thins Original (1 oz)	C -	1.18	140
Stacy's Pita Chips Simply Naked (1 oz)	C -	1.13	130
Nabisco 100 Cal Chips Ahoy! Thin Crisps (1 pack)	D+	1.00	100
Pepperidge Farm Goldfish Cheddar (1 oz)	D+	0.89	140

SNACK FOODS	GRADE	SCORE	CALORIES
Lay's Classic Potato Chips (1 oz)	D+	0.88	160
Quaker Rice Cakes Caramel Corn (1 cake)	D+	0.80	50
Rold Gold Pretzels Sticks (1 oz)	D	0.65	100
Oreos (34 g, 3 cookies)	D	0.63	160
M&M's Milk Chocolate (1.69 ounces)	D	0.58	240
Twix Caramel Cookie Bars (1 pack)	D	0.56	220
Cheez-It Original (1 oz)	D	0.55	150
Nabisco 100 Cal Mr. Salty Yogurt Flavored Pretzels (1 pack)	D	0.40	100
Totino's Pizza Rolls Combination (6 rolls)	D-	0.06	210
Fruit Roll-Ups Blastin' Berry Hot Colors (1 piece)	F	0.00	50
Jell-O Cups (1 cup)	F	0.00	70
Doritos Nacho Cheese (1 oz)	F	-0.07	150
Fig Newtons (1 oz)	F	-0.09	110
Snickers Bar	F	-0.21	280
Nilla Wafers (1 oz)	F	-0.71	140
Cheetos (1 oz)	F	-0.75	160
Little Debbie Oatmeal Creme Pies (1 pie)	F	-0.76	170

THE TRUTH ABOUT SUGAR

Say anything nasty about sugar and folks will swallow it. Sugar caused the recession. Sugar makes your nipples grow. Sugar keyed your car. Sugar's crazy—it knifed my cousin down at the corner bar last Saturday night. Somebody should drop a safe on sugar.

Well, maybe. It's true that sugar is insidious—diabolical, even—and hidden in countless processed foods. It certainly contributes to the obesity crisis. It makes people fat and sometimes even diabetic. These claims are correct—to a limited and oversimplified extent. But sugar doesn't point guns at our heads and force us to eat it. It's only as big a bogeyman as we make it out to be.

We need some truth about sugar. It's too important. The sugar in our bodies, glucose, is a fundamental fuel for body and brain, says David Levitsky, PhD, a professor of psychology and nutritional sciences at Cornell University.

The health threat to the vast American public arises at a very personal level, Levitsky says: "It's that sugars taste good. Sweetened foods tend to make us overeat. And that threatens the energy balance in our bodies."

Read this and learn a few facts about the sweet stuff hiding in some of your favorite meals and drinks. Then, the next time some uninformed punk says sugar's out of line, you won't be tempted to drag sugar behind a dumpster and kick the crap out of it. The fact is, you may be the one who's out of line.

Sugar and Diabetes
SUGAR DOESN'T CAUSE DIABETES

Too much sugar does. Diabetes means your body can't clear glucose from your blood. And when glucose isn't processed quickly enough, it destroys tissue, Levitsky says. People with type 1 diabetes were born that way—sugar didn't cause their diabetes. But weight gain in children and adults can cause metabolic syndrome, which often leads to type 2 diabetes.

"That's what diabetes is all about—being unable to eliminate glucose," says Levitsky. "The negative effect of eating a lot of sugar is a rise in glucose. A normal pancreas and normal insulin receptors can handle it, clear it out, or store it in some packaged form, like fat."

What matters: That "normal" pancreas. Overeating forces your pancreas to work overtime cranking out insulin to clear glucose. Eric Westman, MD, an obesity researcher at the Duke University Medical Center, says that in today's world, "it's certainly possible that the unprecedented increase in sugar and starch consumption leads to pancreatic burnout."

Your job: Drop the pounds if you're overweight, and watch your sugar intake. Research has shown for years that dropping 5 to 7 percent of your body weight can reduce your odds of developing diabetes.

Sugar and High-Fructose Corn Syrup
SIMPLY AVOIDING HIGH-FRUCTOSE CORN SYRUP WON'T SAVE YOU FROM OBESITY

In the 1970s and 1980s, the average American's body weight increased in tandem with the food industry's use of high-fructose corn syrup (HFCS), which has become a staple because it's cheap. But it's not a smoking gun. "This is a correlation, not a causation," says Levitsky.

"Obesity is about consuming too many calories," says Lillian Lien, MD, the medical director of inpatient diabetes management at the Duke University Medical Center. "It just so happens that a lot of overweight people have been drinking HFCS in sodas

and eating foods that are high on the glycemic index—sweet snacks, white bread, and so forth. The calorie totals are huge, and the source just happens to be sugar based."

Dr. Westman notes that the effect of a high-glycemic food can be lessened by adding fat and protein. Spreading peanut butter (protein and fat) on a bagel (starch, which becomes glucose in your body), for example, slows your body's absorption of the sugar.

What matters: We can demonize food manufacturers because they produce crap with enough salt and sugar to make us eat more of it than we should—or even want to. But it comes down to how much we allow down our throats. "A practical guide for anyone is weight," says Dr. Lien. "If your weight is under control, then your calorie intake across the board is reasonable. If your weight rises, it's not. That's more important than paying attention to any specific macronutrient." Still, skinny isn't always safe. (Keep reading.)

Sugar and Fat
TOO MUCH SUGAR FILLS YOUR BLOOD WITH FAT

Studies dating back decades show that eating too much fructose, a sugar found naturally in fruits and also added to processed foods, raises blood lipid levels.

And while the relatively modest quantities in fruit shouldn't worry you, a University of Minnesota study shows that the large amounts of fructose we take in from processed foods may prove especially nasty: Men on high-fructose diets had 32 percent higher triglycerides than men on high-glucose diets.

Why? Your body can't metabolize a sweet snack as fast as you can eat it, says Levitsky. So your liver puts some of the snack's glucose into your bloodstream, or stores it for later use. But if your liver's tank is full, it packages the excess as triglycerides. The snack's fructose goes to your liver as well, but instead of being deposited in your bloodstream, it's stored as glycogen. Your liver can store about 90 to 100 grams of glycogen, so it converts the excess to fat (the triglycerides).

What matters: By maintaining a healthy weight, most people can keep their triglycerides at acceptable levels. "If you're overweight or gaining weight, however, they'll accumulate and become a core predictor of heart disease and stroke," Levitsky says.

If you're one of those overweight people, your first step is to lay off sugary and starchy foods, beer, and sweet drinks. Your body wasn't built to handle all that sugar. Consider this: You'd have to eat four apples in order to ingest roughly the same amount of fructose that's in one large McDonald's Coke.

Avoid Blood Sugar Spikes

FEWER BLOOD SUGAR SPIKES HELP YOU LIVE LONGER

If you live large—big meals, lots of beer, little moderation—you may be shortening your life even if your weight is okay. Repeated blood sugar spikes stress the organs that make up the metabolic engine of your body. That takes a toll.

And you might not notice. "People can live symptom free for years in a prediabetic state even though they've lost as much as 50 percent of their pancreatic function," says Dr. Lien. "And they don't even know it." People with prediabetes share the same health risks, especially for heart disease, that haunt people with full-blown diabetes.

What matters: Moderation. It's simple, yet difficult. Think about what you put in your mouth. Sugar is diabolical; it tastes great and is less filling. Back off on the high-impact glycemics: beer, sugary soft drinks and sport drinks, potatoes, pasta, baked goods, pancakes. "The less sugar stress you put on your system, the longer it will function properly," says Levitsky. And stop blaming sugar for all the world's problems. Even if it is diabolical.

—*Additional reporting by* Men's Health

What's Really in...
Mission Guacamole Fla

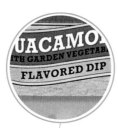

FLAVORED DIP

Mission's tagline is "The Authentic Tradition." So how does the company get away with casting a jar of oil, food dyes, and herpes medication as guacamole? By tacking on the words "flavored dip." Read labels closely and you'll see that Mission isn't the only one guilty of this sleight of hand. In fact, it's just one more euphemism in the growing cocktail-ization of our food industry. "Juice drinks" are often fractionally fruit and predominately lab-engineered sugars. "Bacon-flavored" bits are artificially flavored oil and flour chunks. Regardless of their snake-oil natures, these foods are adhering to federal guidelines, according to the FDA. Other than peanut butter, which the government mandates be at least 90 percent peanuts, most products aren't required to contain the ingredients those foods would customarily be made out of. Scary, huh?

DATEM

If avocados aren't really in here, what is? Datem, to name one odd ingredient. An emulsifier often derived from genetically modified soybean oil, it's largely utilized to strengthen dough in bread. In this jar, it helps retain gas, pumping up the volume to give this otherwise flat, oily paste a guac-like texture.

AVOCADO POWDER

The most striking thing about this ingredients list is what's not included: avocados. Standing in for what should be guacamole's base is something called "avocado powder," which itself accounts for less than 2 percent of the bulk. Mission is mum on this substance, but many Web sites selling the powder say it contains partially hydrogenated oils, sweeteners, and a preservative called BHT (butylated hydroxytoluene), which either increases or decreases cancer risk depending on the study you read and has been used to fight, of all things, herpes. Consumers have not responded well to avocado-less guac, filing class-action lawsuits against Mission and Kraft.

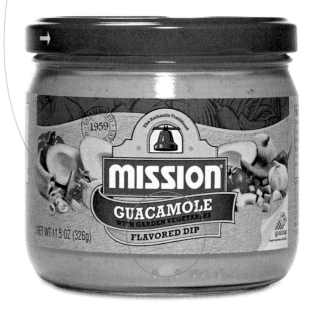

vored Dip

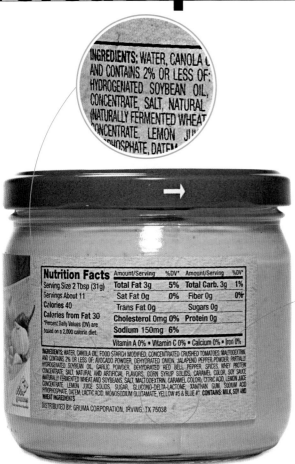

INGREDIENTS: WATER, CANOLA
AND CONTAINS 2% OR LESS OF:
HYDROGENATED SOYBEAN OIL,
CONCENTRATE, SALT, NATURAL
NATURALLY FERMENTED WHEAT
ONCENTRATE, LEMON JI
HOSPHATE, DATE

Nutrition Facts
Serving Size 2 Tbsp (31g)
Servings About 11
Calories 40
Calories from Fat 30
*Percent Daily Values (DV) are
based on a 2,000 calorie diet.

Amount/Serving	%DV*	Amount/Serving	%DV*
Total Fat 3g	5%	Total Carb. 3g	1%
Sat Fat 0g	0%	Fiber 0g	0%
Trans Fat 0g		Sugars 0g	
Cholesterol 0mg 0%		Protein 0g	
Sodium 150mg 6%			

Vitamin A 0% • Vitamin C 0% • Calcium 0% • Iron 0%

INGREDIENTS: WATER, CANOLA OIL, FOOD STARCH MODIFIED, CONCENTRATED CRUSHED TOMATOES; MALTODEXTRIN AND CONTAINS 2% OR LESS OF: AVOCADO POWDER, DEHYDRATED ONION, JALAPEÑO PEPPER POWDER, PARTIALLY HYDROGENATED SOYBEAN OIL, GARLIC POWDER, DEHYDRATED RED BELL PEPPER, SPICES, WHEY PROTEIN CONCENTRATE, SALT, NATURAL AND ARTIFICIAL FLAVORS, CORN SYRUP SOLIDS, CARAMEL COLOR, SOY SAUCE (NATURALLY FERMENTED WHEAT AND SOYBEANS, SALT, MALTODEXTRIN; CARAMEL COLOR), CITRIC ACID, LEMON JUICE CONCENTRATE, LEMON JUICE SOLIDS, SUGAR, GLUCONO-DELTA-LACTONE; XANTHAN GUM, SODIUM ACID PYROPHOSPHATE, DATEM; LACTIC ACID, MONOSODIUM GLUTAMATE, YELLOW #5 & BLUE #*. **CONTAINS: MILK, SOY AND WHEAT INGREDIENTS**

DISTRIBUTED BY: GRUMA CORPORATION, IRVING, TX 75038

PARTIALLY HYDROGE- NATED SOYBEAN OIL

The food industry hydrogenates oils to make more-solid forms of fat. The problem is that partial hydrogenation produces some really dangerous stuff called trans fats. A review of trans fat studies published in the *New England Journal of Medicine* found that "trans fats appear to increase the risk of coronary heart disease more than any other macronutrient." The same review attributed up to 100,000 cardiac deaths in America each year to trans fats. While Mission uses partially hydrogenated oils in this guacamole dip, the company lists 0 grams of trans fats on the label. What gives? Well the FDA only requires disclosure of 0.5 grams of trans fats or more per serving. A product containing 0.49 grams of trans fats could still be listed as trans-fat free. But eat 2 servings of such a food, and you'd consume nearly half of what the American Heart Association warns should be a 2-gram daily limit.

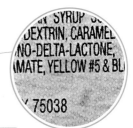

N SYRUP
DEXTRIN, CARAMEL
NO-DELTA-LACTONE,
MATE, YELLOW #5 & BL

75038

YELLOW 5

Without avocados, Mission has to combine Yellow 5 food coloring with Blue 1 to imbue this dip with guacamole's normal green color. In 2008, the United Kingdom's food-safety agency to begin phasing out six food colorings, including Yellow 5. In contrast, the FDA says the dye is safe for consumption, and consequently you can find it in everything from cereals to pickles to, well, guacamole-flavored dip.

What's Really in...
Pringles Ranch

DRIED POTATOES

Consider the classic potato chip:
a slice of potato fried to crispy perfection
and dusted with salt. By no means
is it healthy, but it is relatively straightforward. And Pringles? They're modern
foods' Frankensteinian equivalent.
Comparing a Pringle to a real russet
potato chip is like comparing a Slim Jim
to a New York strip steak. The fresh
ingredients are gone, and in their place
we have dehydrated potatoes pressed
into a chiplike mold alongside rice
flour, wheat starch, and maltodextrin.

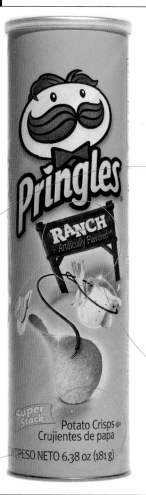

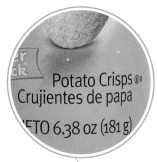

POTATO CRISPS

Pringles' maker Procter & Gamble, hoping
to avoid a mandatory potato chip tax in
England, actually went to court to argue that
these oblong vessels don't qualify as real
potato chips (we've always found the "crisps"
language on the package a bit suspicious).
The foundation of its case was that Pringles
contain only 40 percent potato flour.
The other 60 percent is rice, wheat, corn,
and other additives. The British court
disagreed, forcing Pringles to pay a snack
tax of $160 million.

232

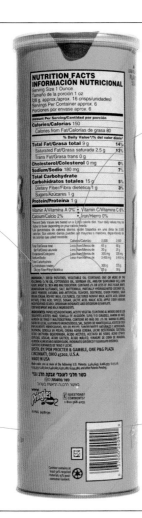

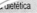

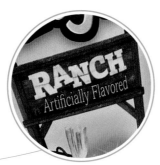

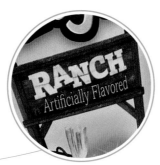

"Natural flavor" may be one of the biggest misnomers in the food industry. Think about it: If a flavor were truly "natural," then why would it need to be artificially added in a factory? And why do they then list "Artificially Flavored" on the front label? The FDA essentially considers a natural ingredient to be any plant- or animal-derived product used for flavoring—as opposed to nutritional—purposes. Perhaps no company takes advantage of the FDA's many vagaries better than Pringles. After all, this is the manufacturer responsible for the most outrageous flavors in the snack industry: prawn cocktail, seaweed, chili cheese dog, and, of course, the ever-popular soft-shell crab. Were these snacks made from ground up crustaceans and dehydrated Ball Park franks? Of course not. But since the FDA allows the company to hide behind a vague term, we'll never know for sure. It could be made from sperm whale blubber, an exotic fungus, or the fingernail shavings of the Dalai Lama. More than likely, it's a complex and proprietary combination of chemicals and fillers that Pringles' scientists handcraft in a laboratory for every canister of crisps.

The Saltiest Foods in the Supermarket

Salty food may seem like the least of your worries, especially if you're among the 40 percent of people who mindlessly shake salt on every dish. An extra dash here, a few sprinkles there—what's the big deal?

A lot, when you consider some of the shocking stats and shady food industry practices we've uncovered. Daily salt consumption is on the rise in the United States, from 2,300 milligrams in the 1970s to more than 3,400 milligrams today—more than double what the American Heart Association recommends we consume.

And according to Monell Chemical Senses Center researchers, 77 percent of that sodium intake comes from processed foods and restaurant fare. The makers' motivation: Pile on the salt so we don't miss natural flavors and fresh ingredients.

Studies show that a high-sodium diet (especially when your potassium intake is low) is linked to a host of maladies, including high blood pressure, stroke, osteoporosis, and asthma. To protect your heart, your bones, your muscles, and your taste buds, we scoured the aisles to expose the 10 saltiest supermarket foods in America. No need to take the information with a grain of salt. These packages provide plenty.

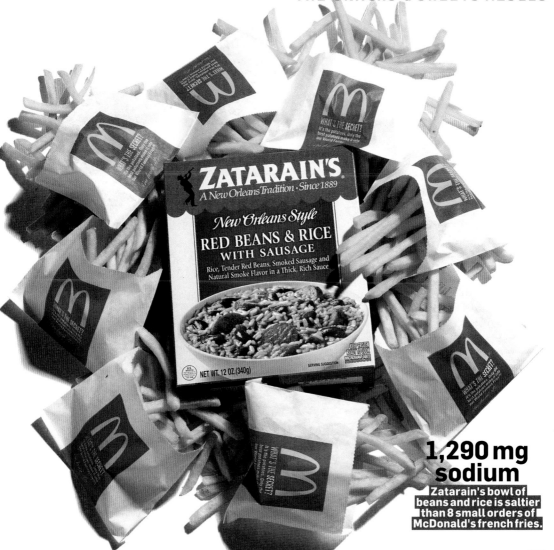

1,290 mg sodium

Zatarain's bowl of beans and rice is saltier than 8 small orders of McDonald's french fries.

SALTIEST SNACK MIX

10 Cheez-It Snack Mix Double Cheese

(30 g, ¼ cup)
470 mg sodium
130 calories
5 g fat (1.5 g saturated)

If the sodium count itself doesn't scare you, how about this: The word "salt" appears in the ingredients list 11 times.

Eat This Instead!
Cheerios Snack Mix

(29 g, ⅔ cup)
240 mg sodium
120 calories
3 g fat (0.5 g saturated)

SALTIEST PRETZELS

9 Rold Gold Tiny Twists Cheddar

(28 g, ≈20 pretzels)
490 mg sodium
110 calories
1 g fat (0 g saturated)

Pretzels are salt magnates regardless of brand, but Rold Gold regularly packs in twice the sodium as its competitors. Each individual Tiny Twist has about 25 milligrams.

Eat This Instead!
Snyder's of Hanover Mini Pretzels

(30 g, 20 minis)
250 mg sodium
110 calories
0 g fat

SALTIEST DELI MEAT

8 Oscar Mayer Shaved Ham

(50 g, 4 slices)
760 mg sodium
50 calories
1.5 g fat (0.5 g saturated)

Deli meats are notoriously high in sodium, and none are worse than ham. In hopes of boosting the flavor and extending the shelf life of deli cuts, manufacturers will inject a sodium solution directly into the meat, turning a few slices of lean protein into a vessel that, in the case of this Oscar Mayer folly, delivers more than half of your day's sodium intake.

Eat This Instead!
Applegate Black Forest Ham

(2 oz, 57 g)
480 mg sodium
50 calories
1.5 g fat (0.5 g saturated)

SALTIEST BURRITO

7 Evol Burritos Egg & Sausage

(227 g, 1 burrito)
870 mg sodium
490 calories
17 g fat (5 g saturated)

We commend Evol for using cage-free hens' eggs and pork from pigs raised without antibiotics, but this burrito's reliance on sodium-rich chorizo casts a dark cloud over an otherwise decent breakfast.

Eat This Instead!
Amy's Light in Sodium Bean & Rice Burrito

(170 g, 1 burrito)
290 mg sodium
320 calories
8 g fat (1 g saturated)

SALTIEST SOUP

6 Campbell's Chunky New England Clam Chowder

(240 ml, 1 cup)
890 mg sodium
210 calories
10 g fat (1.5 g saturated)

Canned soups pack more salt per ounce than almost any other packaged food in the supermarket, and Campbell's regular Chunky line is the most sodium-saturated soup brand of them all. Most varieties top a quarter of your day's sodium with just 1 cup; this chowder chews through nearly 60 percent.

Eat This Instead!
Campbell's Chunky Healthy Request New England Clam Chowder

(1 cup)
410 mg sodium
130 calories
3 g fat (1 g saturated)

1,590 mg sodium

Nuts to this! Jimmy Dean's Breakfast Bowl packs the sodium equivalent of 2 pounds of salted peanuts.

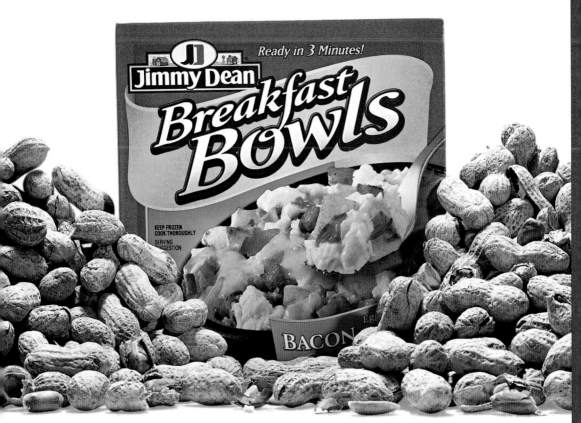

Ready in 3 Minutes!

Jimmy Dean

Breakfast **Bowls**

KEEP FROZEN
COOK THOROUGHLY

SERVING
SUGGESTION

BACON

Egg

5 Zatarain's New Orleans Style Red Beans & Rice with Sausage

(340 g, 1 bowl)
1,290 mg sodium
560 calories
19 g fat (7 g saturated)

The Big Easy didn't make a name for itself by being subtle, and Zatarain's clearly didn't pull any punches when paying homage to one of Cajun Country's most emblematic dishes. The result is a bowl with nearly all of your day's sodium inside.

Eat This Instead!

Amy's Bowls Light in Sodium Mexican Casserole

(269 g, 1 bowl)
390 mg sodium
370 calories
16 g fat (5 g saturated)

4 DiGiorno Cheese Stuffed Crust Pepperoni Pizza

(240 g, 1 pizza)
1,370 mg sodium
670 calories
32 g fat (15 g saturated)

DiGiorno once again proves why its pizzas are the worst in the freezer. Even if you survive the onslaught of sodium you still have 75 percent of your day's saturated fat to grapple with. This pie is wrong in so many ways.

Eat This Instead!

Lean Cuisine French Bread Pepperoni Pizza

(148 g, 1 pizza)
690 mg sodium
310 calories
7 g fat (2 g saturated)

3 P.F. Chang's Home Menu Shrimp Lo Mein

(312 g, ½ package)
1,550 mg sodium
360 calories
12 g fat (1 g saturated)

It's not enough that P.F. Chang's serves the saltiest restaurant food in America, now it has to taint the grocery aisles with its sodium-dense sludge, too? Blame the reliance on three salt-heavy ingredients that are used to make the brackish stir-fry sauce: chicken broth, soy sauce, and oyster-flavored sauce.

Eat This Instead!

Kashi Sweet & Sour Chicken

(283 g, 1 entrée)
380 mg sodium
320 calories
3.5 g fat (0.5 g saturated)

2 Jimmy Dean Breakfast Bowls Bacon

(226 g, 1 bowl)
1,590 mg sodium
460 calories
28 g fat (11 g saturated)

The eggs are salted. The potatoes are salted. The bacon is cured in the stuff, and the processed cheese has it in spades. No wonder this bacon bowl has more than your day's allotment of sodium. You could eat 2 pounds of oil-roasted, salted peanuts and still take in less.

Eat This Instead!

Jimmy Dean D-Lights Turkey Sausage Bowl

(198 g, 1 bowl)
710 mg sodium
230 calories
7 g fat (3 g saturated)

1 Hormel Chili with Beans

(15 oz, 2 cups)
1,800 mg sodium
520 calories
14 g fat (6 g saturated)

Imagine all the other things you could eat that have fewer than 1,800 milligrams of sodium: 1.7 pounds of dry-roasted peanuts, 12 strips of Oscar Mayer Center Cut Bacon, 8 servings of Nacho Cheese Doritos, 39 cups of Jolly Time Better Butter popcorn. Instead, you're going to blow more than a day's worth of sodium on a measly plastic container of chili? We hope you're smarter than that.

Eat This Instead!

Amy's Organic Chili Medium Black Bean

(1 cup)
680 mg sodium
200 calories
3 g fat (0 g saturated)

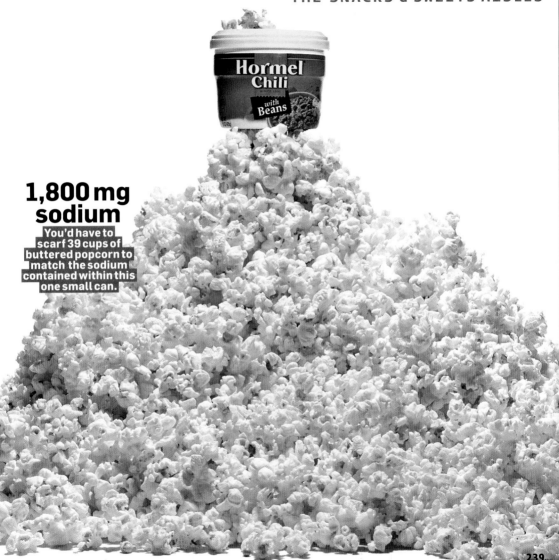

1,800 mg sodium

You'd have to scarf 39 cups of buttered popcorn to match the sodium contained within this one small can.

The Trans-Fattiest Foods in the Supermarket

Way back in the mid-'90s, the *American Journal of Public Health* released a report indicting trans fats for causing no fewer than 30,000 annual deaths from heart disease in the United States.

More than 25 years later, many food producers still haven't gotten the memo. Because the fats are cheap and have long shelf lives, reckless food producers continue to sneak partially hydrogenated oils, the main source of trans fats, into many of America's most popular packaged goods. Until the government decides to outlaw them, it's up to us to protect ourselves. Start by avoiding these dangers lurking in the supermarket.

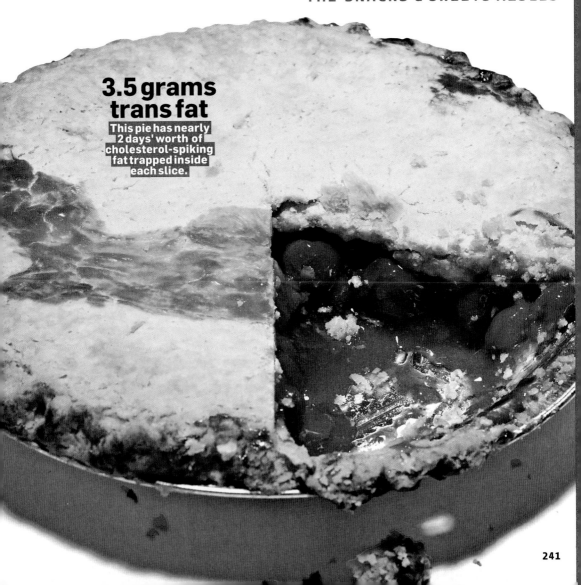

3.5 grams trans fat

This pie has nearly 2 days' worth of cholesterol-spiking fat trapped inside each slice.

Bisquick

(40 g, 1/3 cup mix)
1.5 g trans fats
160 calories
4.5 g fat (1 g saturated)
1 g fiber

The award for Most Shocking Use of Trans Fats goes to Bisquick. Who knew that during all those years of Sunday pancake breakfasts you were consuming your limit of trans fats for a day or more every time you reached for the Bisquick? For those not looking to boost their cholesterol with every bite of pancake, there are excellent alternatives out there, like the fiber-rich mix from Hodgson Mill. Better yet, take the extra 2 minutes to make your pancake batter from scratch.

Eat This Instead!
Hodgson Mill Whole Wheat Buttermilk Pancake Mix

(40 g, 1/3 cup)
130 calories
1 g fat (0 g saturated, 0 g trans)
4 g fiber

Gardetto's Special Request Roasted Garlic Rye Chips

(30 g, 1/2 cup)
3 g trans fats
170 calories
10 g fat (2 g saturated)
320 mg sodium

For this bag, Gardetto's has extracted only the trans-fattiest component of its grease-laden Original Recipe, and the result is a trans-fats travesty. Partially hydrogenated oil is the second ingredient, occurring even before the snack's namesake, rye.

Eat This Instead!
Chex Mix Bold Party Blend

(29 g, 1/2 cup)
120 calories
4 g fat
(1 g saturated, 0 g trans)
190 mg sodium

Pillsbury Grands! Homestyle Buttermilk

(58 g, 1 biscuit)
3 g trans fats
170 calories
6 g fat (1.5 g saturated)
580 mg sodium

Pastry makers prefer semi-solid fats, like trans, because they provide a crispier, flakier texture. Is it worth sacrificing health for? Not to us. A full 15 percent of the calories in this biscuit come from artery-clogging oils.

Eat This Instead!
Pillsbury Grands! Homestyle Buttermilk Reduced Fat

(58 g, 1 biscuit)
160 calories
4.5 g fat
(2 g saturated, 0 g trans)
590 mg sodium

Pop-Secret Butter

(2 Tbsp kernels, 4 1/2 cups popped)
5 g trans fats
180 calories
12 g fat (2.5 g saturated)
310 mg sodium

Microwave popcorn is one of the biggest contributors of trans fats to the American diet. The reason: Popcorn companies still rely on partially hydrogenated oil to pop their kernels. Shovel in this whole bag during your next movie night and you've just put down 15 grams of the bad stuff, 10 times what experts deem safe to consume in a day.

Eat This Instead!
Act II Butter Lover's

(2 cups popped)
50 calories
1.5 g fat
(0 g saturated, 0 g trans)
48 mg sodium

Marie Callender's Cherry Pie

(119 g, 1/10 pie)
3.5 g trans fats
370 calories
25 g sugars
17 g fat (3.5 g saturated)

The box boldly proclaims that Marie uses only "the finest ingredients," but her surreptitious product sourcing has managed to create arguably the single most dangerous piece of food in the entire supermarket. Eat this whole pie and you've just consumed more than

17 days' worth of cholesterol-spiking, heart-threatening trans fats. Marie, we know you think you make a pretty mean slice of pie, and based upon all evidence available, we can't disagree.

Eat This Instead!

Pepperidge Farm Puff Pastry Turnovers Cherry

(89 g, 1 turnover)
260 calories
10 g sugars
13 g fat
(7 g saturated, 0 g trans)

TRANS-FATTIEST FOOD IN THE SUPERMARKET

Celeste Pizza for One Original

(144 g, 1 pizza)
5 g trans fats
340 calories
16 g fat (4 g saturated)
1,020 mg sodium

Notice how Celeste avoids calling this a "cheese" pizza? That's because the topping isn't cheese—it's "imitation mozzarella." Translation: water, partially hydrogenated oil, and a smattering of flavors and binders. Mama Celeste should be ashamed.

Eat This Instead!

Lean Cuisine Traditional Pepperoni Pizza

(170 g, 1 pizza)
380 calories
610 mg sodium
9 g fat
(3 g saturated, 0 g trans)

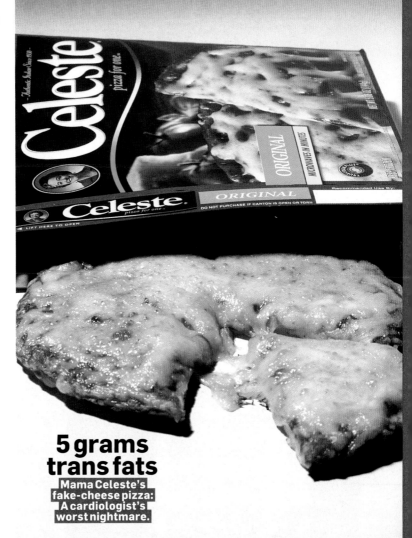

5 grams trans fats

Mama Celeste's fake-cheese pizza: A cardiologist's worst nightmare.

Potato Chips
Eat This

*Popchips represent the perfect
middle ground between
the two extremes of the chip world:
the crunch and character of
a fried chip and the calories
and fat of a baked one.
What more could you want?*

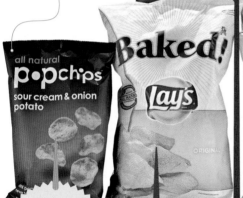

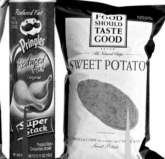

Not That!

Lay's Kettle Cooked Original
(1 oz, 16 chips)

160 calories
9 g fat
(1 g saturated)
90 mg sodium

"Kettle" cooking seems to imply a connection to a bygone era when food was simpler. Too bad a serving of these spuds contains nearly as much fat as a small order of McDonald's fries.

T.G.I. Friday's Potato Skins Jalapeño Cheddar
(1 oz, 16 chips)

150 calories
8 g fat
(1 g saturated)
340 mg sodium

A full 40 ingredients, the first of which is not potatoes, but rather vegetable oil.

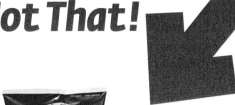

This classic bag of Lay's punishes careless snackers with an excessive amount of calories and fat.

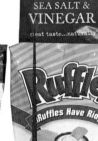
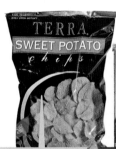
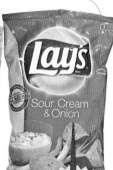

Terra Sweet Potato Chips
(1 oz, 17 chips)

160 calories
11 g fat
(1 g saturated)
10 mg sodium

These chips support our stance that the healthy reputation of sweet potatoes has been somewhat overhyped.

Pringles Light Original
(1 oz, 15 crisps)

70 calories
0 g fat
160 mg sodium

No fat here, but this crisp's olestra may flush your body of a bevy of vital fat-soluble nutrients in the loose stools it will generate.

Kettle Sea Salt & Vinegar
(1 oz, 13 chips)

150 calories
9 g fat
(1 g saturated)
210 mg sodium

A thoroughly mediocre bag of fried potatoes.

Ruffles Reduced Fat
(1 oz, 13 chips)

140 calories
7 g fat
(1 g saturated)
180 mg sodium

Reduced-fat chips might trump their ultra-oily siblings, but they still fall short when compared to the low fat content of a well-made baked chip.

Lay's Sour Cream & Onion
(1 oz, 17 chips)

160 calories
10 g fat
(1 g saturated)
160 mg sodium

245

Corn Chips
Eat This

No matter who makes the chip or how they make it, 120 calories per serving is about as low as it goes. Consider this the healthiest salsa scooper in the supermarket.

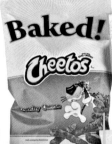

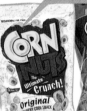
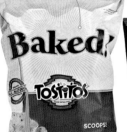
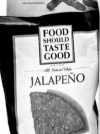
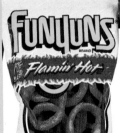
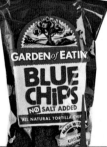

CornNuts Original
(1 oz, ⅓ cup)

130 calories
4.5 g fat
(0.5 g saturated)
160 mg sodium

We're fans of simple foods. Here, you're literally eating a corn kernel cooked with a little corn oil and salt.

Guiltless Gourmet Chipotle Tortilla Chips
(1 oz, 18 chips)

123 calories
3 g fat
(0 g saturated)
250 mg sodium

Fewer calories, fewer ingredients, and half the fat of the Doritos.

Tostitos Baked! Scoops
(1 oz, 14 chips)

120 calories
3 g fat
(0.5 g saturated)
140 mg sodium

Food Should Taste Good Jalapeño with Cheddar Tortilla Chips
(1 oz, 12 chips)

140 calories
6 g fat
(1 g saturated)
190 mg sodium

These fiber-packed chips are baked before frying, which minimizes oil absorption.

Baked! Cheetos Crunchy Cheese
(1 oz, 34 pieces)

130 calories
5 g fat
(1 g saturated)
240 mg sodium

Baked chips require less oil to turn crispy, and less oil on your chips potentially results in less flab on your belly.

Funyuns Flamin' Hot Onion Flavored Rings
(1 oz, 13 rings)

130 calories
7 g fat
(1 g saturated)
300 mg sodium

The resemblance to onion rings hides the fact that these are a surprisingly moderate snack choice.

Garden of Eatin' Blue Chips No Salt Added
(1 oz, 12 chips)

140 calories
7 g fat
(0.5 g saturated)
10 mg sodium

This is the lowest-sodium chip of any kind in the supermarket.

Not That!

Doritos Spicy Sweet Chili
(1 oz, 11 chips)

140 calories
7 g fat
(1 g saturated)
270 mg sodium

Ever wonder why Doritos are so addictive? Perhaps having MSG as the fifth item on the ingredients list has something to do with it.

Bugles Original Flavor
(30 g, 1 ⅓ cups)

160 calories
9 g fat
(8 g saturated)
310 mg sodium

Each serving of these little horns contains 40 percent of your day's saturated fat limit.

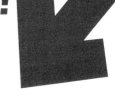

Don't fall for the "multigrain" hype. By weight, this chip contains nearly four times more fat than fiber.

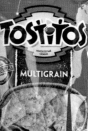

El Sabroso Original Guacachip
(1 oz, 28 g)

150 calories
9 g fat
(1 g saturated)
160 mg sodium

The bag says "real avocados," but the ingredients statement says "avocado powder."

Cheetos Flamin' Hot Crunchy
(1 oz, 21 pieces)

170 calories
11 g fat
(1.5 g saturated)
250 mg sodium

Nearly 100 of these calories come from oil.

Chester's Puffcorn Cheese
(1 oz, 46 pieces)

160 calories
11 g fat
(1.5 g saturated)
290 mg sodium

Nearly two-thirds of these calories come from the frying oil.

Fritos Chili Cheese Flavored Corn Chips
(1 oz, 31 chips)

160 calories
10 g fat
(1.5 g saturated)
260 mg sodium

It takes Frito-Lay 31 ingredients to make these chips, partially hydrogenated soybean oil being the most nefarious of the lot.

Tostitos Multigrain Tortilla Chips
(1 oz, 8 chips)

150 calories
7 g fat
(1 g saturated)
110 mg sodium

Wheat, Soy, Bean & R

Eat This

Genisoy Soy Crisps Rich Cheddar Cheese
(1 oz, 17 crisps)

120 calories
4 g fat
(1 g saturated)
180 mg sodium
1 g fiber

A full third of these calories are derived from protein and fiber.

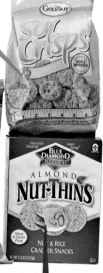

Kashi turns its whole-grain wisdom to crisps and turns out one with 5 grams of fiber per serving.

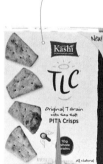

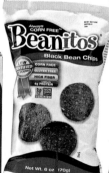

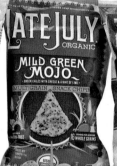

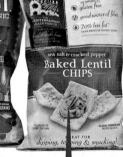

Kashi TLC Pita Crisps Original 7 Grain with Sea Salt
(1 oz, 11 crisps)

120 calories
3 g fat
(0 g saturated)
180 mg sodium
5 g fiber

Beanitos Black Bean Chips
(1 oz)

140 calories
7 g fat
(0.5 g saturated)
55 mg sodium
5 g fiber

The chip champion! The black beans not only add 5 grams of fiber, but also, in combination with the chip's brown rice, create 4 grams of complete protein.

Late July Mild Green Mojo Multigrain Snack Chips
(1 oz, 13 chips)

110 calories
4.5 g fat
(0 g saturated)
210 mg sodium
2 g fiber

Chia and flax seeds help each serving earn a potent 280 milligrams of omega-3s.

Mediterranean Snacks Baked Lentil Chips Sea Salt & Pepper
(1 oz, 22 chips)

110 calories
3 g fat
(0 g saturated)
250 mg sodium
3 g fiber

This chip earns 3 grams of fiber from lentil, garbanzo, and adzuki bean flour.

Blue Diamond Almond Nut Thins
(30 g, 16 chips)

130 calories
2.5 g fat
(0 g saturated)
115 mg sodium
<1 g fiber

Almonds, the second ingredient in these chips, are teeming with vitamin E.

Not That!

Quaker Quakes Rice Snacks Cheddar Cheese
(30 g, 18 mini cakes)

140 calories
5 g fat
(0.5 g saturated)
410 mg sodium
1 g fiber

These crisps have scarcely any protein or fiber, but they do contain MSG and partially hydrogenated oil.

A fiberless chip such as this one will spike your blood sugar and signal your body to store fat.

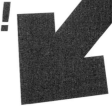

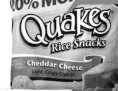

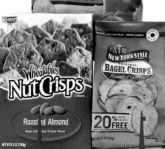

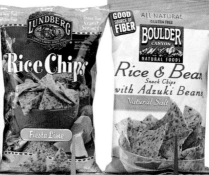

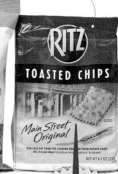

Keebler Wheatables Nut Crisps Roasted Almond
(30 g, 16 crackers)

140 calories
6 g fat
(1 g saturated)
220 mg sodium
1 g fiber

On the ingredients list, flour, soybean oil, and sugar all appear well before almonds.

New York Style Bagel Crisps Roasted Garlic
(1 oz, 6 crisps)

130 calories
5 g fat
(2.5 g saturated)
320 mg sodium
1 g fiber

Loaded with palm oil, which has been shown to have the same effect on cholesterol as partially hydrogenated oils.

Lundberg Rice Chips Fiesta Lime
(1 oz, 10 chips)

140 calories
7 g fat
(0.5 g saturated)
270 mg sodium
1 g fiber

When it comes to rice, Lundberg is head of the class, but its chips are simultaneously heavy on fat and light on fiber.

Boulder Canyon Rice & Bean Snack Chips with Adzuki Beans Natural Salt
(1 oz, 20 chips)

120 calories
7 g fat
(1 g saturated)
130 mg sodium
3 g fiber

Made up mostly of lackluster rice flour and modified corn starch.

Ritz Toasted Chips Main Street Original
(1 oz, 13 chips)

130 calories
4.5 g fat
(0.5 g saturated)
250 mg sodium
1 g fiber

249

Pretzels & Snack Mix
Eat This

Rold Gold Tiny Twists Honey Mustard
(28 g, 20 pieces)

110 calories
1 g fat (0 g saturated)
430 mg sodium

Nowhere else in the snack aisle will you find this much flavor for so few calories. Still, keep yourself to a single serving to avoid sodium overload.

Chex Mix Dark Chocolate
(30 g, ½ cup)

140 calories
4.5 g fat
(2 g saturated)
60 mg sodium

Made with actual dark chocolate, which has been shown to decrease the risk of heart disease.

A serving from this Bold bag is actually 10 calories lighter than Chex Traditional Party Mix.

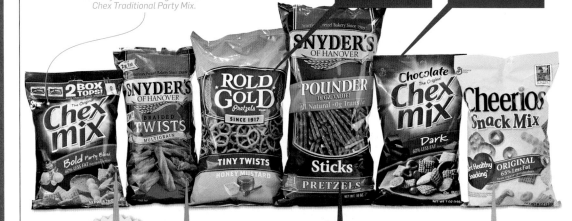

Chex Mix Bold Party Blend
(29 g, ½ cup)

120 calories
4 g fat (1 g saturated)
190 mg sodium

Snyder's Braided Twists Multigrain
(30 g, 9 twists)

120 calories
2 g fat (0 g saturated)
160 mg sodium

The 3 grams of fiber in each serving make this a snack with hunger-quashing capabilities.

Snyder's of Hanover Pretzel Sticks
(30 g, 28 sticks)

110 calories
1 g fat (0 g saturated)
300 mg sodium

Want to turn this into a more substantial snack? Pair it with a tablespoon of peanut butter and you can squash afternoon hunger for around 200 calories.

Cheerios Snack Mix Original
(29 g, ½ cup)

120 calories
3 g fat
(0.5 g saturated)
240 mg sodium

Thankfully, Cheerios Snack Mix doesn't suffer from the same sugar blight that afflicts some of the brand's cereal products. Plus, each serving packs a few grams of fiber.

Not That!

Bugles Sweet & Salty Chocolate Peanut Butter
(32 g, ⅔ cup)

170 calories
9 g fat (6 g saturated)
150 mg sodium

Four different kinds of oil give this mix as much saturated fat as six strips of bacon.

Snyder's of Hanover Honey Mustard & Onion Pretzel Pieces
(28 g, ⅓ cup)

140 calories
7 g fat (3 g saturated)
240 mg sodium

A thick application of palm oil gives this bag considerably more fat than Rold Gold's.

The gratuitous use of partially hydrogenated oils makes this line one dangerous snack. Each serving has nearly as much trans fats as the American Heart Association recommends as the maximum to consume in a day.

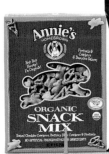
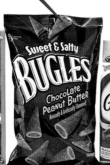
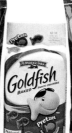
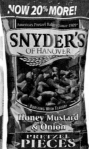
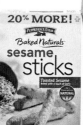
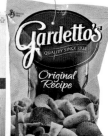

Annie's Homegrown Organic Snack Mix
(28 g, ½ cup)

130 calories
5 g fat
(0.5 g saturated)
250 mg sodium

Organic is good, but a fiberless snack is not.

Pepperidge Farm Goldfish Baked Snack Crackers Pretzel
(30 g, 43 pieces)

130 calories
2.5 g fat
(0.5 g saturated)
430 mg sodium

These fish are swimming in sodium and oil.

Pepperidge Farm Baked Naturals Snack Sticks Toasted Sesame
(12 sticks)

140 calories
5 g fat (1 g saturated)
290 mg sodium

Better than a bag of standard chips, but not quite as good as pretzels or baked chips.

Gardetto's Original Recipe Snack Mix
(30 g, ½ cup)

150 calories
7 g fat
(1.5 g saturated,
1.5 g trans)
260 mg sodium

Popcorn
Eat This

In its ideal state, popcorn can be a perfect snack: low calorie, whole grain, and with a good hit of fiber. This bag takes the nutritional high road with four simple ingredients and zero trans fats.

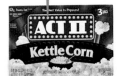

Smart Balance Deluxe Microwave Popcorn Smart N' Healthy!
(2 cups popped)

50 calories
0 g fat
0 mg sodium

With this Smart Balance bag, you control the sodium level. Add a pinch of sea salt or a sprinkle of Parmesan cheese before diving in.

Act II Kettle Corn
(2 cups popped)

60 calories
3 g fat
(1 g saturated)
40 mg sodium

Act II cuts calories by swapping out sugar for sucralose.

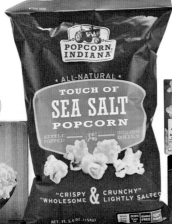

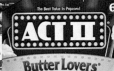

Orville Redenbacher's Natural Simply Salted
(2 cups popped)

60 calories
4 g fat
(2 g saturated)
130 mg sodium

Popcorn, Indiana Touch of Sea Salt
(2 cups)

85 calories
4 g fat
(0 g saturated)
125 mg sodium

Nothing but popcorn, canola oil, and sea salt. Oh, and 2 grams of fiber per serving. You won't find a more unadulterated bag anywhere.

Orville Redenbacher's Spicy Nacho
(2 cups popped)

60 calories
4 g fat
(2 g saturated)
100 mg sodium

Kudos to Mr. Redenbacher, who derives his nacho flavor from real jalapeños.

Cracker Jack The Original
(28 g, ½ cup)

120 calories
2 g fat
(0 g saturated)
70 mg sodium
15 g sugars

It's not the most wholesome snack around, but it's 75 percent lower in fat than Orville's version.

Act II Butter Lovers
(2 cups popped)

50 calories
2 g fat
(0 g saturated)
90 mg sodium

Act II achieves a rich butter flavor without the dangerous load of fat.

252

Not That!

Jolly Time KettleMania Kettle Corn
(2 cups popped)

90 calories
6 g fat
(2 g saturated,
2 g trans)
80 mg sodium

"Mania" is correct. You'd have to be a maniac to eat this much trans fats in one sitting.

Newman's Own Popcorn Light Butter
(2 cups popped)

70 calories
2 g fat
(1 g saturated)
97 mg sodium

Not a terrible choice, but if you're looking for a "light" popcorn, there are better bags to buy.

The reckless use of partially hydrogenated oils imbues each bag with 12 grams of trans fats, which have a firm link to heart disease. Pop-Secret should be ashamed of itself.

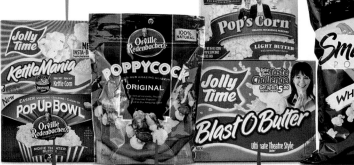
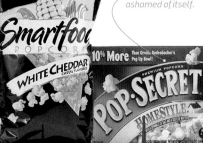

Orville Redenbacher's Pop Up Bowl Movie Theater Butter
(2 cups popped)

70 calories
5 g fat
(2 g saturated)
80 mg sodium

Don't let a gimmicky "Pop Up Bowl" influence the quality of the popcorn you eat.

Orville Redenbacher's Poppycock Original
(31 g, ⅓ cup)

160 calories
8 g fat
(2 g saturated)
120 mg sodium
13 g sugars

The heavy application of glaze puts this one in the candy category.

Jolly Time Blast O Butter
(2 cups popped)

90 calories
6 g fat
(2 g saturated,
2 g trans)
170 mg sodium

Jolly Time isn't shy about pouring on the partially hydrogenated oils. One serving has more trans fats than you should consume in a day.

Smartfood White Cheddar
(2 cups)

183 calories
11 g fat
(2.5 g saturated)
331 mg sodium

Smart? Hardly. This bag earns a heavy glut of fat from oils, cheese, and buttermilk.

Pop-Secret Homestyle
(2 cups popped)

60 calories
4 g fat
(0 g saturated,
2 g trans)
140 mg sodium

Dips and Spreads
Eat This

Wholly Guacamole Guaca Salsa
(30 g, 2 Tbsp)

35 calories
3 g fat
(0 g saturated)
110 mg sodium

Avocados are the first of only seven ingredients, all of which you likely keep stocked in your kitchen.

Desert Pepper Black Bean Dip Spicy
(31 g, 2 Tbsp)

25 calories
0 g fat
300 mg sodium

This jar contains a trio of nutritional A-listers: black beans, tomatoes, and sweet green peppers.

Cheese dips, by nature, tend to be heavy with calories, but On the Border lightens the load by blending in tomatoes, peppers, water, and nonfat milk.

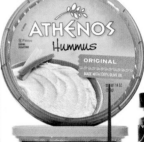

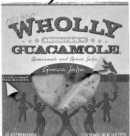

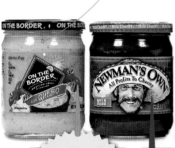

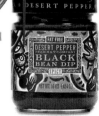

On the Border Salsa con Queso
(34 g, 2 Tbsp)

45 calories
3 g fat
(0.5 g saturated)
260 mg sodium

Newman's Own Chunky Bandito Mild Salsa
(32 g, 2 Tbsp)

10 calories
0 g fat
65 mg sodium

We balked when Ronald Reagan tried to turn ketchup into a vegetable, but if someone did the same for salsa, a legitimate nutritional superpower, we'd throw our support behind it.

Tribe All Natural Hummus Sweet Roasted Red Peppers
(28 g, 2 Tbsp)

40 calories
2.5 g fat
(0 g saturated)
125 mg sodium

Based on chickpeas and sesame seeds, hummus makes for an incredible vegetable dip and sandwich spread.

Athenos Hummus Original
(27 g, 2 Tbsp)

50 calories
3 g fat
(0 g saturated)
160 mg sodium

Made with real olive oil, which lends an authentic flavor and more heart-healthy fats.

Not That!

Tostitos Zesty Bean & Cheese Dip Medium
(33 g, 2 Tbsp)

45 calories
2 g fat
(0.5 g saturated)
230 mg sodium

Contains more than 25 ingredients, including corn oil, monosodium glutamate, DATEM (an emulsifier), and two artificial shades of yellow.

Mission Guacamole Flavored Dip
(31 g, 2 Tbsp)

40 calories
3 g fat
(0 g saturated)
150 mg sodium

"Flavored" is the key word. This imposter is made mostly of water, oil, and cornstarch.

After water, soybean oil is the number-one ingredient in this jar. If you're going to blow 90 calories on a cheese dip, you should at least be eating, you know, actual cheese.

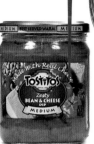
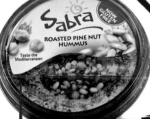
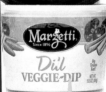

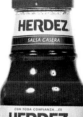
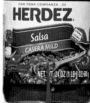
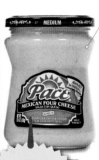

Sabra Roasted Pine Nut Hummus
(28 g, 2 Tbsp)

80 calories
7 g fat
(1 g saturated)
125 mg sodium
4 g carbohydrates

Instead of the traditional olive oil, Sabra's ingredients statement lists "soybean and/or canola."

Marzetti Dill Veggie Dip
(29 g, 2 Tbsp)

110 calories
11 g fat
(3 g saturated)
200 mg sodium

This dip is mostly sour cream. The only "veggies" are dehydrated onion and garlic, and they're buried deep in the ingredients list.

Herdez Salsa Casera Mild
(31 g, 2 Tbsp)

10 calories
0 g fat
270 mg sodium

Be on the watch for elevated sodium in salsa. By the time you finish this jar, you'll have taken in 3,780 milligrams, more than double the daily limit for most people.

Pace Mexican Four Cheese Salsa con Queso
(30 g, 2 Tbsp)

90 calories
7 g fat
(1.5 g saturated)
430 mg sodium

Fruits, Nuts & Seeds

Eat This

Dried fruits and vegetables have been flooding the supermarket of late, which can be a great thing if you choose carefully. Bare Fruit apples have no added sweeteners or artificial anything. Just organic apples and a pinch of cinnamon.

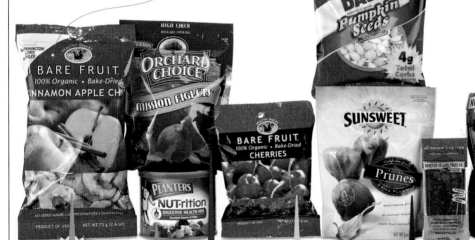

David Pumpkin Seeds Roasted & Salted
(30 g, ¼ cup)

160 calories
12 g fat
(2.5 g saturated)
10 mg sodium
1 g fiber

Among the most magnesium-rich foods on the planet.

Emerald Cinnamon Roast Almonds
(28 g, ¼ cup)

150 calories
13 g fat
(1 g saturated)
40 mg sodium
3 g fiber

Cinnamon can help ease blood sugar spikes.

Bare Fruit Bake-Dried Cinnamon Apple Chips
(12 g)

29 calories
0 g fat
7 g sugars
1 g fiber

Planters NUTrition Digestive Health Mix
(32 g, ¼ cup)

150 calories
8 g fat
(1 g saturated)
40 mg sodium
5 g fiber

The fiber and healthy fats in nuts squash hunger.

Blue Ribbon Orchard Choice Mission Figlets
(40 g, ¼ cup, 5 figs)

110 calories
0 g fat
20 g sugars
5 g fiber

Loads of fiber and no added sugar.

Bare Fruit Bake-Dried Cherries
(36 g)

108 calories
0 g fat
16 g sugars
2 g fiber

Bare Fruit specializes in slow-cooked fruit with zero added sugars. This is one pristine fruit snack.

Sunsweet California Pitted Prunes
(40 g, ¼ cup)

100 calories
0 g fat
15 g sugars
3 g fiber

Diced prunes mixed with mandarin oranges, baby spinach, and feta make for a tasty salad.

Stretch Island Fruit Co. All Natural Fruit Strip Summer Strawberry
(14 g, 1 strip)

45 calories
0 g fat
9 g sugars
1 g fiber

Just fruit purees and juice.

Not That!

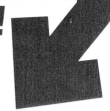

Blue Diamond Natural Oven Roasted Almonds Butter Toffee
(28 g, 24 nuts)

160 calories
12 g fat
(1 g saturated)
35 mg sodium
3 g fiber

Three of the first four ingredients are forms of sugar.

David Sunflower Kernels Roasted & Salted
(30 g, ¼ cup)

190 calories
15 g fat
(2 g saturated)
220 mg sodium
3 g fiber

Doused in partially hydrogenated oil.

"Snack healthier," Seneca implores eaters on the label (then proceeds to dip its apples in oil and corn syrup).

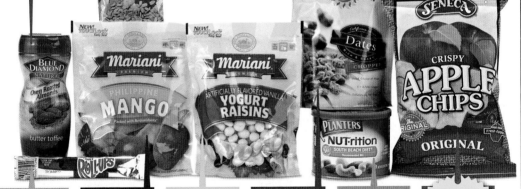

Fruit Roll-Ups Strawberry
(14 g, 1 roll)

50 calories
1 g fat
(0 g saturated)
7 g sugars
0 g fiber

Made from 14 ingredients including partially hydrogenated oils. The one ingredient missing? Fruit.

Mariani Philippine Mango
(40 g, 6 slices)

130 calories
0 g fat
27 g sugars
1 g fiber

Mangoes natural sugars intensify in the drying process, which makes the added sugar all the more puzzling.

Mariani Vanilla Flavored Yogurt Raisins
(30 g, 2 Tbsp)

150 calories
7 g fat
(6 g saturated)
17 g sugars
1 g fiber

The yogurt is really partially hydrogenated oil.

Sunsweet California Grown Dates Chopped
(40 g, ¼ cup)

120 calories
0 g fat
27 g sugars
3 g fiber

The sugar coating pushes these dates dangerously close to candy status.

Planters NUTrition South Beach Diet Recommended Mix
(28 g, 18 pieces)

170 calories
15 g fat
(2 g saturated)
50 mg sodium
2 g fiber

Seneca Crispy Apple Chips Original
(28 g, 12 chips)

140 calories
7 g fat
(1 g saturated)
12 g sugars
2 g fiber

257

Cookies
Eat This

Kashi TLC Oatmeal Dark Chocolate Soft-Baked Cookies
(30 g, 1 cookie)

130 calories
5 g fat
(1.5 g saturated)
65 mg sodium
8 g sugars

Thanks to oats barley, and buckwheat, Kashi's cookie has more fiber (4 grams) than a standard slice of whole-wheat bread.

Nabisco Ginger Snaps
(28 g, 4 cookies)

120 calories
2.5 g fat
(0.5 g saturated)
190 mg sodium
11 g sugars

Small cookies are a good strategy—they can help you feel like you're eating more than you actually are.

This cookie isn't just the best of the Chips Ahoy! line, it's also one of the lowest-calorie cookies on the shelf.

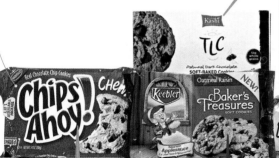
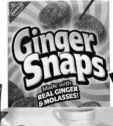
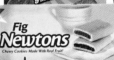
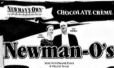

Chips Ahoy! Chewy
(27 g, 2 cookies)

120 calories
5 g fat
(2.5 g saturated)
85 mg sodium
10 g sugars

Keebler Baker's Treasures Soft Oatmeal Raisin
(32 g, 2 cookies)

130 calories
4.5 g fat
(1.5 g saturated)
105 mg sodium
10 g sugars

Keebler's newest creation displaces some of the oil calories with applesauce, a strategy we'd like to see applied to more cookies in the elves' catalog.

Nabisco Fig Newtons Original
(31 g, 2 cookies)

110 calories
2 g fat
(0 g saturated)
130 mg sodium
12 g sugars

Yes, it's made with real figs. That doesn't make it "healthy," but it's nice to have some real fruit to offset the processed sugar.

Newman's Own Newman-O's Chocolate Crème Filled Chocolate Cookies
(28 g, 2 cookies)

130 calories
5 g fat
(1.5 g saturated)
110 mg sodium
11 g sugars

Compared with Oreo, Newman takes a moderate approach to oil and sugar.

Not That!

Keebler Sandies Simply Shortbread
(31 g, 2 cookies)

160 calories
9 g fat
(4 g saturated)
90 mg sodium
7 g sugars

We applaud the low sugar count, but not the heavy deposits of soybean and palm oils.

Mrs. Fields Milk Chocolate Chip
(34 g, 1 cookie)

160 calories
8 g fat
(4 g saturated)
160 mg sodium
15 g sugars

The dearth of fiber ensures that this will pass straight through your belly, spike your blood sugar, and convert quickly to flab.

This cookie has more fat, more sodium, and more sugar than the same cookie from Chips Ahoy!

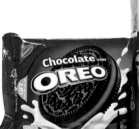
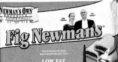
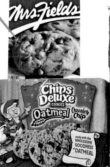
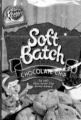

Nabisco Chocolate Creme Oreo
(30 g, 2 cookies)

150 calories
7 g fat
(2.5 g saturated)
110 mg sodium
13 g sugars

And the regular Oreos are even worse—they deliver an extra gram of sugar and 10 extra calories per serving.

Newman's Own Fig Newmans Low Fat
(38 g, 2 bars)

140 calories
2 g fat
(1 g saturated)
170 mg sodium
13 g sugars

Surprisingly enough, the Fig Newmans low-fat cookie has more calories than the original Newtons. Blame the extra rush of refined carbs.

Keebler Chips Deluxe Oatmeal Chocolate Chip
(31 g, 2 cookies)

150 calories
7 g fat
(3 g saturated)
105 mg sodium
10 g sugars

Add just one of these 75-calorie Keebler cookies to your daily diet and you'll gain nearly 8 pounds this year.

Keebler Soft Batch Chocolate Chip
(32 g, 2 cookies)

160 calories
7 g fat (3 g saturated)
110 mg sodium
12 g sugars

Snack Cakes
Eat This

There's nothing nutritionally worthwhile about any ingredient listed on this package, but a Twinkie does a decent job of delivering sweet, squishy indulgence without inflicting too much damage.

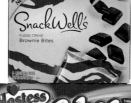

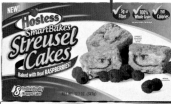

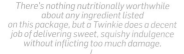

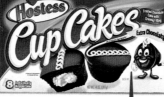

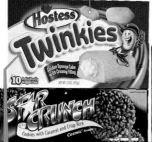

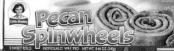

Hostess Twinkies
(43 g, 1 cake)

150 calories
4.5 g fat
(2.5 g saturated)
18 g sugars

Little Debbie Star Crunch
(31 g, 1 cookie)

150 calories
6 g fat
(3.5 g saturated)
13 g sugars

Star Crunch's puffed-rice approach keeps the cake sufficiently light and airy.

Hostess CupCakes
(50 g, 1 cake)

180 calories
7 g fat
(3.5 g saturated)
20 g sugars

One of these is permissible. Two are likely to sabotage your weight-loss efforts.

Little Debbie Pecan Spinwheels
(30 g, 1 roll)

100 calories
3.5 g fat
(1 g saturated)
7 g sugars

This is one of the lowest-calorie products in the entire Little Debbie catalog.

Not That!

Little Debbie Strawberry Shortcake Rolls
(61 g, 1 roll)

240 calories
9 g fat (3 g saturated)
27 g sugars

The only reference to fruit in the ingredient list is to "artificial strawberry," i.e., an additive engineered in a lab to look and taste like the real thing. No thanks, Debbie.

Entenmann's Little Bites Fudge Brownies
(62 g, 1 pack)

270 calories
14 g fat
(4 g saturated)
25 g sugars

Entenmann's brownies are only slightly better than its doughnuts.

Each Ding Dong has double the fat of the Twinkie, and because it comes in a two-pack, you have to practice restraint to avoid bingeing.

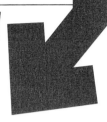

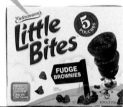

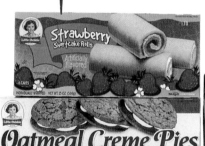

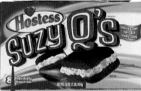

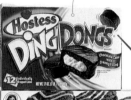

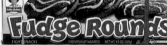

Little Debbie Oatmeal Crème Pies
(38 g, 1 pie)

170 calories
7 g fat (2 g saturated)
12 g sugars

Don't be fooled; the oatmeal is nothing more than the vehicle for fat and sugar.

Hostess Suzy Q's
(57 g, 1 cake)

220 calories
9 g fat
(4.5 g saturated)
24 g sugars

One Suzy Q has 50 more calories than a Wendy's Jr. Original Chocolate Frosty.

Little Debbie Fudge Rounds
(Big Pack)
(67 g, 1 round)

310 calories
12 g fat
(4.5 g saturated)
30 g sugars

Little Debbie's Big Packs are woeful not just for the content of their cakes but also for the Flintstonian portion size. This one has more calories than 8 strips of bacon.

Hostess Ding Dongs
(40 g, 1 cake)

180 calories
9 g fat
(7 g saturated)
18 g sugars

Pudding
Eat This

Royal Flan with Caramel Sauce
(19 g dry mix, ⅓ cup prepared with 2% milk)

130 calories
1 g fat
(0 g saturated)
18 g sugars

You can control your sugar intake by reducing your use of the caramel sauce.

Mousse Temptations by Jell-O Sugar Free Dark Chocolate Decadence
(65 g, 1 snack)

60 calories
2.5 g fat
(1.5 g saturated)
0 g sugars

Half the calories and fat of Jell-O's box version.

Given the choice between sugar free and fat free, we'll take sugar free every time.

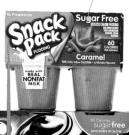

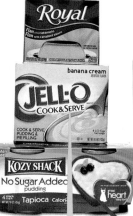

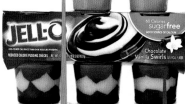

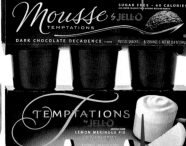

Snack Pack Pudding Caramel Sugar-Free
(99 g, 1 pudding cup)

60 calories
3 g fat
(1.5 g saturated)
0 g sugars

Jell-O Sugar Free Chocolate Vanilla Swirls
(106 g, 1 snack)

60 calories
1.5 g fat
(1 g saturated)
0 g sugars

Concern yourself less with a pudding's fat content than its sugar load.

Jell-O Cook & Serve Banana Cream
(½ cup prepared with 2% milk)

140 calories
0 g fat
15 g sugars

Not the lightest pudding on the market, but made with low-fat milk, this makes for a reasonable (and decadent) dessert.

Kozy Shack No Sugar Added Pudding Tapioca
(113 g, 1 snack cup)

70 calories
0.5 g fat
(0 g saturated)
5 g sugars

Chicory root powder pads this cup with 4 grams of fiber, which is as much as you'd find in a bowl of Quaker Quick Oats.

Temptations by Jell-O Lemon Meringue Pie
(111 g, 1 snack)

100 calories
2 g fat
(2 g saturated)
15 g sugars

Not all of Jell-O's Temptations are equally commendable, but this one finds the middle ground between prudence and indulgence.

Not That!

Temptations by Jell-O Chocolate Truffle Indulgence (box)
(½ cup prepared with fat-free milk)

130 calories
6 g fat
(4 g saturated)
9 g sugars

Two of the first three ingredients are oils.

Kozy Shack Restaurant Style Flan Crème
(113 g, 1 flan)

150 calories
4 g fat
(2 g saturated)
20 g sugars

Every tablespoon packs nearly 3 grams of sugar and 18 calories.

Unless they're sugar free, Snack Pack puddings are not to be trusted.

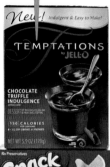
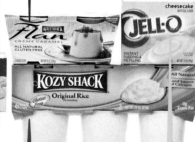

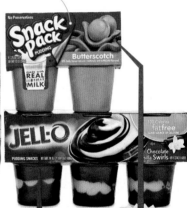

Snack Pack Lemon Pudding
(99 g, 1 cup)

130 calories
2.5 g fat
(1.5 g saturated)
20 g sugars

Sugar accounts for nearly two-thirds of these calories.

Kozy Shack Original Rice Pudding
(113 g, 1 snack cup)

130 calories
3 g fat
(2 g saturated)
14 g sugars

White rice is a nutritionally subpar grain, so anything made with it (milk, pudding) is likely to be something you should avoid.

Jell-O Instant Pudding Cheesecake
(½ cup prepared with 2% milk)

160 calories
0 g fat
20 g sugars

It's no surprise that one of the worst desserts also is the star of one of the worst puddings in the supermarket.

Jell-O Fat Free Chocolate Vanilla Swirls
(113 g, 1 snack)

100 calories
0 g fat
17 g sugars

Beware the bait and switch: Fat-free products are frequently saddled with egregious amounts of sugar and salt.

Snack Pack Pudding Butterscotch
(92 g, 1 pudding cup)

110 calories
2.5 g fat
(1 g saturated)
14 g sugars

263

Meal Replacement &

Eat This

Kashi folds whey and soy proteins into a blend of seven whole grains to give this low-calorie bar a phenomenal nutritional profile.

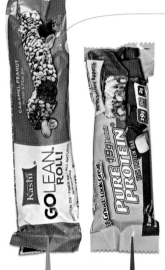

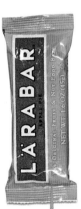

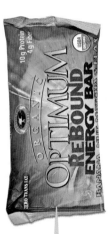

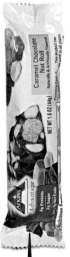

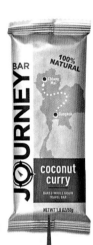

Kashi GoLean Roll! Caramel Peanut
(55 g, 1 bar)

190 calories
5 g fat
(1.5 g saturated)
6 g fiber
14 g sugars
12 g protein

Pure Protein S'mores
(50 g, 1 bar)

180 calories
5 g fat
(3.5 g saturated)
0 g fiber
2 g sugars
19 g protein

You won't find another bar with so much protein for so few calories.

Lärabar Apple Pie
(45 g, 1 bar)

190 calories
10 g fat
(1 g saturated)
5 g fiber
18 g sugars
4 g protein

Made from just six ingredients, and all of them whole foods you might have in your pantry.

Nature's Path Optimum Rebound Banana, Nut, Matcha & Flax
(56 g, 1 bar)

190 calories
4 g fat
(0.5 g saturated)
4 g fiber
20 g sugars
10 g protein

Atkins Advantage Caramel Chocolate Nut Roll
(44 g, 1 bar)

170 calories
12 g fat
(4.5 g saturated)
8 g fiber
2 g sugars
8 g protein

Journey Bar Coconut Curry
(50 g, 1 bar)

220 calories
11 g fat
(4 g saturated)
5 g fiber
10 g sugars
5 g protein

All of Journey bars are long on fiber and short on added sugars.

Protein Bars

Not That!

Of the first 12 ingredients in this bar, fully half are some form of sugar or oil.

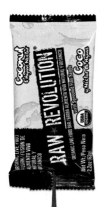

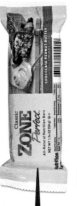

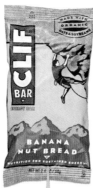

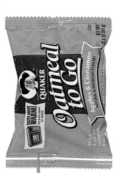

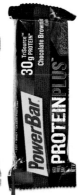

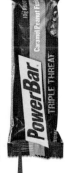

Raw Revolution Coconut & Agave Nectar
(62 g, 1 bar)

280 calories
18 g fat
(6 g saturated)
5 g fiber
20 g sugars
6 g protein

Same fiber count, double the sugar.

Zone Perfect Classic Nutrition Bar Chocolate Peanut Butter
(50 g, 1 bar)

210 calories
7 g fat
(4 g saturated)
3 g fiber
15 g sugars
14 g protein

Clif Banana Nut Bread
(68 g, 1 bar)

240 calories
6 g fat
(1 g saturated)
4 g fiber
22 g sugars
9 g protein

First ingredient: organic brown rice syrup. Sounds fancy, but it's basically sugar.

Quaker Oatmeal to Go Apples with Cinnamon
(60 g, 1 bar)

220 calories
4 g fat
(1 g saturated)
200 mg sodium
5 g fiber
22 g sugars
4 g protein

PowerBar ProteinPlus Chocolate Brownie
(90 g, 1 bar)

360 calories
11 g fat
(4.5 g saturated)
<1 g fiber
30 g sugars
30 g protein

Body builders only.

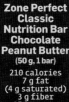

PowerBar Triple Threat Caramel Peanut Fusion
(45 g, 1 bar)

230 calories
9 g fat
(4.5 g saturated)
3 g fiber
15 g sugars
10 g protein

Individually Packag

Eat This

One of the best grab-and-go snacks around. The 15 grams of protein go a long way toward snuffing out midday hunger.

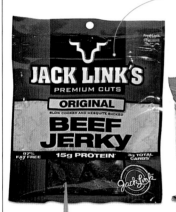

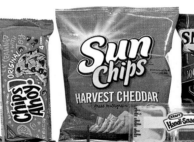

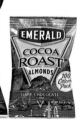

Jack Link's Original Beef Jerky
(1 oz, 28 g)

80 calories
1 g fat
(0 g saturated)
590 mg sodium
15 g protein

Chips Ahoy! Chocolate Chip Cookies
(40 g, 1 package)

190 calories
9 g fat
(3 g saturated)
13 g sugars

Nutritious? No, but the small serving size makes them safer than most packaged sweets.

SunChips Harvest Cheddar
(28 g, 15 chips, 1 package)

140 calories
6 g fat
(1 g saturated)
200 mg sodium

SunChips uses whole grains to add an impressive 3 grams of fiber to this bag.

Kraft Handi-Snacks Ritz Crackers 'n Cheese Dip
(27 g, 1 package)

100 calories
6 g fat
(1.5 g saturated)
330 mg sodium

This dip is made with Cheddar and whey protein.

Snyder's of Hanover Mini Pretzels
(0.9 oz, 1 package)

100 calories
0 g fat
220 mg sodium

Pretzels are baked, not fried, making them a better choice than chips for a midday snack.

Emerald 100 Calorie Pack Cocoa Roast Almonds
(18 g, 1 pack)

100 calories
8 g fat
(0.5 g saturated)
1 g sugars

Two grams of fiber and a load of healthy fats make this a guilt-free indulgence.

ed Snacks

Not That!

There's nothing slim about this product. More than 75 percent of its calories are derived from fat. By comparison, 75 percent of Jack Link's calories come from protein.

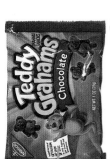

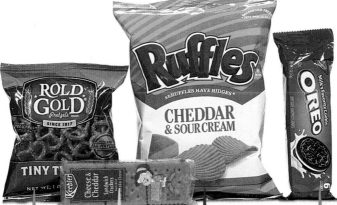

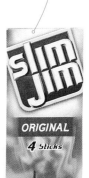

Teddy Grahams Chocolate
(28 g, 1 package)

120 calories
4 g fat
(1 g saturated)
8 g sugars

Unlike an almond's slow-burning fuel, these are mostly blood-sugar-spiking flour.

Rold Gold Tiny Twists
(1 oz, 1 package)

110 calories
1 g fat
(0 g saturated)
450 mg sodium

Snyder's makes a similar product with half as much sodium.

Keebler Cheese & Cheddar Sandwich Crackers
(39 g, 1 package)

190 calories
9 g fat
(2.5 g saturated)
290 mg sodium

Keebler products tend to pack more calories and fat than their rivals.

Ruffles Cheddar & Sour Cream
(53 g, 1 pouch)

300 calories
21 g fat
(3 g saturated)
440 mg sodium

There's no reason to settle for a fat-heavy chip like this.

Oreos
(57 g, 1 package)

270 calories
11 g fat
(3 g saturated)
23 g sugars

Serving size is king in the snack world. Add just one of these packages to your daily routine and you'll gain more than 2 pounds in a month.

Slim Jim Original
(1 oz)

150 calories
13 g fat
(5 g saturated)
430 mg sodium
6 g protein

Candy
Eat This

Nearly every calorie on this page comes from sugar, so the key to mitigating the damage is to find a candy that has less-concentrated sweetness. Jujubes, containing about a third of a gram of sugar in each piece, qualifies as one of the better candy bargains.

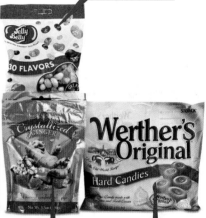

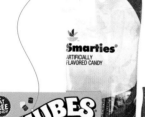

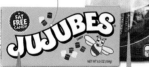

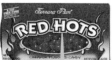

Jujubes
(40 g, 52 pieces)

110 calories
0 g fat
18 g sugars

Smarties Candy Rolls
(42 g, 6 rolls)

150 calories
0 g fat
36 g sugars

Use Smarties to quell a sweet tooth and you'll likely be satisfied by the time you finish one roll. That's not too bad considering that each roll has only 25 calories.

Red Hots
(34 g, 40 pieces)

120 calories
0 g fat
28 g sugars

Half the size of a Hot Tamale, so you get to munch on more for less.

The Ginger People Crystallized Ginger
(24 g, 4 pieces)

80 calories
0 g fat
18 g sugars

Studies have linked ginger with a host of potential health benefits, including alleviating arthritis and fighting nausea.

Werther's Original Hard Candy
(16 g, 3 pieces)

70 calories
1.5 g fat
(1 g saturated)
10 g sugars

Hard candies make for longer-lasting treats with fewer calories.

Not That!

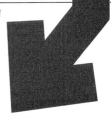

Skittles Original
(42 g, ¼ cup)

170 calories
2 g fat
(2 g saturated)
32 g sugars

Skittles hit all the dangers of candy: a deluge of sugar, a layer of saturated fat, and an absurd number of artificial colors—several of which have been linked to hyperactivity in children.

The problem with candy is that it's concentrated sugar with no fat, fiber, or protein to slow its passage through your body. Plus the more you eat, the more you crave. That puts pounds on your body, and over time, it puts you at risk for diabetes.

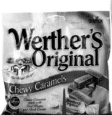
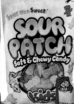
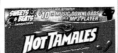
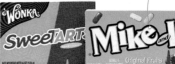

Werther's Original Chewy Caramels
(19 g, 3 pieces)

85 calories
3 g fat
(1.5 g saturated)
7 g sugars

You can put down about 10 of these in the time it takes you to get through one Werther's hard candy.

Sour Patch Kids
(40 g, 16 pieces)

150 calories
0 g fat
26 g sugars

Eat 1 serving a day and you'll put on nearly 15 pounds in a year.

Hot Tamales
(40 g, 20 pieces)

140 calories
0 g fat
25 g sugars

Advertised as "fat free," but nearly all candy is.

SweeTARTS
(45 g, 39 pieces)

180 calories
0 g fat
36 g sugars

Few producers are capable of packing so many calories into so tiny a package. You might as well eat 2 heaping spoonfuls of table sugar.

Mike and Ike Original Fruits
(40 g, 23 pieces)

150 calories
0 g fat
23 g sugars

Candy Bars
Eat This

York Peppermint Pattie
(39 g, 1 patty)

140 calories
2.5 g fat
(1.5 g saturated)
25 g sugars

For a smaller treat, go with York Miniatures. You can have three for about the same number of calories.

Hershey's Kit Kat
(43 g, 1 package)

210 calories
11 g fat
(7 g saturated)
21 g sugars

The wafer core is light and porous, which saves you calories over the denser bars.

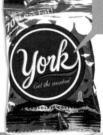

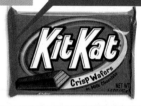

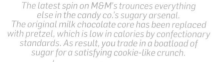

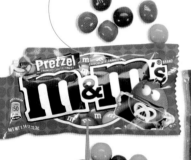

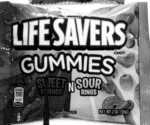

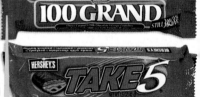

Pretzel M&M's
(32 g, 1 bag)

150 calories
5 g fat (3 g saturated)
16 g sugars

Life Savers Gummies
(40 g, 10 pieces)

130 calories
0 g fat
25 g sugars

The secret to the chew: gelatin. Starburst uses the same trick, but spoils it with a strange mix of oils.

Nestlé 100 Grand
(43 g, 1 package)

190 calories
8 g fat
(5 g saturated)
30 g carbohydrates
22 g sugars

This is an *Eat This, Not That!* Hall of Famer, routinely beating out more common chocolate bars by 80 or more calories.

Hershey's Take 5
(42 g, 1 package)

200 calories
11 g fat
(5 g saturated)
18 g sugars

The pretzel core saves you a boatload of calories.

Not That!

Nestlé Butterfinger
(60 g, 1 bar)

270 calories
11 g fat
(6 g saturated)
28 g sugars

Nobody better lay a finger on this Butterfinger.

Andes Creme de Menthe Thins
(38 g, 8 pieces)

200 calories
13 g fat
(11 g saturated)
20 g sugars

This is one of the worst candies in the supermarket. The first two ingredients are sugar and partially hydrogenated oil.

M&M's pack in a lot of sugar even by candy-bar standards. This little bag packs in more sweetness than two Little Debbie Chocolate Marshmallow Pies.

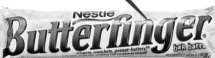
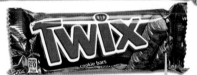
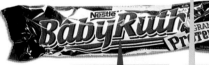
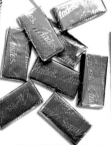

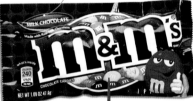

Nestlé Baby Ruth
(44 g, 1 bar)

280 calories
14 g fat
(8 g saturated)
33 g sugars

Together, saturated fat and sugar account for more than 200 of the calories in this package.

Mars Twix Caramel
(51 g, 1 package)

250 calories
12 g fat
(9 g saturated)
33 g carbohydrates
24 g sugars

This package contains nearly as much saturated fat as two Snickers bars.

Starburst Original Fruit Chews
(40 g, 8 pieces)

160 calories
3.5 g fat
(3 g saturated)
23 g sugars

The firmness of the chew owes to the third ingredient: hydrogenated palm kernel oil.

Milk Chocolate M&M's
(48 g, 1 bag)

240 calories
10 g fat
(6 g saturated)
31 g sugars

271

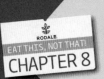

THE FREEZER SECTION

**EAT
THIS
NOT
THAT!**
SUPERMARKET
SURVIVAL GUIDE

Welcome to the Big Chill.

It is the gathering place of overworked bachelorettes, newly divorced dads, starving college students, harried moms, recent parolees, and other folks who just can't muster the physical and mental energy it takes to keep up with Rachael Ray. It is the frozen-foods section of the supermarket or, as it's also known, the pick-up aisle. It is a cold and, yes, a lonely place.

Yet despite its reputation as the last respite of sad singletons on their way home from church basements, the frozen-foods aisle can—and should—be a place where you stock up on nutritional reinforcements, where you build your own personal armory of appetite appeasers. When it's one of those it's-getting-late/I'm-tired/the-game's-on/I'm-hungry/whoa-where'd-my-beer-go? kind of nights, you could reach for the phone and dial up a pepperoni pie from Pizza Hut, quickly setting yourself back $10 and 720 calories for just two slices. Or you could go to your own freezer to extract, having made a wise food choice in a sounder state of mind, a Kashi Mediterranean Pizza that you could heat up even more quickly, two slices of which would cost you more like 290 calories and about half the price. Make a swap like that twice a week and you'd drop 12½ pounds this year alone!

So think of smart shopping in the freezer section as the equivalent of hiring a squad of nutritional bodyguards. Would you rather be eating a home-cooked meal of tortiglioni alla norma with a nice frisée salad and a glass of merlot on the side? Sure, and you'd probably rather be eating it in the sprawling dining room of your Greek Revival mansion overlooking Malibu Beach. But guess what: Sometimes you gotta settle for the best of two mediocre choices. And that's where frozen foods come in. The average American eats frozen foods about 71 times a year, and in almost every case, it's a better deal than ordering takeout.

That said, there's one area where the frozen-foods aisle is actually the best of all worlds: the fruits and vegetables section. While your instinct may be to buy fresh produce, you can save time and boost the nutrition factor of your fruits and vegetables by spending more time chilling in the freezer case. Sure, locally grown produce is the best bet in season, but the frozen version is often just as nutritious, sometimes even more so. Most frozen produce hits the deep freeze within hours of harvest. The "fresh" stuff, on the other hand, has often been flown in from Mexico or Chile, probably shedding a trail of nutrients along the way to your kitchen table. A study published in the journal *Food Chemistry* found that the nutrient statuses of frozen peas, broccoli, carrots, and green beans were equal to those of their "fresh" counterparts in the supermarket produce aisle, while frozen spinach was actually nutritionally superior.

Even better: Those subzero snacks are cheaper, too. A recent survey found that fresh broccoli, snap peas, squash, and green peppers ran $3 or more a pound, while the frozen versions were $1.50 or less a pound. (To maximize your savings, look for bags of frozen vegetables, which tend to cost less than the boxed variety.)

Here are some more tricks to keep in mind when you're facing the big chill:

ADD 8 PERCENT.

To the food's caloric content, that is, when choosing frozen meals. Coming up with exact calorie counts for full dinners is trickier than averaging out what you'll get from a serving of a single food, like a cereal or a soda. And since packagers want to look as nutritionally appealing as possible, they're likely to err on the low side: When Tufts University researchers looked at 10 frozen supermarket meals, they found that the calorie counts reported by the food companies averaged 8 percent less than the researchers' nutritional analyses.

IF YOU'RE NOT EATING IT TOMORROW, BUY IT FROZEN.

This is especially true of fruits, vegetables, and juices. One study found that green beans and spinach lose as much as 75 percent of their vitamin C after being stored in the fridge for a week. And at Arizona State University, an analysis found that ready-to-drink orange juice has significantly lower amounts of vitamin C than frozen juice—and that it loses almost all of its vitamin C within 4 weeks of opening the package.

PLAY MIX AND MATCH WITH WHAT'S ON OFFER.

Why choose between prepackaged meals when you can pick out everything you want to eat and have it all be ready at the same time? Maybe you like sweet peas, chicken cordon blue, and garlic bread. If there's no complete dinner that meets your criteria, just buy all the ingredients separately and heat them up all at once. Buying a bunch of frozen ingredients will keep your palate entertained, and save you money in the long haul.

DON'T BURN YOURSELF.

When scientists found the intact bodies of woolly mammoths frozen in the Siberian ice, they were astounded to discover that the flesh was still edible—no freezer burn

here. Why? Because unlike your leftover T-bones, the mammoth meat was completely enclosed and protected from the air. When meat is exposed to air, even in the freezer, it allows the water molecules to sneak out of the steak like a deadbeat sneaking out on a restaurant tab. To keep your steaks tasty until 2525, remove the fresh meat from its package, wrap it snugly in plastic wrap, and then slip it into a freezer bag, squeezing out as much air as possible.

SKIP THE SODIUM.

Sodium is a good preservative, so it should come as no surprise the freezer is the saltiest section in the supermarket. Read labels carefully to make sure you're not getting more salt than you would with fresh foods. And be sure to factor in the suspicious serving sizes used by frozen food manufacturers to make their products look healthier than they are—there's a good chance you'll be eating more than one serving worth of that pizza, that mac and cheese, or that pot pie.

STOCK UP TO SAVE UP.

It takes more energy to keep air chilled than it does to keep solid food chilled. So the more you pack in your freezer, the cheaper it is to keep it running. Neat trick, huh?

What's Really in...
Hot Pockets Ham & Cheese

L-CYSTEINE

Some combos just can't be beat: PB&J, pizza and beer, cheese and waterfowl feathers... Wait, you've never tried that one? If you've had a Ham & Cheese Hot Pocket you have. Sure, some of that smoky-sweet ham flavor is authentic (presumably), but some of it comes courtesy of the duck feather–derived amino acid L-cysteine. In its role as a food additive, its purpose is to emulate certain flavors. For example, when L-cysteine reacts with sugar, the combination creates a meaty flavor. Disturbing as the idea of fake ham flavoring may be, however, it doesn't even compare to the absurd fact that it requires duck feathers for Hot Pockets to achieve it.

ANNATTO

Yes, even the insides of the Hot Pocket are dyed to look more appealing. Annatto is a natural colorant derived from the South American achiote tree, and it's often used in processed cheese products to impart a rich, golden hue. But hey—at least it's not Yellow 5, right? Well, not so quick; annatto might actually be just as bad as the chemical dyes. A study published in *Archives of Toxicology Supplement* found that the dye caused allergic responses as frequently as artificial dyes did.

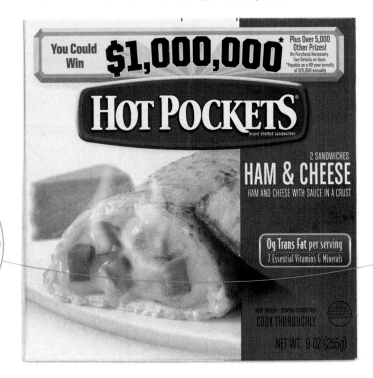

...AINS 2% OR ... bread crumbs [wheat ... arlic powder, reduced lactos ... aprika & annatto), **SUGAR**, P ... ides, salt, L-cysteine hydro ... **'D EGG WHITES.**

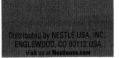

43320792-10

Ingredients: **UNBLEACHED ENRICHED FLOUR** (wheat-flour, malted barley flour, niacin, reduced iron, thiamin mononitrate, riboflavin, folic acid), **WATER, HAM WATER ADDED GROUND AND FORMED, NATURAL SMOKE FLAVOR ADDED** (cured with water, sugar, salt, sodium phosphates, natural smoke flavor, sodium erythorbate, sodium nitrite), **PART SKIM MOZZARELLA CHEESE WITH MODIFIED FOOD STARCH** (part skim mozzarella cheese [pasteurized milk, cultures, salt, enzymes], modified food starch, potassium chloride, flavors, annatto), **SEASONING** (palm oil, maltodextrin, corn syrup solids, wheat flour, salt, cheddar cheese [milk, cheese cultures, salt, enzymes], sodium caseinate, artificial color [titanium dioxide, yellow 6 lake, yellow 5 lake, yellow 5, yellow 6], dipotassium phosphate, lactic acid, natural and artificial flavor, buttermilk powder, calcium lactate, reduced lactose whey, autolyzed yeast extract, butter [cream, salt], whey, disodium phosphate, disodium guanylate, disodium inosinate, whey protein concentrate, sodium citrate), **CONTAINS 2% OR LESS OF: PARTIALLY HYDROGENATED SOYBEAN OIL, PALM OIL** (with soy lecithin, artificial flavor, beta carotene), **MODIFIED FOOD STARCH, SEASONING** (toasted bread crumbs [wheat flour, sugar, yeast, soybean oil, salt], cheddar cheese [milk, cheese cultures, salt, enzymes], salt, whey, dextrose, dehydrated onion, natural flavor, soybean oil, garlic powder, reduced lactose whey, disodium phosphate, citric acid, lactic acid, disodium inosinate & guanylate, spice, blue-cheese [milk, cheese cultures, salt, enzymes], extractives of paprika & annatto), **SUGAR, PARTIALLY HYDROGENATED PALM KERNEL OIL** (with soy lecithin, citric acid as preservative), **DOUGH CONDITIONER** (calcium sulfate, distilled monoglycerides, salt, L-cysteine hydrochloride, garlic powder, tricalcium phosphate, enzymes, ascorbic acid, citric acid, BHT), **DRIED EGG YOLKS, SALT, YEAST, DRIED WHEY, SOY FLOUR, DRIED EGG WHITES. CONTAINS WHEAT, MILK, EGG & SOY INGREDIENTS.**

43320792-10

Distributed by NESTLÉ USA, INC.
ENGLEWOOD, CO 80112 USA
Visit us at Nestleusa.com

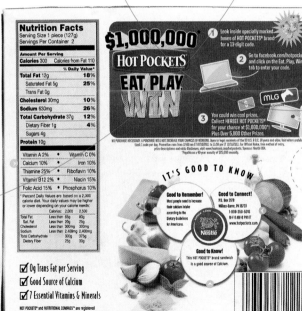

Nutrition Facts
Serving Size 1 piece (127g)
Servings Per Container 2

Amount Per Serving	
Calories 300	Calories from Fat 110

	% Daily Value*
Total Fat 12g	18%
Saturated Fat 5g	25%
Trans Fat 0g	
Cholesterol 30mg	10%
Sodium 630mg	26%
Total Carbohydrate 37g	12%
Dietary Fiber 1g	4%
Sugars 4g	
Protein 10g	

Vitamin A 2%	•	Vitamin C 0%	
Calcium 10%	•	Iron 10%	
Thiamine 25%	•	Riboflavin 10%	
Vitamin B12 2%	•	Niacin 15%	
Folic Acid 15%	•	Phosphorus 10%	

* Percent Daily Values are based on a 2,000 calorie diet. Your daily values may be higher or lower depending on your calorie needs:

	Calories:	2,000	2,500
Total Fat	Less than	65g	80g
Sat. Fat	Less than	20g	25g
Cholesterol	Less than	300mg	300mg
Sodium	Less than	2,400mg	2,400mg
Total Carbohydrate		300g	375g
Dietary Fiber		25g	30g

$1,000,000*
HOT POCKETS
EAT, PLAY WIN

1 Look inside specially marked boxes of HOT POCKETS® brand for a 13-digit code.

2 Go to facebook.com/hotpockets and click on the Eat, Play, Win tab to enter your code.

3 You could win cool prizes. Collect HERBIE HOT POCKETS® for your chance at $1,000,000*! Plus Over 5,000 Other Prizes.

NO PURCHASE NECESSARY. A PURCHASE WILL NOT INCREASE YOUR CHANCES OF WINNING. Open to legal residents of the 50 U.S. & D.C. 18 years and older. Void where prohibited. Limit 1 code per day. Promotion runs from 12:00 am ET 01/16/2012 to 11:59 pm ET 07/15/2012. For Official Rules, free method of entry, prize descriptions and odds disclosure, visit www.facebook.com/hotpockets. Sponsor: Nestlé USA. *Payable as a 40-year annuity of $25,000 annually.

IT'S GOOD TO KNOW

Good to Remember!
Most people need to increase their calcium intake according to the Dietary Guidelines for Americans.

Good to Connect!
P.O. Box 2178
Wilkes-Barre, PA 18703
1-800-350-5016
M-F 8 AM-8 PM ET
www.hotpockets.com

Good to Know!
This HOT POCKETS® brand sandwich is a good source of Calcium.

☑ 0g Trans Fat per Serving
☑ Good Source of Calcium
☑ 7 Essential Vitamins & Minerals

HOT POCKETS® and NUTRITIONAL COMPASS™ are registered trademarks of Société des Produits Nestlé S.A., Vevey, Switzerland. MLG, MAJOR LEAGUE GAMING, and the MLG logo are trademarks of Major League Gaming, Inc.

0 43695 07112 2

RCH (part skim n
up solids, wheat flour, sa
otassium phosphate, lactic a
nate, disodium guanylate, d
h soy lecithin, artificial flave
ultures, salt, enzymes], s
& guanylate, spi

DISODIUM GUANYLATE

Fish and seaweed have a place in your diet. Take the sushi bar, for instance; it's a great place to get both. But in your Hot Pocket? That doesn't sound so good. But essentially, that's what you're getting here. Disodium guanylate is made from dehydrated sardines or seaweed. It's used to imbue a smoky, meaty flavor that apparently Hot Pockets' pork, noted here by the unsavory moniker "ham water added ground and formed," simply can't match.

Skinny Cow French Vanilla

MICROCRYSTALLINE CELLULOSE

Sure, we love the idea of produce at the dessert table, but this is a little extreme. Microcrystalline cellulose, the main ingredient in this "ice cream" bar, is actually finely ground wood pulp. Its intended purpose is to absorb water and prevent ice crystal formation, but what's odd is that it appears even before dairy in the hierarchy of ingredients. Is it dangerous? Probably not, but it's one of the ways Skinny Cow achieves a large serving size with so few calories. It also may be one of the reasons diet desserts can feel so unfulfilling. Either way, it's a little strange to think that a fudge-drizzled frozen dessert started out as a tree before it landed in the freezer aisle.

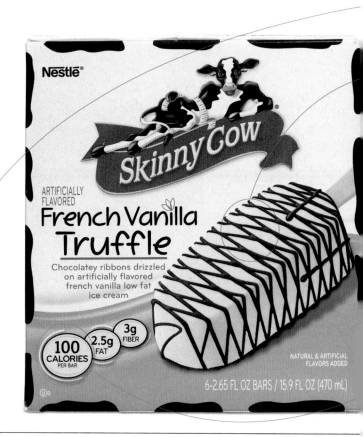

per gram:
• Carbohydrate 4 •

P, CHOCOLATEY RIBBONS (COCONUT OIL,
ILK, CHOCOLATE, ARTIFICIAL FLAVOR, SOY L
IN, CALCIUM CARBONATE, INULIN (DIETARY
MICROCRYSTALLINE CELLULOSE,
AM, MONOGLYCERIDES, SORBITOL, CAROB BE
E, ANNATTO COLOR, CARRAGEENAN, NATURA

5929 COLLEGE AVE., OAK
by Société d

Nestlé

Skinny Cow

ARTIFICIALLY FLAVORED
French Vanilla Truffle

Chocolatey ribbons drizzled on artificially flavored french vanilla low fat ice cream

100 CALORIES PER BAR

2.5g FAT

3g FIBER

NATURAL & ARTIFICIAL FLAVORS ADDED

6-2.65 FL OZ BARS / 15.9 FL OZ (470 mL)

Truffle Bars

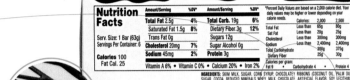

Nutrition Facts

Serv. Size: 1 Bar (63g)
Servings Per Container: 6

Calories 100
Fat Cal. 25

Amount/Serving	%DV*	Amount/Serving	%DV*
Total Fat 2.5g	4%	Total Carb. 19g	6%
Saturated Fat 1.5g	8%	Dietary Fiber 3g	12%
Trans Fat 0g		Sugars 12g	
Cholesterol 20mg	7%	Sugar Alcohol 0g	
Sodium 45mg	2%	Protein 3g	

Vitamin A 6% • Vitamin C 0% • Calcium 20% • Iron 2%

*Percent Daily Values are based on a 2,000 calorie diet. Your daily values may be higher or lower depending on your calorie needs.

		2,000	2,500
Total Fat	Less than	65g	80g
Sat Fat	Less than	20g	25g
Cholesterol	Less than	300mg	300mg
Sodium	Less than	2,400mg	2,400mg
Total Carbohydrate		300g	375g
Dietary Fiber		25g	30g

Calories per gram:
Fat 9 • Carbohydrate 4 • Protein 4

INGREDIENTS: SKIM MILK, SUGAR, CORN SYRUP, CHOCOLATEY RIBBONS (COCONUT OIL, PALM OIL, SUGAR, COCOA, REDUCED MINERALS WHEY, MILK, CHOCOLATE, ARTIFICIAL FLAVOR, SOY LECITHIN), POLYDEXTROSE, EGG YOLKS, WHEY PROTEIN, CALCIUM CARBONATE, INULIN (DIETARY FIBER), PROPYLENE GLYCOL MONOSTEARATE, MICROCRYSTALLINE CELLULOSE, SODIUM CARBOXYMETHYLCELLULOSE, GUAR GUM, CREAM, MONOGLYCERIDES, SORBITOL, CAROB BEAN GUM, GROUND VANILLA BEANS, VITAMIN A PALMITATE, ANNATTO COLOR, CARRAGEENAN, NATURAL FLAVOR, INVERT SUGAR, SALT.

DISTRIBUTED BY: DREYER'S GRAND ICE CREAM, INC., 5929 COLLEGE AVE., OAKLAND, CA 94618
Unless noted to the contrary, all trademarks are owned by Société des Produits Nestlé S.A., Vevey, Switzerland.
KEEP FROZEN UNTIL SERVED   INNER UNITS NOT LABELED FOR RETAIL SALE

PointsPlus 3

The PointsPlus™ value for this product was calculated by Dreyer's Grand Ice Cream, Inc. and is provided for informational purposes only. This is not an endorsement, sponsorship or approval of this product or its manufacturer by Weight Watchers International, Inc., the owner of the Weight Watchers® and PointsPlus™ trademarks.

"CHOCOLATEY RIBBONS"

Chocolate and chocolatey are two very different substances, especially in the world of processed food. Chocolate is comprised of cocoa butter and cocoa solids; "chocolatey ribbons" are made mostly from low-grade oils, sugar, and artificial flavors. Which would you prefer for dessert tonight?

100 CALORIES PER BAR

"100 CALORIES"

Sweets and snacks manufacturers love to display this number on their packages, as if it were a seal of approval from the American Diatetic Association. Not quite. Hostess cupcakes, Oreos, Chips Ahoy—all are offered in 100-calorie packs and are all potent reminders that low calorie doesn't mean healthy.

CARRAGEENAN

This is a thickener, stabilizer, and emulsifier extracted from red seaweed. It boasts some impressive benefits, but some troubling effects as well. On one hand, carrageenan may have some antiviral and virus-inhibiting capabilities. But conversely, in animal studies, the compound has been shown to cause ulcers, colon inflammation, and digestive tract cancers. The negative effects seem limited to degraded carrageenen—a class that has been treated with heat and chemicals—but a University of Iowa study concluded that even undegraded carrageenan could become degraded in the human digestive system.

Frozen Breakfast Ent

Eat This

An ideal breakfast includes a substantial load of protein, and this bowl has that nailed. Protein accounts for 40 percent of the calories, which increases your odds of making it to lunch without snacking.

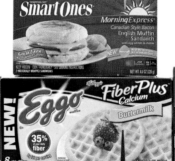

Smart Ones Morning Express Canadian Style Bacon English Muffin Sandwich
(113 g, 1 sandwich)

210 calories
6 g fat
(2.5 g saturated)
510 mg sodium
2 g fiber
13 g protein

Next to ham, Canadian bacon is the leanest of the breakfast meats.

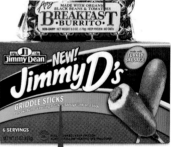

Amy's Black Beans & Tomatoes Breakfast Burrito
(170 g, 1 burrito)

270 calories
8 g fat
(1 g saturated)
540 mg sodium
5 g fiber
11 g protein

Black beans are one of the most antioxidant-rich, fiber-packed foods on the planet.

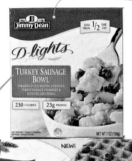

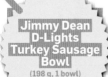

Jimmy Dean D-Lights Turkey Sausage Bowl
(198 g, 1 bowl)

230 calories
7 g fat (3 g saturated)
710 mg sodium
2 g fiber
23 g protein

Kashi Blueberry Waffles
(72 g, 2 waffles)

150 calories
5 g fat
(0.5 g saturated)
340 mg sodium
6 g fiber
4 g protein

Kashi lists whole grains and blueberries prominently on the ingredients list, hence the huge hit of fiber found in these first-rate waffles.

Kellogg's Eggo FiberPlus Calcium Buttermilk Waffles
(70 g, 2 waffles)

160 calories
6 g fat
(1.5 g saturated)
390 mg sodium
9 g fiber
3 g protein

The most fiber-packed waffles in the freezer, guaranteed to beat back hunger for hours.

Jimmy D's Griddle Sticks
(71 g, 1 stick)

160 calories
6 g fat
(1.5 g saturated)
410 mg sodium
0 g fiber
7 g protein

Even the most finicky eater can be won over with this meal, and the fact that it's made with low-fat turkey sausage prevents it from doing too much damage.

Not That!

Evol Egg & Potato Burrito
(227 g, 1 burrito)

440 calories
13 g fat (4 g saturated)
820 mg sodium
4 g fiber
17 g protein

Evol makes some decent burritos, but this isn't one of them. It features more potatoes than eggs, resulting in an oversized cargo of carbohydrates.

Aunt Jemima Griddlecake Sandwiches Sausage, Egg & Cheese
(125 g, 1 sandwich)

350 calories
20 g fat
(7 g saturated)
900 mg sodium
<1 g fiber
13 g protein

Teeming with saturated fat. Plus, sugar is the second ingredient.

More than 150 of these calories are carbohydrates, which is not how you want to start your day.

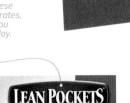

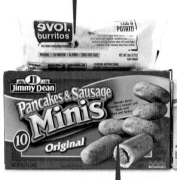

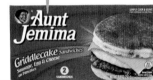

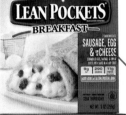

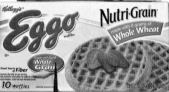

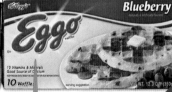

Jimmy Dean Original Pancake & Sausage Minis
(96 g, 4 pieces)

320 calories
19 g fat
(6 g saturated)
800 mg sodium
1 g fiber
9 g protein

Speckled with fat and saddled with sodium, sausage is the bane of the breakfast table.

Kellogg's Eggo Nutri-Grain Whole Wheat Waffles
(70 g, 2 waffles)

170 calories
6 g fat
(1.5 g saturated)
400 mg sodium
3 g fiber
5 g protein

A big improvement over regular Eggos, but they still can't compete with the best in the freezer.

Kellogg's Eggo Blueberry Waffles
(70 g, 2 waffles)

190 calories
6 g fat
(1.5 g saturated)
370 mg sodium
<1 g fiber
4 g protein

Blueberries are the 11th ingredient on the list. Switch to Kashi's waffles and the superfruit jumps up to the third position.

Lean Pockets Sausage, Egg & Cheese
(127 g, 1 piece)

290 calories
9 g fat (4 g saturated)
470 mg sodium
2 g fiber
11 g protein

Frozen Quick Bites &

Eat This

Ian's Natural Foods Fish Sticks
(93 g, 5 sticks)

190 calories
6 g fat
(1 g saturated)
310 mg sodium

Ian's sticks are made with pollock, and they contain no ingredients you wouldn't use in your own kitchen.

Ling Ling All Natural Mini Spring Rolls Vegetable
(156 g, 3 pieces and sauce)

210 calories
7 g fat
(0 g saturated)
630 mg sodium

Each vegetable-stuffed roll provides nearly a quarter of your day's vitamin A.

The corn tortillas help keep the calorie and fat counts in check. Plus, each individual taquito delivers 5 grams of protein and 2 grams of fiber.

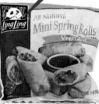

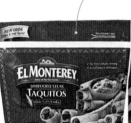
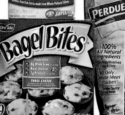
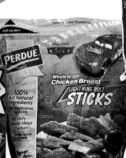

El Monterey Shredded Steak Corn Taquitos
(85 g, 2 taquitos)

160 calories
4 g fat
(1 g saturated)
250 mg sodium

Ore-Ida Bagel Bites Three Cheese
(88 g, 4 pieces)

190 calories
5 g fat
(2.5 g saturated)
370 mg sodium

Add a slice of deli ham before baking to boost the protein in these mini pizzas.

Perdue Whole Grain Chicken Breast Lightning Bolt Sticks
(88 g, 5 pieces)

290 calories
9 g fat
(2 g saturated)
460 mg sodium

The whole-wheat flour used to encase these nuggets helps add a full gram of fiber to each.

Lean Pockets Stuffed Quesadilla Grilled Chicken Fajita
(92 g, 1 piece)

170 calories
4 g fat
(1.5 g saturated)
340 mg sodium

White-meat chicken, onions and peppers all work to provide maximum flavor for minumum calories.

Health Is Wealth Jalapeño & Cheese Munchees
(99 g, 7 pieces)

198 calories
3.5 g fat
(1 g saturated)
595 mg sodium

The sodium is high, but each popper has less than 30 calories. You could do worse.

Appetizers

THE FREEZER SECTION

Not That!

Ling Ling All Natural Potstickers Vegetable Dumpling
(166 g, 5 pieces and sauce)

300 calories
4 g fat
(0.5 g saturated)
1,110 mg sodium

Each small sticker has about 10 percent of your day's sodium intake.

Gorton's Classic Breaded Fish Sticks (104 g, 6 sticks)

250 calories
15 g fat
(4 g saturated)
360 mg sodium

The hefty ingredients list contains both MSG and TBHQ (tertbutyl-hydro-quinone), an additive that has been reported to cause hyperactivity and behavioral problems in children.

It's not the extra 100 calories and 230 milligrams of sodium that bother us the most. It's the inexplicable appearance of trans fats in these mini miscreants.

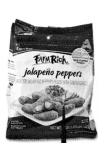
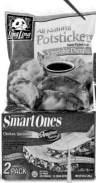
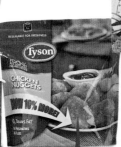
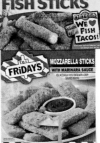
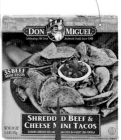

Farm Rich Stuffed Jalapeño Peppers
(96 g, 4 pieces)

240 calories
16 g fat
(6 g saturated)
820 mg sodium

Farm Rich's poppers contain no fiber and trace amounts of protein, which means they'll have a negligible impact on your hunger.

Smart Ones Anytime Selections Quesadilla Chicken
(113 g, 1 piece)

210 calories
6 g fat
(2.5 g saturated)
470 mg sodium

Too meager to constitute a meal, but too caloric and sodium-riddled to serve as a snack.

Tyson Chicken Nuggets
(90 g, 5 pieces)

270 calories
17 g fat
(4 g saturated)
470 mg sodium

If you're going to feed your kids fried chicken, the least you can do is make sure they get some fiber out of it. Perdue's new sticks pack 5 grams per serving. Tyson's? Zilch.

T.G.I. Friday's Mozzarella Sticks
(no sauce)
(96 g, 3 pieces)

300 calories
13.5 g fat
(4.5 g saturated)
510 mg sodium

It's never a good idea to wrap cheese in breading and drop it in a deep fryer.

Don Miguel El Charrito Beef & Cheese Mini Tacos
(79 g, 4 mini tacos)

260 calories
13 g fat
(4 g saturated, 1 g trans)
480 mg sodium

285

Frozen Pizzas
Eat This

This pie features more pesto than cheese, which means you end up with more monounsaturated fat from olive oil than saturated fat from dairy. That's a healthy swap.

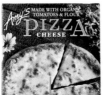
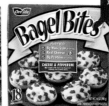
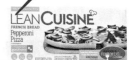

New!

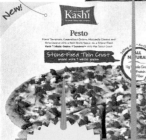

Kashi Pesto Stone-Fired Thin Crust
(113 g, ⅓ pie)

240 calories
9 g fat (3.5 g saturated)
590 mg sodium
27 g carbohydrates
14 g protein

Amy's Cheese Pizza
(167 g, 1 pie)

420 calories
17 g fat (6 g saturated)
720 mg sodium
56 g carbohydrates
18 g protein

For the rare times when you allow yourself the privilege of eating a whole pizza, this is where you should turn. Exactly what a personal serving size should be.

Newman's Own Uncured Pepperoni Thin & Crispy
(125 g, ⅓ pie)

320 calories
16 g fat (6 g saturated)
800 mg sodium
31 g carbohydrates
15 g protein

Newman's eschews chemical nitrates and nitrites in favor of sea salt and celery juice for their uncured pepperoni.

Tofurky Vegan Cheese
(113 g, ¼ pie)

240 calories
8 g fat
(2.5 g saturated)
350 mg sodium
39 g carbohydrates
6 g protein

Tofurky's "cheese" is made using a combination of protein, flour, and oils. It's a great alternative for those who are lactose intolerant.

Not That!

Red Baron Singles Pepperoni French Bread Pizza
(153 g, 1 pizza)

380 calories
15 g fat (7 g saturated)
1,090 mg sodium
43 g carbohydrates
16 g protein

After bread, the next two ingredients are water and soybean oil—not exactly a recipe for a delicious (or nutritious) pizza.

Michelina's Lean Gourmet Pepperoni Pizza Snackers
(85 g, 11 pieces)

200 calories
8 g fat (1.5 g saturated)
290 mg sodium
26 g carbohydrates
7 g protein

Blame the fatty pastry crust. After flour and water, the first two ingredients are shortening and sugar.

The crust is the least nutritious part of any pie, and unfortunately, the heft of Amy's outweighs the fact that it's made with whole wheat flour.

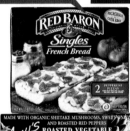
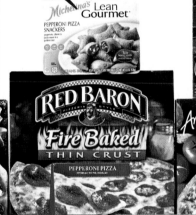
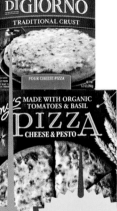
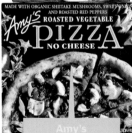

Amy's Roasted Vegetable No Cheese
(113 g, ⅓ pie)

280 calories
9 g fat (1.5 g saturated)
540 mg sodium
42 g carbohydrates
7 g protein

Not bad if you're looking for a cheeseless flatbread, but for the lactose intolerant, why not enjoy something closer to the real thing?

Red Baron Fire Baked Thin Crust Pepperoni Pizza
(149 g, ½ pie)

400 calories
19 g fat (9 g saturated)
960 mg sodium
40 g carbohydrates
17 g protein

We hate to pick on the Baron, but even his thin crust pies pack too much of the bad stuff to win our approval.

DiGiorno Traditional Crust Four Cheese
(260 g, 1 pie)

710 calories
30 g fat (11 g saturated, 3.5 g trans)
1,190 mg sodium
85 g carbohydrates
26 g protein

DiGiorno's personal pie is swamped with sodium, sugar, and trans fats, making it easily the worst in the freezer.

Amy's Whole Wheat Crust Cheese & Pesto
(132 g, ⅓ pie)

360 calories
18 g fat (4 g saturated)
680 mg sodium
37 g carbohydrates
13 g protein

Frozen Pasta Entrées
Eat This

If you do it daily, the 40 calories you save by eating Kashi's Chicken Pasta Pomodoro instead of Smart Ones' Three Cheese Ziti will help you shed more than 4 pounds in a year. And you'll be less hungry while you do it, too, because Kashi's meal provides more protein and fiber.

Kashi Chicken Pasta Pomodoro
(283 g, 1 entrée)

280 calories
6 g fat (1.5 g saturated)
470 mg sodium
38 g carbohydrates
19 g protein

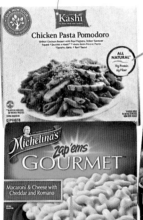

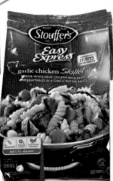

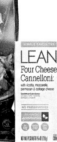

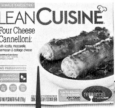

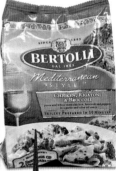

Michelina's Zap'ems Gourmet Macaroni & Cheese with Cheddar and Romano
(213 g, 1 package)

260 calories
6 g fat (2.5 g saturated)
500 mg sodium
39 g carbohydrates
10 g protein

Diffuse the comfort food's flab-producing potential with this light rendition.

Stouffer's Easy Express Garlic Chicken Skillet
(326 g, ½ package)

330 calories
6 g fat (2.5 g saturated)
990 mg sodium
45 g carbohydrates
24 g protein

Budding chefs take note: The more vegetables you use, the less sauce and pasta you'll need.

Lean Cuisine Four Cheese Cannelloni
(258 g, 1 package)

240 calories
6 g fat (3 g saturated)
690 mg sodium
30 g carbohydrates
17 g protein

Swap out white sauce for red sauce and you'll save calories every time, no exception.

Bertolli Mediterranean Style Chicken, Rigatoni & Broccoli
(340 g, ½ package)

380 calories
15 g fat (4 g saturated)
970 mg sodium
37 g carbohydrates
22 g protein

After pasta, the first two ingredients are broccoli and chicken.

Not That!

Smart Ones Three Cheese Ziti Marinara
(255 g, 1 entrée)

Marinara is typically the safest of the pasta sauces, but that rule fails to hold as soon as Smart Ones buries the plate under a rubbery quilt of cheese.

300 calories
8 g fat (3.5 g saturated)
580 mg sodium
44 g carbohydrates
14 g protein

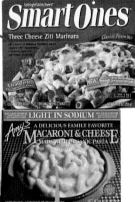

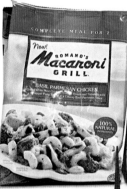

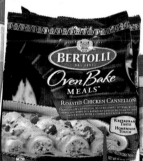

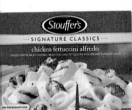

Romano's Macaroni Grill Basil Parmesan Chicken
(340 g, ½ package)

460 calories
20 g fat
(12 g saturated)
1,050 mg sodium
42 g carbohydrates
29 g protein

A heavy hand with the cream laces this pasta with more than half a day of saturated fat.

Bertolli Oven Bake Meals Roasted Chicken Cannelloni
(298 g, ½ package)

490 calories
28 g fat
(11 g saturated)
1,030 mg sodium
37 g carbohydrates
23 g protein

These noodles are stuffed with cheese and covered with cream. Call it dairy fat overload.

Stouffer's Chicken Fettuccini Alfredo
(297 g, 1 package)

570 calories
27 g fat
(10 g saturated)
850 mg sodium
55 g carbohydrates
26 g protein

Alfredo sauce contains any of the following: oil, butter, cheese, cream, and egg yolk. In other words, it's a full-fat assault.

Amy's Light in Sodium Macaroni & Cheese
(255 g, 1 entrée)

400 calories
16 g fat
(10 g saturated)
290 mg sodium
47 g carbohydrates
16 g protein

We've seen worse mac out there, but Amy's packages its pasta as a healthy alternative, and we're just not buying it.

289

Frozen Fish Entrées
Eat This

The smoky, spicy finesse of a blackening rub can imbue any fillet with massive flavor at no caloric cost. It's easily one of the healthiest ways to prepare meat and fish.

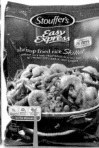

SeaPak Salmon Burgers
(91 g, 1 burger)

110 calories
5 g fat
(1 g saturated)
340 mg sodium
16 g protein

Toss this on the grill, then sandwich it between a toasted bun with arugula, grilled onions, and Greek yogurt spiked with olive oil, garlic, and fresh dill.

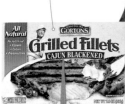

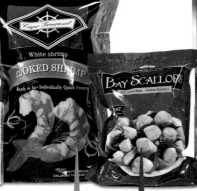

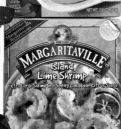

Gorton's Cajun Blackened Grilled Fillets
(108 g, 1 fillet)

90 calories
3 g fat
(0.5 g saturated)
400 mg sodium
16 g protein

Cape Gourmet Cooked Shrimp
(3 oz)

50 calories
0.5 g fat
330 mg sodium
10 g protein

Unadulterated shrimp are one of the leanest sources of protein on the planet.

Northern King Bay Scallops
(4 oz)

150 calories
1 g fat
(0 g saturated)
155 mg sodium
29 g protein

Scallops are teeming with the amino acid tryptophan, which bolsters feelings of wellbeing and helps regulate sleep cycles.

Margaritaville Island Lime Shrimp
(4 oz, 6 shrimp)

240 calories
11 g fat
(3 g saturated)
330 mg sodium
12 g protein

These shrimp have also been tossed in butter. The difference is quantity; here it's a light bath, but in SeaPak's scampi it's a tidal wave.

Stouffer's Easy Express Shrimp Fried Rice Skillet
(354 g, ½ package)

290 calories
3 g fat
(0.5 g saturated)
980 mg sodium
14 g protein

American interpretations of Asian cuisine tend to be high in sodium, but 13 grams of fiber more than make up for it.

Not That!

SeaPak Seasoned Ahi Tuna Steaks
(128 g, 1 steak)

240 calories
14 g fat
(1 g saturated)
840 mg sodium
24 g protein

SeaPak goes heavy on both the oil and the salt to weaken an otherwise solid hunk of fish. Buy your tuna unadulterated.

You know what makes the breading crispy? The same thing that makes it 150 percent more caloric and 267 percent fattier: oil.

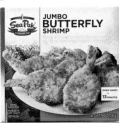

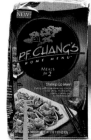

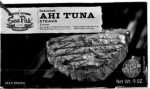

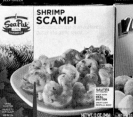

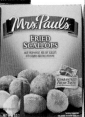

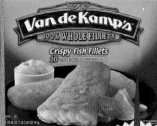

PF Chang's Home Menu Shrimp Lo Mein
(312 g, ½ package)

360 calories
12 g fat
(1 g saturated)
1,550 mg sodium
22 g protein

Chang's sauce is polluted with three kinds of oil.

SeaPak Shrimp Scampi
(4 oz, 113 g, 6 shrimp)

340 calories
31 g fat
(14 g saturated)
540 mg sodium
11 g protein

Shrimp are essentially pure protein, so it's puzzling to find that protein accounts for just 13 percent of this entrée's calories.

Mrs. Paul's Fried Scallops
(13 scallops)

260 calories
11 g fat
(4 g saturated)
700 mg sodium
12 g protein

Scallops are one of the sea's greatest gifts to man. Spoiling them with the fry treatment is an abomination. You end up with more calories from fat than protein.

SeaPak Jumbo Butterfly Shrimp
(3 oz, 84 g, 4 shrimp)

210 calories
10 g fat
(1.5 g saturated)
480 mg sodium
10 g protein

Each shrimp delivers more than 50 calories, and nearly half of that comes from unnecessary fats.

Van de Kamp's Crispy Fish Fillets
(110 g, 2 fillets)

210 calories
10 g fat
(3.5 g saturated)
690 mg sodium
9 g protein

Frozen Chicken Entré

Eat This

Kashi Lemongrass Coconut Chicken
(283 g, 1 entrée)

300 calories
8 g fat
(4 g saturated)
680 mg sodium
38 g carbohydrates
18 g protein

Kashi makes the best frozen dinners in the supermarket.

Evol's teriyaki bowl is made with brown rice, free-range chicken, and enough produce to meet 90 percent of your day's vitamin A needs.

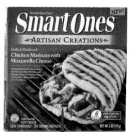

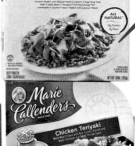

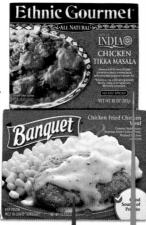

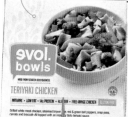

Evol Bowls Teriyaki Chicken
(255 g, 1 bowl)

250 calories
6 g fat
(1 g saturated)
490 mg sodium
34 g carbohydrates
14 g protein

Banquet Chicken Fried Chicken Meal (286 g, 1 entrée)

350 calories
17 g fat
(4 g saturated)
930 mg sodium
35 g carbohydrates
12 g protein

A thinner coating of breading and a heavier reliance on sides saves you 90 calories over Banquet's "premium" take on the same meal.

Ethnic Gourmet Chicken Tikka Masala (283 g, 1 package)

260 calories
6 g fat
(2 g saturated)
680 mg sodium
32 g carbohydrates
19 g protein

The sauce is created with nonfat yogurt, which provides the thick heft of cream without all the calories.

Marie Callender's Fresh Flavor Steamer Chicken Teriyaki (283 g, 1 entrée)

280 calories
3.5 g fat
(1 g saturated)
890 mg sodium
44 g carbohydrates
17 g protein

At it's best, this new line from Marie can compete with anyone in the freezer.

Smart Ones Artisan Creations Grilled Flatbread Chicken Marinara with Mozzarella Cheese (170 g, 1 flatbread)

290 calories
6 g fat
(1.5 g saturated)
640 mg sodium
41 g carbohydrates
18 g protein

es

Not That!

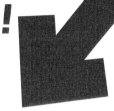

Marie Callender's Fresh Flavor Steamer Sesame Chicken
(291 g, 1 meal)

400 calories
12 g fat
(2 g saturated)
710 mg sodium
54 g carbohydrates
18 g protein

Get as much protein and more fiber for 100 fewer calories.

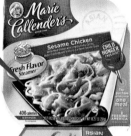

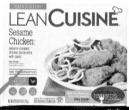

Another Healthy Choice dessert masquerading as dinner. This bowl contains 29 grams of sugar, as much as you'd find in two scoops of Breyers All Natural Chocolate Ice Cream.

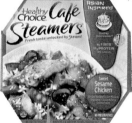

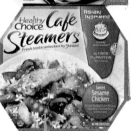

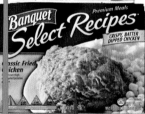

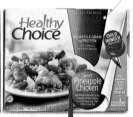

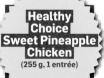

Lean Cuisine Chicken Club Panini
(170 g, 1 panini)

360 calories
9 g fat
(3.5 g saturated)
675 mg sodium
45 g carbohydrates
24 g protein

Saving 70 calories might not seem like much, but do it once a day and you'll lose 7 pounds this year.

Healthy Choice Café Steamers Sweet Sesame Chicken
(292 g, 1 meal)

340 calories
5 g fat
(1 g saturated)
330 mg sodium
55 g carbohydrates
17 g protein

Packs as much sugar as a two-pack of peanut butter Twix.

Lean Cuisine Sesame Chicken
(255 g, 1 package)

330 calories
9 g fat
(1 g saturated)
650 mg sodium
47 g carbohydrates
16 g protein

There's nothing lean about breaded chicken tossed with 14 grams of sugar.

Banquet Select Recipes Classic Fried Chicken Meal (228 g, 1 entrée)

440 calories
26 g fat
(6 g saturated,
1.5 g trans)
1,140 mg sodium
30 g carbohydrates
22 g protein

This is one of the worst in Banquet's line of freezer entrées.

Healthy Choice Sweet Pineapple Chicken
(255 g, 1 entrée)

380 calories
7 g fat
(1 g saturated)
190 mg sodium
70 g carbohydrates
9 g protein

293

Frozen Beef Entrées

Eat This

If you'd rather eat a potpie, just pour this into a bowl and eat it with a piece of toasted whole-grain bread. There, all the potpie perks without the fat.

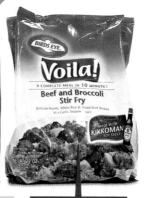

Hot Pockets Sideshots Cheeseburgers
(127 g, 2 buns)

290 calories
10 g fat (4 g saturated)
660 mg sodium
37 g carbohydrates
12 g protein

A fairly innocuous snack to set in front of a group of hungry kids.

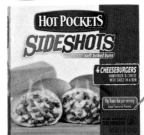

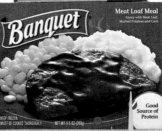

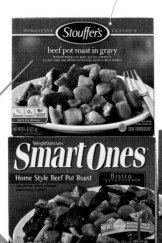

Stouffer's Homestyle Classics Beef Pot Roast
(251 g, 1 entrée)

230 calories
7 g fat (2 g saturated)
820 mg sodium
26 g carbohydrates
16 g protein

Smart Ones Home Style Beef Roast
(255 g, 1 meal)

180 calories
4.5 g fat (2 g saturated)
670 mg sodium
18 g carbohydrates
17 g protein

Most protein bars can't deliver this dose for so few calories. Tack on 4 g of fiber and you have an amazing 180-calorie package.

Banquet Meat Loaf Meal
(269 g, 1 meal)

280 calories
13 g fat (5 g saturated)
1,000 mg sodium
28 g carbohydrates
12 g protein

When it comes to delivering comfort dishes for a reasonable number of calories, Banquet's regular line of entrées is among the best in the freezer.

Birds Eye Voila! Beef and Broccoli Stir Fry
(218 g, 1¾ cup)

210 calories
6 g fat (1.5 g saturated)
700 mg sodium
27 g carbohydrates
10 g protein

The first ingredient in this bag is broccoli. In the cost-conscious world of processed foods, that's exceedingly rare.

Not That!

A potpie crust is essentially an oversized pastry, which is to say lots of carbohydrates glued together with saturated fat.

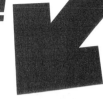

Smart Ones Mini Cheeseburgers
(140 g, 2 mini-burgers)

400 calories
18 g fat (8 g saturated)
720 mg sodium
40 g carbohydrates
20 g protein

Each burger has 20 percent of your day's saturated fat.

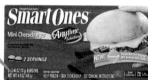

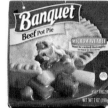

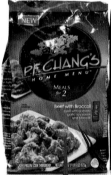

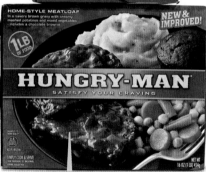

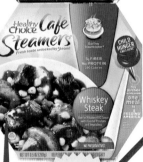

PF Chang's Home Menu Beef with Broccoli
(312 g, ½ package)

360 calories
18 g fat (3 g saturated)
1,330 mg sodium
26 g carbohydrates
21 g protein

Chang's bagged meals suffer from the same malady as its restaurant fare, which is to say far too much sodium.

Hungry-Man Home-Style Meatloaf
(484 g, 1 package)

660 calories
35 g fat (12 g saturated)
1,660 mg sodium
61 g carbohydrates
26 g protein

Word of advice to the calorie conscious: Purge Hungry-Man from your freezer for good. This is the worst brand in the frozen-foods aisle.

Healthy Choice Café Steamers Grilled Whiskey Steak
(269 g, 1 meal)

290 calories
4 g fat (1.5 g saturated)
480 mg sodium
47 g carbohydrates
16 g protein

More than a quarter of the calories in this box come from added sugars.

Banquet Beef Pot Pie
(198 g, 1 pie)

390 calories
22 g fat (9 g saturated, 0.5 g trans)
1,010 mg sodium
36 g carbohydrates
10 g protein

Frozen Meatless Entr

Eat This

Eggplant parm is normally a ruse, a greasy, cheesy gut bomb masquerading as vegetarian virtue. But Cedarlane's version is the real deal; the first four ingredients are eggplant, tomatoes, tomato puree, and onions.

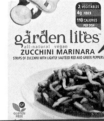
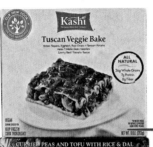

Garden Lites Zucchini Marinara
(198 g, 1 package)

110 calories
4 g fat
(0.5 g saturated)
390 mg sodium

Garden Lites cuts out the carb overload of regular pasta by replacing the noodles with thick strands of zucchini.

Kashi Tuscan Veggie Bake
(283 g, 1 meal)

260 calories
9 g fat
(1.5 g saturated)
700 mg sodium

This dish packs an impressive 8 grams of fiber, thanks to the potent collaboration of whole-grain noodles, beans, squash, eggplant, tomatoes, sweet potatoes, and lentils.

Cedarlane Eggplant Parmesan
(282 g, 1 package)

320 calories
16 g fat
(6 g saturated)
780 mg sodium

MorningStar Farms Lasagna with Sausage-Style Crumbles
(284 g, 1 entrée)

270 calories
6 g fat
(2.5 g saturated)
590 mg sodium

Twenty grams of protein, 6 grams of fiber, and relatively low sodium. Not bad for a meatless microwave dinner.

Amy's Indian Mattar Tofu
(269 g, 1 entrée)

280 calories
8 g fat
(1 g saturated)
680 mg sodium

Indian cuisine's potent flavors are derived primarily from antioxidant-rich spices like turmeric, cardamom, and coriander.

Amy's Burrito Beans, Rice, and Cheddar Cheese
(170 g, 1 burrito)

310 calories
9 g fat
(2.5 g saturated)
580 mg sodium

Make this burrito a quick weekday lunch and the 7 grams of fiber will help beat back those late-afternoon hunger pangs.

Lean Cuisine Cheddar Potatoes with Broccoli
(289 g, 1 meal)

210 calories
4 g fat
(1.5 g saturated)
600 mg sodium

The potatoes and broccoli in this dish help add 820 milligrams of potassium, which go a long way toward negating the negative effect of sodium.

Not That!

This is more along the lines of what you'd expect from a breaded, fried, and cheesed entrée. Even if you sawed this meal in half, you'd still be left with more than 20 grams of fat.

Healthy Choice Roasted Red Pepper Marinara
(241 g, 1 meal)

270 calories
6 g fat
(2 g saturated)
560 mg sodium

Aside from the lycopene in the marinara sauce, this meal contributes little nutritionally.

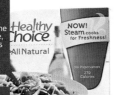

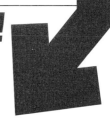

Stouffer's Farmers' Harvest Vegetable Lasagna
(298 g, 1 meal)

400 calories
19 g fat
(7 g saturated)
680 mg sodium

Stouffer's lasagna delivers a nice array of produce, but unfortunately that doesn't protect you from the excessive use of cheese and soybean oil.

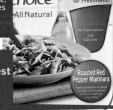

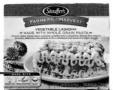

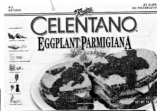

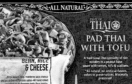

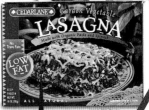

Amy's Bowls Country Cheddar
(269 g, 1 bowl)

430 calories
21 g fat
(6 g saturated)
690 mg sodium

The noodles may be organic, but they're still drowning in a sea of molten cheese.

Evol Bean, Rice, and Cheese
(227 g, 1 burrito)

460 calories
8 g fat
(2.5 g saturated)
650 mg sodium

EVOL's biggest slip here is with the oversized tortilla, which helps push the carb count up to 78 grams.

Ethnic Gourmet Bowl Pad Thai with Tofu
(283 g, 1 entrée)

420 calories
8 g fat
(1.5 g saturated)
720 mg sodium

At 25 grams per serving, this dish has more sugar than a scoop of Ben & Jerry's Peanut Butter Cup Ice Cream.

Cedarlane Low Fat Garden Vegetable Lasagna
(284 g, 1 package)

360 calories
6 g fat
(4 g saturated)
780 mg sodium

Even with 90 more calories, Cedarlane's lasagna has half the protein and a third the fiber as MorningStar's.

Celentano Eggplant Parmigiana
(396 g, 1 package)

660 calories
44 g fat
(10 g saturated)
960 mg sodium

Frozen Sides
Eat This

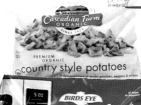

Cascadian Farm Country Style Potatoes
(85 g, ¾ cup)

50 calories
0 g fat
10 mg sodium

This bag contains a total of four ingredients: potatoes, onions, green peppers, and red peppers. Perfect.

Shoestring fries typically soak up more fat, but these skinny-cut spuds are the exception to that rule. Cascadian Farm dips them in apple juice before bagging, which helps them brown up nice in the oven. No deep-frying required.

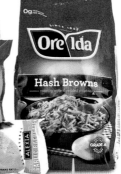

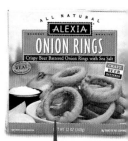

Cascadian Farm Shoe String French Fries
(85 g, 3 oz)

110 calories
5 g fat
(1 g saturated)
10 mg sodium

Alexia Garlic Baguette
(43 g, 2 pieces)

130 calories
4.5 g fat
(2.5 g saturated)
240 mg sodium

This is the lowest-calorie garlic bread on the market.

Birds Eye Steamfresh Vegetables Italian Blend
(100 g, 1 cup)

40 calories
0 g fat
47 mg sodium

Birds Eye's blend comes ready to steam in a microwaveable bag. That makes it both healthy and simple.

Ore-Ida Country Style Hash Browns
(87 g)

70 calories
0 g fat
20 mg sodium

These hash browns are pure potato, and they make a perfect low-cal accompaniment for eggs.

Alexia Onion Rings Beer Battered
(85 g, 6 rings)

180 calories
8 g fat
(1 g saturated)
240 mg sodium

Alexia's beer-battered rings have less breading, which means fewer carbs and less fat-absorbing potential.

Not That!

Alexia
Sauté Reds
(1 cup, 182 g)

200 calories
12 g fat
(1.5 g saturated)
180 mg sodium

Sauteing is normally
a pretty healthy form of
cooking, but these
spuds emerge with
more calories than most
fried potatoes
in the freezer section.

These fries come predunked in oil to help them crisp up. Switch to Cascadian Farm's and you get the same effect at just more than half the calories.

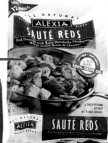

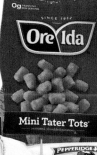

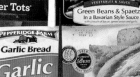

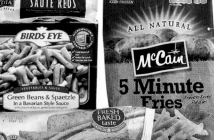

Alexia
Onion Rings
Panko Breaded
(85 g, 6 rings)

240 calories
13 g fat
(2 g fat)
(2 g saturated)
150 mg sodium

Choose your rings
wisely. With a heavy
panko shell and three
types of oil, these
onions contain a third
more calories than
Alexia's other variety.

Ore-Ida
Mini Tater Tots
Seasoned,
Shredded
Potatoes
(87 g)

170 calories
9 g fat
(1.5 g saturated)
420 mg sodium

This is one of
the easiest and most
effective swaps
in the supermarket.

Birds Eye
Green Beans &
Spaetzle in
a Bavarian Style
Sauce
(128 g, 1 cup)

150 calories
7 g fat
(3.5 g saturated)
390 mg sodium

Noodles, bacon,
and butter overshadow
the benefits of
the green beans.

Pepperidge Farm
Garlic Bread
Garlic
(47 g, 2.5" slice)

180 calories
8 g fat
(3 g saturated)
270 mg sodium

Pepperidge Farm
slathers this
nutrient-devoid white
bread with
gratuitous amounts
of soybean oil.

McCain
5 Minute Fries
(85 g)

200 calories
8 g fat
(1 g saturated)
220 mg sodium

Ice Creams
Eat This

Breyers's Original line is impressive not only for keeping the calorie counts reasonable, but also for doing so with a minimal number of ingredients. Make this your go-to ice cream brand.

Breyers Blasts! Waffle Cone with Hershey's Semi-Sweet Chocolate Chips
(½ cup)

140 calories
4.5 g fat
(3.5 g saturated)
16 g sugars

Häagen-Dazs Five Milk Chocolate
(½ cup)

220 calories
12 g fat
(7 g saturated)
20 g sugars

If you must go with a highly indulgent "premium" ice cream, choose one from Häagen-Dazs's Five line.

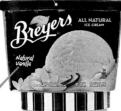

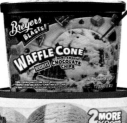
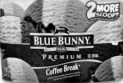
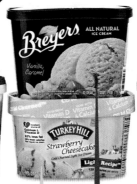
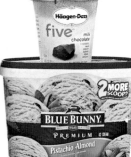

Breyers Natural Vanilla
(½ cup)

130 calories
7 g fat
(4 g saturated)
14 g sugars

Edy's Slow Churned Mint Chocolate Chip
(½ cup)

120 calories
4.5 g fat
(3 g saturated)
13 g sugars

Edy's keeps the calories down by using more fat-free milk than cream.

Blue Bunny Coffee Break
(½ cup)

130 calories
7 g fat
(4.5 g saturated)
15 g sugars

This carton contains an indulgent trio of coffee-infused flavors: vanilla coffee bean, dark espresso, and coffee liqueur.

Light Recipe Turkey Hill Strawberry Cheesecake
(½ cup)

120 calories
3.5 g fat
(2 g saturated)
15 g sugars

Cheesecake chunks and strawberry swirls for 120 calories? Yes!

Breyers Original Vanilla Caramel
(½ cup)

130 calories
6 g fat
(4 g saturated)
15 g sugars

Breyers deploys its caramel swirls in moderation to keep calories in check.

Blue Bunny Pistachio Almond
(½ cup)

150 calories
8 g fat
(4 g saturated)
13 g sugars

The fact that this cream contains real almonds doesn't make it a health food, but it sure doesn't hurt.

Not That!

Graeters Chocolate Chocolate Chip
(½ cup, 114 g)

300 cal
18 fat (10 sat)
30 g sugars

With 30 grams of sugar, Graeters qualifies as one of the sweetest ice creams in the freezer.

Häagen-Dazs Caramel Cone
(½ cup)

320 calories
19 g fat
(10 g saturated,
0.5 g trans)
27 g sugars

One pint has 30 percent more calories than an entire bag of Jet-Puffed Marshmallows.

This one falls firmly in the so-called premium category, where sugar and fat reign supreme.

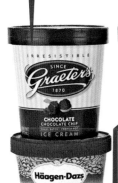

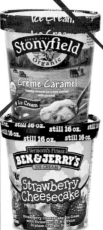

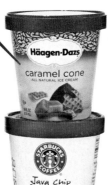

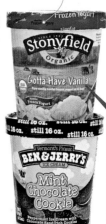

Häagen-Dazs Pistachio
(¾ cup)

290 calories
20 g fat
(11 g saturated,
0.5 g trans)
19 g sugars

The healthy fat from the pistachios is more than canceled out by the saturated and trans fat totals.

Stonyfield Organic Crème Caramel
(½ cup)

260 calories
14 g fat
(9 g saturated)
28 g sugars

Don't be fooled by the pastoral label. This is an invitation for trouble.

Ben & Jerry's Strawberry Cheesecake
(½ cup)

250 calories
15 g fat
(7 g saturated)
22 g sugars

Ben & Jerry may avoid artificial ingredients, but they sure love sugar and fat.

Starbucks Java Chip Frappuccino
(½ cup)

250 calories
15 g fat
(10 g saturated)
22 g sugars

Starbucks' Frappuccinos are dangerous in any form—liquid or solid.

Ben & Jerry's Mint Chocolate Cookie
(½ cup)

260 calories
14 g fat
(8 g saturated)
22 g sugars

You'd have to eat 8 strips of bacon to equal this saturated fat level.

Stonyfield Organic Gotta Have Vanilla
(½ cup)

250 calories
16 g fat
(10 g saturated)
20 g sugars

301

Frozen Yogurts & Sorbets

Eat This

Häagen-Dazs Chocolate Sorbet
(½ cup)

130 calories
0.5 g fat
(0 g saturated)
20 g sugars

Häagen-Dazs's sorbet gets its deep chocolate flavor courtesy of low-fat cocoa powder.

Ciao Bella Sorbet Wild Blueberry
(½ cup)

70 calories
0 g fat
16 g sugars

By virtue of its fruit-first approach, Ciao Bella makes some of the lowest-calorie sorbets out there. This shaves calories off the toll, and the blueberries in this carton contain brain-boosting antioxidants.

It's no surprise that Stonyfield's frozen yogurt is better than its ice cream, but it is a surprise that it's also better than the company's regular nonfrozen yogurt.

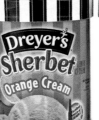

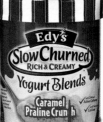

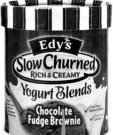

Stonyfield Nonfat Frozen Yogurt Gotta Have Java
(½ cup)

100 calories
0 g fat
18 g sugars

Blue Bunny Frozen Yogurt Bordeaux Cherry Chocolate
(½ cup)

120 calories
3 g fat
(1.5 g saturated)
17 g sugars

Milk and cherries are two of the first three ingredients, which is just as it should be.

Dreyer's Sherbet Orange Cream
(½ cup)

120 cal
2 fat (1 g saturated)
19 g sugars

Sherbet is a perfect middle point between ice cream and sorbet: a touch of fat gives it the creaminess we crave without all the excess calories.

Edy's Slow Churned Yogurt Blends Caramel Praline Crunch
(½ cup)

120 calories
4 g fat
(2 g saturated)
16 g sugars

Edy's yogurts are every bit as upstanding as its ice cream counterparts.

Edy's Slow Churned Yogurt Blends Chocolate Fudge Brownie
(½ cup)

120 calories
3.5 g fat
(1.5 g saturated)
14 g sugars

Impressively low in calories, considering it packs fudge swirls and brownie pieces.

Not That!

Luigi's Real Italian Ice
(1 cup)

100 cal
0 fat
20 g sugars

Fruit juice falls squarely below sugar and corn syrup on the ingredient statement.

Ciao Bella Sorbet Dark Chocolate
(½ cup)

200 calories
10 g fat
(6 g saturated)
19 g sugars

Ciao Bella is the nutritional gold standard of sorbets—with the exception of this fat-packed pint, courtesy of gratuitous amounts of cocoa powder.

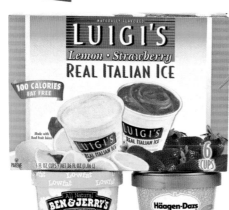

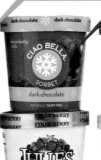

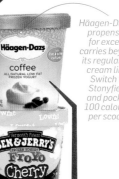

Häagen-Dazs's propensity for excess carries beyond its regular ice cream line. Switch to Stonyfield and pocket 100 calories per scoop.

Ben & Jerry's Fro Yo Frozen Yogurt Chocolate Fudge Brownie
(½ cup)

180 calories
2.5 g fat
(1.5 g saturated)
25 g sugars

Contains more sugar than you'd find in an entire Hershey's Milk Chocolate Bar.

Häagen-Dazs Low-Fat Frozen Yogurt Dulce de Leche
(½ cup)

190 calories
2.5 g fat
(2 g saturated)
25 g sugars

The reduced fat count is a nice start, but we can't recommend this yogurt until the sugar number drops, too.

Julie's Sorbet & Cream Strawberry
(½ cup)

160 calories
6 g fat
(3.5 g saturated)
24 g sugars

Julie's mashup of sorbet and ice cream contains more full-fat cream than some of the regular ice cream cartons on the previous page.

Ben & Jerry's Fro Yo Frozen Yogurt Cherry Garcia
(½ cup)

200 calories
3 g fat
(2 g saturated)
27 g sugars

For all the feel-good mantra extolled by Ben & Jerry's, it still doesn't know how to make a reasonably healthy frozen treat.

Häagen-Dazs Low-Fat Frozen Yogurt Coffee
(½ cup)

200 calories
4.5 g fat
(2.5 g saturated)
20 g sugars

Nondairy Creams
Eat This

Lifeway Frozen Kefir Strawberry
(½ cup)

90 calories
1 g fat
(0 g saturated)
16 g sugars

Kefir contains friendly bacteria that break down lactose, making this a safe option for all but the most severely lactose intolerant.

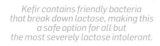

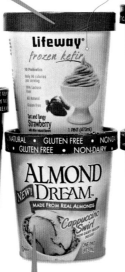

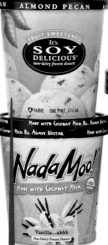

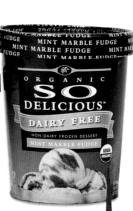

So Delicious Creamy Vanilla

130 cal
3 fat (0 saturated)
13 g sugars

So Delicious makes some of the best nondairy creams in the freezer: low in fat, light on the sugar, easy on the waistline.

Almond Dream Cappuccino Swirl
(½ cup)

140 calories
7 g fat
(0 g saturated)
15 g sugars

Almonds are a primary source of fat in this carton, which means it contains a high concentration of heart-healthy, monounsaturated fatty acids.

It's Soy Delicious Almond Pecan
(½ cup)

139 calories
4.5 g fat
(0.5 g saturated)
12 g sugars

It's Soy Delicious tends to lace its creams with chicory root fiber, which tempers blood sugar spikes by slowing the digestion of sugar. Each scoop here contains 3 grams of fiber.

NadaMoo! Vanilla...ahhh!
(½ cup, 76 g)

130 calories
7 g fat
(6 g saturated)
10 g sugars

Despite the crazy name, this nondairy cream displays a soberminded approach with the sugar, keeping the overall calories down to a respectable level.

So Delicious Dairy Free Mint Marble Fudge
(½ cup)

140 calories
3 g fat
(0.5 g saturated)
17 g sugars

The first ingredient is organic soy milk and the supporting cast includes organic cocoa and organic chocolate sauce. All in all, a solid way to indulge.

Not That!

When a product has a name like Tofutti, you have every right to expect mostly tofu. Alas, the top four ingredients are water, sugar, corn oil, and corn syrup solids.

Tofutti Wild Berry Supreme
(½ cup)

190 calories
9 g fat
(2 g saturated)
19 g sugars

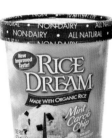
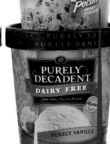
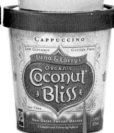
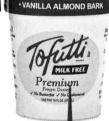

Rice Dream Mint Carob Chip
(½ cup)

180 calories
7 g fat
(1.5 g saturated)
16 g sugars

Not all rice-based desserts like this one are terrible, but they do contain more carbohydrates than some of the other nondairy frozen desserts. This one has 28 grams per scoop.

Purely Decadent Purely Vanilla
(½ cup)

170 calories
5 g fat
(0.5 g saturated)
17 g sugars

The fewer calories you have in your vanilla, the more caloric space you save for toppings.

Soy Dream Butter Pecan
(½ cup)

190 calories
11 g fat
(2 g saturated)
14 g sugars

This carton contains more vegetable oil than pecans.

Luna & Larry's Coconut Bliss Cappuccino
(½ cup)

210 calories
14 g fat
(13 g saturated)
12 g sugars

Fifty-six percent of the calories in this dessert come from saturated fat.

Tofutti Vanilla Almond Bark
(½ cup)

240 calories
15 g fat
(13 g saturated)
16 g sugars

Contains more saturated fat than 5 Taco Bell Fresco Bean Burritos.

Frozen Pies

Eat This

Premade supermarket pies are infamously robust with dangerous fats and inflated sugar levels, but Sara Lee's pumpkin is surprisingly safe. Plus it benefits from pumpkin's beta-carotene, a provitamin that is converted into vitamin A.

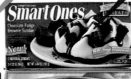

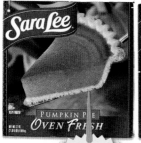

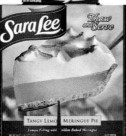

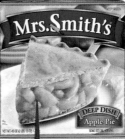

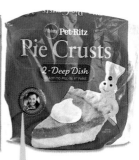

Sara Lee Pumpkin Pie Oven Fresh
(131 g, ⅙ pie)

260 calories
10 g fat
(4 g saturated)
20 g sugars

Sara Lee Tangy Lemon Meringue Pie
(120 g, ⅙ pie)

310 calories
12 g fat
(6 g saturated)
30 g sugars

Keep in mind that you don't have to eat a full slice. It takes only a few bites to satisfy a sweet tooth.

Mrs. Smith's Deep Dish Apple Pie
(128 g, 1/10 pie)

290 calories
13 g fat
(6 g saturated)
18 g sugars

Unlike pizza, deep-dish dessert pie can be a good thing, since you end up with a better ratio of filling to crust.

Pillsbury Pet-Ritz Pie Crusts Deep Dish 9"
(21 g, ⅛ shell)

90 calories
5 g fat (2 g saturated)
1 g sugars

Kudos to Pillsbury for finally removing the trans fats from most of its frozen crusts. The only one still laced with the troublesome lipid is the "all-vegetable" crust.

Not That!

Edwards Singles Hershey's Chocolate Crème Pie
(76 g, 1 piece)

280 calories
17 g fat
(11 g saturated)
21 g sugars

This slice has all the same chocolatey flavors as the Smart Ones sundae. Too bad it takes twice as many calories to achieve the effect.

Edwards Singles Cherry Pie
(120 g, 1 pie)

390 calories
20 g fat
(10 g saturated)
19 g sugars

Edwards' heavy applications of palm and soybean oils in the crust give this pie 50 percent of your day's saturated fat.

The cost for the "PreBaked" convenience is extra fat and sugar—that's not a trade you should be willing to make.

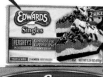

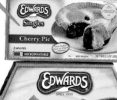

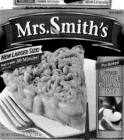

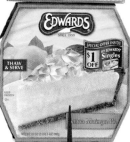

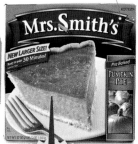

Keebler Ready Crust Graham 10"
(28 g, 1/10 crust)

130 calories
6 g fat
(1.5 g saturated)
7 g sugars

Switch crusts and you eliminate about 40 calories per slice.

Mrs. Smith's PreBaked Dutch Apple Crumb Pie
(131 g, 1/8 pie)

390 calories
18 g fat
(8 g saturated)
19 g sugars

Apparently Mrs. Smith's crumbs are little fat pellets.

Edwards Lemon Meringue Pie
(124 g, 1/8 pie)

350 calories
8 g fat (4 g saturated)
52 g sugars

Yowza! This entire pie has more sugar than 34 servings of Kellogg's Froot Loops.

Mrs. Smith's PreBaked Pumpkin Pie
(131 g, 1/8 pie)

320 calories
12 g fat
(5 g saturated)
27 g sugars

Fruit Bars & Frozen Tr

Eat This

In a box of five flavors, you'll find five different fruit juices. Not bad for silly novelty bars.

Natural Choice Full of Fruit Organic Coconut Fruit Bars
(78 g, 1 bar)
90 calories
3.5 g fat
(3 g saturated)
15 g sugars

The organic coconut contributes a gram of fiber. It's not much, but it helps.

Palapa Azul Fruit Bars Grapefruit
(83 g, 1 bar)
60 calories
0 g fat
(0 g saturated)
12 g sugars

The streets of Mexico are filled with vendors selling fresh fruit paletas. Palapa Azul builds off of that excellent tradition.

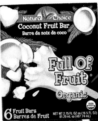
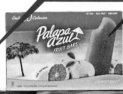
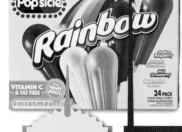

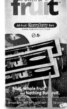
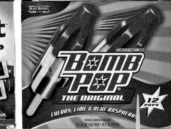
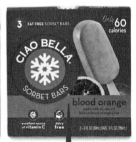

Popsicle Rainbow Ice Pops
(53 g, 1 piece)
45 calories
0 g fat
8 g sugars

Edy's Smoothie Strawberry Banana
(with milk)
190 calories
0 g fat
33 g sugars

Stacked up next to a novelty bar from Good Humor's, this fruit-loaded smoothie looks downright healthy.

Power of Fruit Cherry Berry
(1 tube, 1.7oz)
35 cal
0 g fat
5 g sugars

Made from tart cherries, apples, blueberries, and not a single gram of added sugar.

Blue Bunny Original Bomb Pops
(52 g, 1 bar)
40 calories
0 g fat
8 g sugars

There's nothing nutritionally redeeming about this bar, but on a hot day, it will cool you down without inflicting any serious harm.

Ciao Bella Blood Orange Sorbet Bar
(76 g, 1 bar)
60 calories
0 g fat
11 g sugars

Blood orange juice is the first ingredient after water.

Not That!

Edy's Fruit Bars Tangerine
(85 g, 1 bar)

80 calories
0 g fat
(0 g saturated)
19 g sugars

We like that Edy's uses real tangerine juice, we just wish it used more of it—and less added sugar.

Whole Fruit Coconut Fruit Bars
(78 g, 1 bar)

140 calories
7 g fat
(5 g saturated)
16 g sugars

Coconut is the fattiest denizen of the fruit kingdom. By no means is it unhealthy, but the calories add up very quickly.

Three of the first four ingredients listed are sugar, corn syrup, and cream.

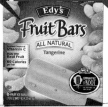

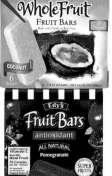

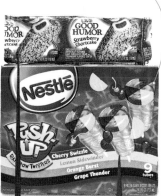

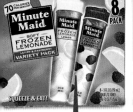

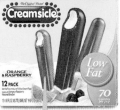

Minute Maid Frozen Lemonade Squeezes
(3 fl oz, 1 tube)

70 calories
0 g fat
(0 g saturated)
14 g sugars

This bar gives sugar a far more prominent role than it gives fruit.

Creamsicle Low-Fat Bars
(43 g, 1 bar)

70 calories
1 g fat
(0 g saturated)
8 g sugars

If you're going to eat a faux-fruit bar, you're best off choosing the one with the fewest calories. This one packs 75 percent more calories than the Bomb Pops.

Edy's Antioxidant Pomegranate
(2.5 oz, 1 bar)

70 calories
0 g fat
16 g sugars

Not a terrible option, but we prefer a bar that is mainly fruit juice, not sugar water.

Good Humor Strawberry Shortcake
(4 fl oz, 1 bar)

230 calories
12 g fat
(5 g saturated)
17 g sugars

True, there are strawberries in this bar, but there are 16 ingredients that feature more prominently—mostly funky additives.

Nestlé Push-Up Rainbow Twisters
(52 g, 1 piece)

70 calories
1 g fat
(0 g saturated)
11 g sugars

Ice Cream Novelties
Eat This

Breyers Smooth & Dreamy Chocolate Caramel Brownie Sandwich
(62 g, 1 sandwich)

160 calories
4 g fat (2 g saturated)
16 g sugars

This is a massive sandwich for only 160 calories. The secret, as with all low-cal ice cream treats, is keeping cream off the top of the ingredients list. Bonus: It packs 3 grams of fiber.

Nestlé Caramel Trio Ice Cream Sandwich
(97 g, 1 sandwich)

160 calories
4 g fat (2 g saturated)
14 g sugars

Classic ice cream sandwiches tend to be among the most reliably safe novelties in the freezer section.

This cookie-laced bar is the lightest offering from Good Humor. If you want an affordable indulgence, look no further.

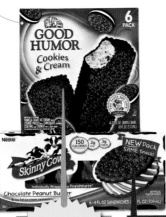

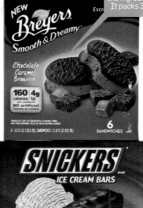

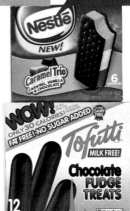

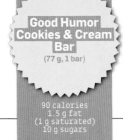

Good Humor Cookies & Cream Bar
(77 g, 1 bar)

90 calories
1.5 g fat
(1 g saturated)
10 g sugars

Skinny Cow Chocolate Peanut Butter Ice Cream Sandwich
(71 g, 1 sandwich)

150 calories
2 g fat (1 g saturated)
15 g sugars

The fat-free milk in this ice cream keeps the calories in check, and the 3 grams of fiber keep your blood sugar stable.

Snickers Ice Cream Bar
(50 g, 1 bar)

180 calories
11 g fat
(6 g saturated)
15 g sugars

Believe it or not, this decadent frozen treat has a full 100 calories fewer than an actual Snickers bar.

Tofutti Chocolate Fudge Treats
(40 g, 1 bar)

30 calories
1.5 g fat
(0 g saturated)
0 g sugars

A reliance on sugar alcohols helps keep the sugar calories out of these bars.

Not That!

Magnum Double Caramel Ice Cream Bar
(90 g, 1 bar)

320 calories
20 g fat
(14 g saturated)
29 g sugars

Not one bar in the Magnum line has fewer than 240 calories.

Klondike Choco Taco
(88 g, 1 taco)

290 calories
15 g fat
(11 g saturated)
25 g sugars

Don't get caught up in the novelty of an ice cream taco. Ultimately, this frozen package still contains more saturated fat than four Taco Bell Chicken Soft Tacos.

It's the same concept (ice cream and cookies in bar form) and the same size as the Good Humor bar, yet the Klondike will saddle you with double the sugar, 10 times the fat, and 160 excess calories.

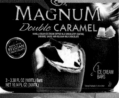

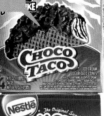

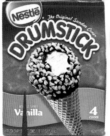

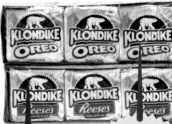

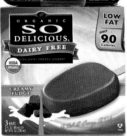

So Delicious Creamy Fudge Bar
(62 g, 1 bar)

90 calories
2 g fat
(0 g saturated)
12 g sugars

This bar contains four different forms of sugar.

Nestlé Drumstick Vanilla Ice Cream Cone

290 calories
16 g fat
(9 g saturated)
20 g sugars

The freezer section has never been better stocked with excellent options for indulging. There's no need to settle for something as crummy as these cones.

Klondike Reese's Bar
(76 g, 1 bar)

260 calories
16 g fat
(11 g saturated)
20 g sugars

Peanut butter contains very little saturated fat. Most of the 11 grams here come from milk fat.

Klondike Oreo Cookies & Cream Bar
(75 g, 1 bar)

250 calories
15 g fat
(11 g saturated)
20 g sugars

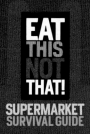

EAT
THIS
NOT
THAT!
**SUPERMARKET
SURVIVAL GUIDE**

DRINK THIS, NOT THAT!

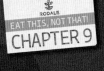

RODALE
EAT THIS, NOT THAT!
CHAPTER 9

Imagine you are a Wizard,

and that with a wave of your hand you can magically change your body, and your health.

You can reduce your risk of diabetes by as much as 26 percent, your risk of overweight or obesity by more than 30 percent, and your calorie intake at any given meal by nearly one-fifth. And imagine you can do it all without having to hunt up some eye of newt, tiger bone, or newborn-dragon blood.

Well, you are that wizard. All you have to do, the next time someone offers you a soda, a sweetened iced tea, or an energy drink, is simply wave it away.

It sounds like fantasy, but it's not—it's science. In a review study published in the journal *Diabetes Care*, people who frequently consumed just one or two sugar-sweetened beverages a day were 26 percent more likely to develop type 2 diabetes than those who drank none. And, according to a 2010 review of studies, drinking a sugar-sweetened beverage instead of water before a meal increases overall calorie intake by an average of 7.8 percent, and by as much as 18.9 percent. That's right: A bottle of sweetened iced tea could add up to 240 calories to your meal, and on top of that, you'd be eating even more calories off your plate than you would without it. No wonder a study showed that people who drink a can of soda a day are 30.4 percent more likely to be overweight or obese and those who drink more than two cans daily are at a 47.2 percent greater risk.

As a population, the United States has a drinking problem that makes Charlie Sheen look like a teetotaler. The average American now drinks as much as 450 calories a day, and about 21 percent of our daily calories now come from sugared drinks. (To put that in perspective, imagine tossing two slices of Domino's sausage pizza into a blender, pressing "puree," and then guzzling it down—once a day, every day of the year.)

Now, let's say you are a wizard, and you wave away 240 calories of soft drinks once a day. Just by switching to an unsweetened beverage, you'd lose a little more than 24 pounds this year—and that's before considering the additional impact of sweetened drinks on your hunger.

Want more magic tricks? You can also:

BURN MORE CALORIES.

In one study, researchers from the University of Utah found that people who drank at least 8 cups of water a day had higher metabolisms and burned calories at higher rates than those who drank just 4 cups. The 8-cup-a-day crew also reported having better concentration and more energy.

LOSE WEIGHT FASTER.

A recent study at Johns Hopkins University found that people who cut liquid calories from their diets lost more weight—and kept it off longer—than people who cut food calories. That's right, watching what you drink is far more effective—and easier—than watching what you eat.

EARN MORE MONEY.

Researchers at Purdue University found that regular soda drinkers had incomes averaging $35,640; people who abstained from soda earned an average of more than $40,000. Maybe that greater energy and better concentration paid off!

LOSE YOUR BEER BELLY.

Fructose can cause your body to build new fat cells around your heart, liver, and digestive organs. In 2010, Robert Lustig, MD, professor of clinical pediatrics at the University of California—San Francisco, reported that fructose has a similar impact on the human body as alcohol does, causing the same kind of liver damage that is found in alcoholics.

LOWER YOUR RISK OF HEART ATTACK.

Visceral fat around your internal organs unleashes compounds within your body that cause inflammation and higher triglyceride and LDL cholesterol levels—the bad stuff that leads to heart disease and stroke.

So, how do you start reaping all these benefits? Remember that almost all sodas, bottled teas, energy drinks, sports drinks, juice drinks, and "vitamin" waters contain sugar. Your goal is to replace these spare-tire-pumping potations with lean liquids. So, what should you be drinking?

WATER. You'll burn more calories and boost overall energy and concentration. Keep a pitcher by your bed and at your desk, and you'll drink up naturally.

COFFEE. But not the sweet, syrupy specialty drinks. Coffee can rev up your metabolism in moderation, but gourmet coffee drinkers consume 206 more calories on average than folks who drink regular joe.

TEA. It not only contains antioxidants that may help protect against heart disease and cancer, but also is nearly calorie free, as long as you don't fall for the sugary kind.

MILK. About 73 percent of the calcium in the American food supply comes from dairy foods, and calcium is critical for fending off weight gain and keeping bones and muscles healthy.

The Anatomy of America's Most Popular Beverages

DISCOVER THE SECRET (AND NOT-SO-SECRET) FORMULAS OF THE DRINKS AMERICANS LOVE MOST

Ever wonder what you're really drinking? The FDA has approved 3,000 food additives, and no doubt more than a few of them are floating around in your favorite beverage. Find out how 10 popular drinks are made, from the healthy and straightforward to the disturbingly scientific.

317

Cola

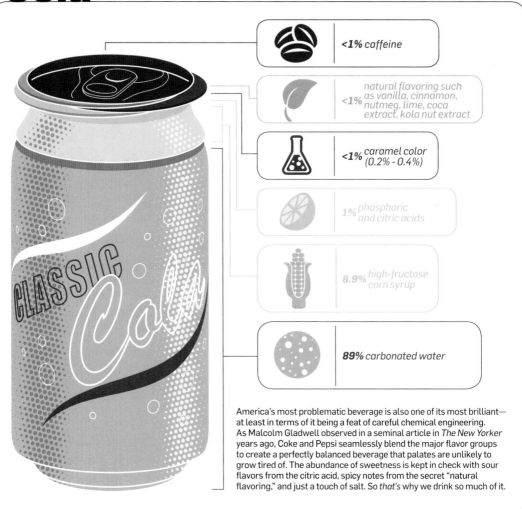

<1% *caffeine*

<1% *natural flavoring such as vanilla, cinnamon, nutmeg, lime, coca extract, kola nut extract*

<1% *caramel color (0.2% - 0.4%)*

1% *phosphoric and citric acids*

8.9% *high-fructose corn syrup*

89% *carbonated water*

America's most problematic beverage is also one of its most brilliant—at least in terms of it being a feat of careful chemical engineering. As Malcolm Gladwell observed in a seminal article in *The New Yorker* years ago, Coke and Pepsi seamlessly blend the major flavor groups to create a perfectly balanced beverage that palates are unlikely to grow tired of. The abundance of sweetness is kept in check with sour flavors from the citric acid, spicy notes from the secret "natural flavoring," and just a touch of salt. So *that's* why we drink so much of it.

Beer

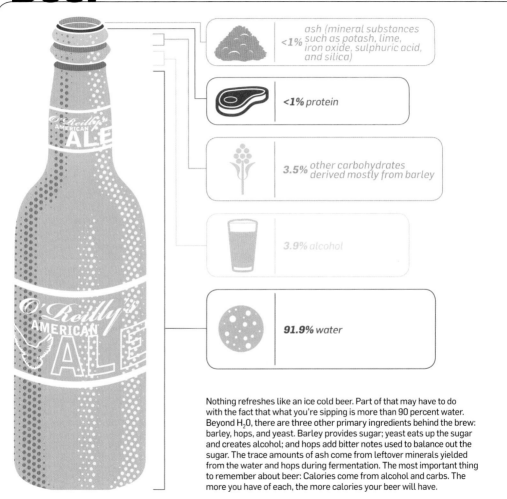

ash (mineral substances such as potash, lime, iron oxide, sulphuric acid, and silica) **<1%**

<1% protein

3.5% other carbohydrates derived mostly from barley

3.9% alcohol

91.9% water

Nothing refreshes like an ice cold beer. Part of that may have to do with the fact that what you're sipping is more than 90 percent water. Beyond H_2O, there are three other primary ingredients behind the brew: barley, hops, and yeast. Barley provides sugar; yeast eats up the sugar and creates alcohol; and hops add bitter notes used to balance out the sugar. The trace amounts of ash come from leftover minerals yielded from the water and hops during fermentation. The most important thing to remember about beer: Calories come from alcohol and carbs. The more you have of each, the more calories your beer will have.

Bottled Coffee Drink

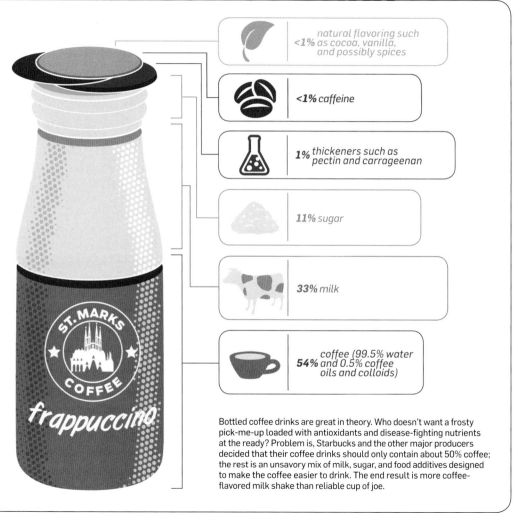

<1% natural flavoring such as cocoa, vanilla, and possibly spices

<1% caffeine

1% thickeners such as pectin and carrageenan

11% sugar

33% milk

54% coffee (99.5% water and 0.5% coffee oils and colloids)

Bottled coffee drinks are great in theory. Who doesn't want a frosty pick-me-up loaded with antioxidants and disease-fighting nutrients at the ready? Problem is, Starbucks and the other major producers decided that their coffee drinks should only contain about 50% coffee; the rest is an unsavory mix of milk, sugar, and food additives designed to make the coffee easier to drink. The end result is more coffee-flavored milk shake than reliable cup of joe.

Cranberry Juice Cocktail

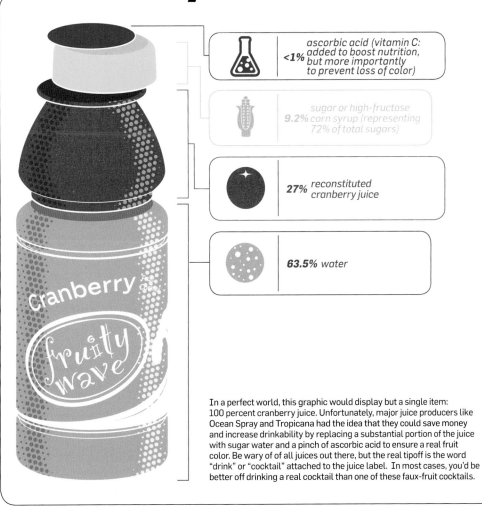

<1% ascorbic acid (vitamin C: added to boost nutrition, but more importantly to prevent loss of color)

9.2% sugar or high-fructose corn syrup (representing 72% of total sugars)

27% reconstituted cranberry juice

63.5% water

Cranberry

fruity wave

In a perfect world, this graphic would display but a single item: 100 percent cranberry juice. Unfortunately, major juice producers like Ocean Spray and Tropicana had the idea that they could save money and increase drinkability by replacing a substantial portion of the juice with sugar water and a pinch of ascorbic acid to ensure a real fruit color. Be wary of of all juices out there, but the real tipoff is the word "drink" or "cocktail" attached to the juice label. In most cases, you'd be better off drinking a real cocktail than one of these faux-fruit cocktails.

Vegetable Juice Blend

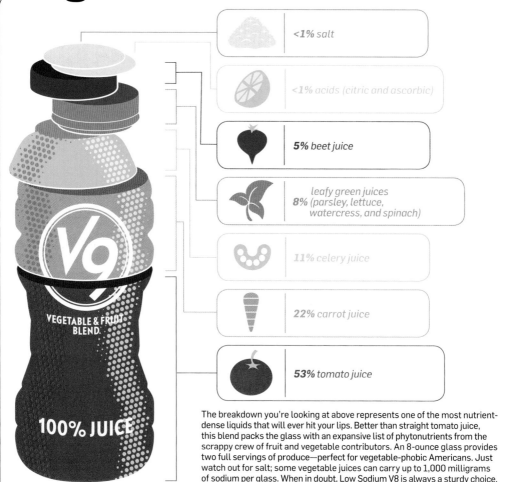

<1% salt

<1% acids (citric and ascorbic)

5% beet juice

8% leafy green juices (parsley, lettuce, watercress, and spinach)

11% celery juice

22% carrot juice

53% tomato juice

The breakdown you're looking at above represents one of the most nutrient-dense liquids that will ever hit your lips. Better than straight tomato juice, this blend packs the glass with an expansive list of phytonutrients from the scrappy crew of fruit and vegetable contributors. An 8-ounce glass provides two full servings of produce—perfect for vegetable-phobic Americans. Just watch out for salt; some vegetable juices can carry up to 1,000 milligrams of sodium per glass. When in doubt, Low Sodium V8 is always a sturdy choice.

Lemonade

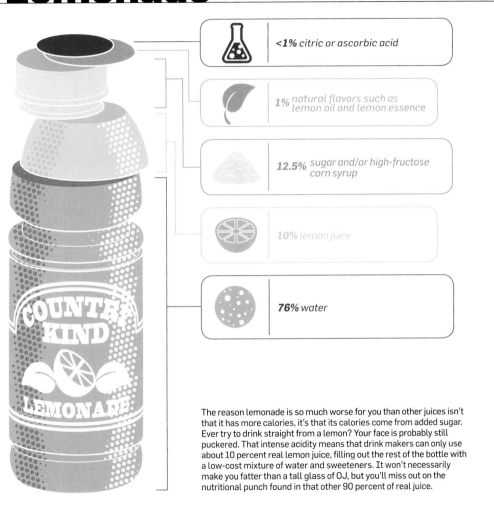

<1% citric or ascorbic acid

1% natural flavors such as lemon oil and lemon essence

12.5% sugar and/or high-fructose corn syrup

10% lemon juice

76% water

The reason lemonade is so much worse for you than other juices isn't that it has more calories, it's that its calories come from added sugar. Ever try to drink straight from a lemon? Your face is probably still puckered. That intense acidity means that drink makers can only use about 10 percent real lemon juice, filling out the rest of the bottle with a low-cost mixture of water and sweeteners. It won't necessarily make you fatter than a tall glass of OJ, but you'll miss out on the nutritional punch found in that other 90 percent of real juice.

Energy Drink

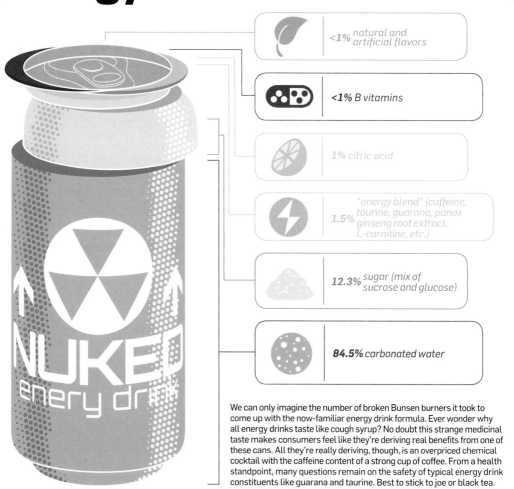

<1% natural and artificial flavors

<1% B vitamins

1% citric acid

1.5% "energy blend" (caffeine, taurine, guarana, panax ginseng root extract, L-carnitine, etc.)

12.3% sugar (mix of sucrose and glucose)

84.5% carbonated water

We can only imagine the number of broken Bunsen burners it took to come up with the now-familiar energy drink formula. Ever wonder why all energy drinks taste like cough syrup? No doubt this strange medicinal taste makes consumers feel like they're deriving real benefits from one of these cans. All they're really deriving, though, is an overpriced chemical cocktail with the caffeine content of a strong cup of coffee. From a health standpoint, many questions remain on the safety of typical energy drink constituents like guarana and taurine. Best to stick to joe or black tea.

Flavored Iced Tea

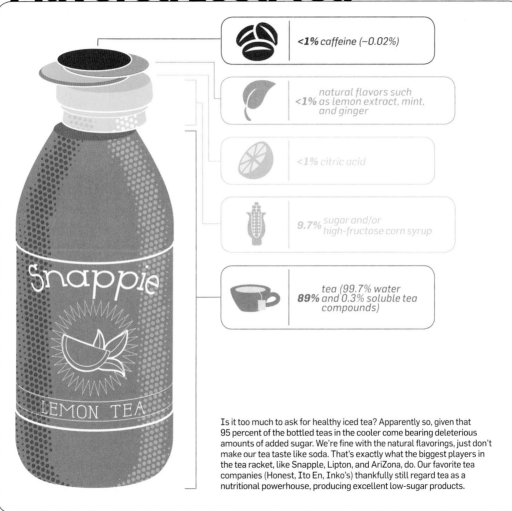

<1% *caffeine (~0.02%)*

<1% *natural flavors such as lemon extract, mint, and ginger*

<1% *citric acid*

9.7% *sugar and/or high-fructose corn syrup*

89% *tea (99.7% water and 0.3% soluble tea compounds)*

Is it too much to ask for healthy iced tea? Apparently so, given that 95 percent of the bottled teas in the cooler come bearing deleterious amounts of added sugar. We're fine with the natural flavorings, just don't make our tea taste like soda. That's exactly what the biggest players in the tea racket, like Snapple, Lipton, and AriZona, do. Our favorite tea companies (Honest, Ito En, Inko's) thankfully still regard tea as a nutritional powerhouse, producing excellent low-sugar products.

Vitamin-Enhanced Water

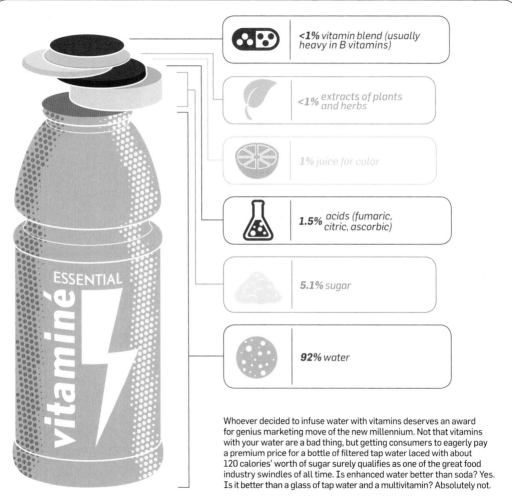

<1% *vitamin blend (usually heavy in B vitamins)*

<1% *extracts of plants and herbs*

1% *juice for color*

1.5% *acids (fumaric, citric, ascorbic)*

5.1% *sugar*

92% *water*

ESSENTIAL

vitaminé

Whoever decided to infuse water with vitamins deserves an award for genius marketing move of the new millennium. Not that vitamins with your water are a bad thing, but getting consumers to eagerly pay a premium price for a bottle of filtered tap water laced with about 120 calories' worth of sugar surely qualifies as one of the great food industry swindles of all time. Is enhanced water better than soda? Yes. Is it better than a glass of tap water and a multivitamin? Absolutely not.

Shelf-stable
Chocolate "Milk" Drink

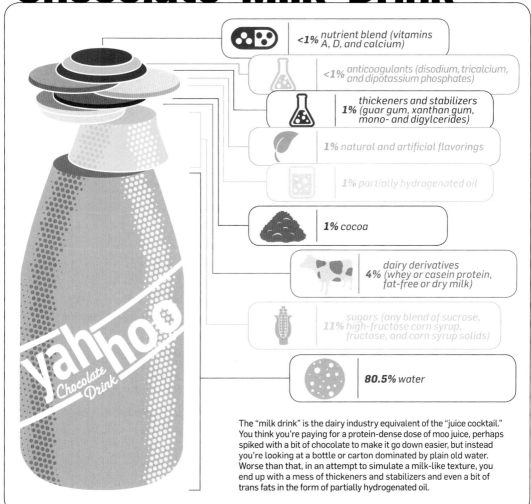

<1% nutrient blend (vitamins A, D, and calcium)

<1% anticoagulants (disodium, tricalcium, and dipotassium phosphates)

1% thickeners and stabilizers (guar gum, xanthan gum, mono- and digylcerides)

1% natural and artificial flavorings

1% partially hydrogenated oil

1% cocoa

4% dairy derivatives (whey or casein protein, fat-free or dry milk)

11% sugars (any blend of sucrose, high-fructose corn syrup, fructose, and corn syrup solids)

80.5% water

The "milk drink" is the dairy industry equivalent of the "juice cocktail." You think you're paying for a protein-dense dose of moo juice, perhaps spiked with a bit of chocolate to make it go down easier, but instead you're looking at a bottle or carton dominated by plain old water. Worse than that, in an attempt to simulate a milk-like texture, you end up with a mess of thickeners and stabilizers and even a bit of trans fats in the form of partially hydrogenated oil.

Juices
Eat This

Tropicana Trop50 Some Pulp
(8 fl oz)

50 calories
0 g fat
10 g sugars

This lightened-up OJ is still 42 percent real juice.

V8 V-Fusion + Tea Pineapple Mango Green Tea
(8 fl oz)

50 calories
0 g fat
10 g sugars

V8's V-Fusion + Tea line uses metabolism-boosting green tea to cut through calorie-dense fruit juices.

Mix equal parts of this and unsweetened iced tea for an Arnold Palmer with a mere 25 calories per cup.

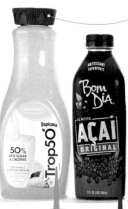
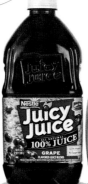
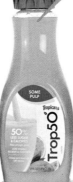
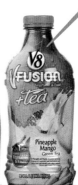
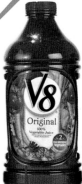
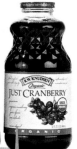

Tropicana Trop50 Lemonade
(8 fl oz)

50 calories
0 g fat
12 g sugars

Bom Dia Açaí Original
(8 fl oz)

100 calories
0 g fat
23 g sugars

Bom Dia's açaí berries are juiced within 12 hours of picking to preserve delicate nutrients.

Juicy Juice 100% Juice Grape
(8 fl oz)

120 calories
0 g fat
28 g sugars

Juicy Juice manages to cut 8 grams of sugar from each cup by adding apple juice to cut through grape's sweetness. That said, this is still pretty sweet, and should be consumed only in moderation.

V8 100% Vegetable Juice
(8 fl oz)

50 calories
0 g fat
420 mg sodium

The best way to slash a produce deficit in your diet. Each 8-ounce glass contains 2 servings of vegetables.

R.W. Knudsen Family Just Cranberry
(8 fl oz)

70 calories
0 g fat
9 g sugars

One ingredient: cranberries. By R.W. Knudsen's estimation, there are 1,150 in every bottle.

Not That!

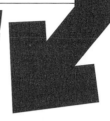

V8 V-Fusion Peach Mango
(8 fl oz)

120 calories
0 g fat
26 g sugars

We commend the fact that V8 sticks to 100 percent juice, but 120 calories for an 8-ounce glass is steep by any measure—especially when there's a great alternative made by the same brand.

SunnyD Tangy Original
(8 fl oz)

120 calories
0 g fat
27 g sugars

Actual juice makes up only 5 percent of this bottle. The rest is mostly high-fructose corn syrup, water, thickeners, and artificial colors.

Lemons are too tart to drink straight, which is why 99 percent of the bottles on the market contain no more than 10 to 20 percent real juice. The rest is just sugar water.

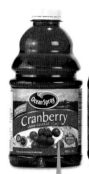
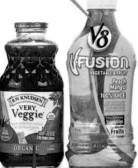
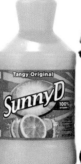
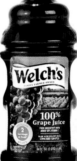
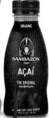
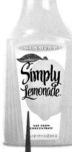

Ocean Spray Cranberry Juice Cocktail
(8 fl oz)

120 calories
0 g fat
30 g sugars

"Juice cocktails" are just excuses for bottlers to stick premium price tags on cheap juices with added sweeteners.

R.W. Knudsen Family Organic Very Veggie
(8 fl oz)

70 calories
0 g fat
630 mg sodium

One cup has as much sodium as four small orders of McDonald's french fries.

Welch's 100% Grape Juice
(8 fl oz)

140 calories
0 g fat
36 g sugars

Grape juice delivers an impressive cache of antioxidants, but it's also one of the most sugar-heavy beverages on the planet. For daily nutrition, there's nothing better than real fruit.

Sambazon Açaí The Original
(8 fl oz)

140 calories
3 g fat
(1 g saturated)
24 g sugars

Switch to Bom Dia and save 40 calories per cup. Do that a couple times a day and you'll drop more than 4 pounds in 6 months.

Simply Lemonade
(8 fl oz)

120 calories
0 g fat
28 g sugars

Single-Serving Juices

Eat This

A strategic splash of coconut water helps Bolthouse Farms keep the calories low and the flavor profile strong.

Honest Kids Super Fruit Punch
(6.75 fl oz)

40 calories
0 g fat
10 g sugars

This organic juice fits in a whole day's worth of vitamin C at a fraction of the others' caloric costs.

Ocean Spray Cran-Energy Cranberry
(12 fl oz)

50 calories
0 g fat
12 g sugars

This lighter version of cranberry juice is packed with energizing B vitamins and green tea extracts.

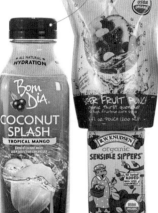

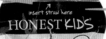

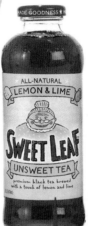

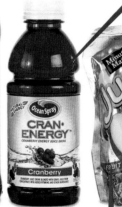

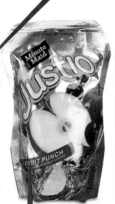

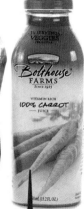

Bom Dia Coconut Splash Tropical Mango
(16 fl oz)

120 calories
0 g fat
28 g sugars

R.W. Knudsen Family Organic Sensible Sippers Apple
(4.23 fl oz)

30 calories
0 g fat
7 g sugars

R.W. Knudsen uses a splash of water to cut through apple juice's naturally concentrated sugar load.

Sweet Leaf Unsweet Tea Lemon & Lime
(16 fl oz)

0 calories
0 fat
0 sugars

Sweet Leaf's citrus–iced tea blend is as refreshing as any calorie-free beverage you'll find.

Minute Maid Just 10 Fruit Punch
(6.75 fl oz)

10 calories
0 g fat
2 g sugars

This pouch limits calories with a blend of natural and artificial sweeteners.

Bolthouse Farms 100% Carrot Juice
(16 fl oz)

140 calories
0 g fat
28 g sugars

Unadulterated carrot juice is surprisingly sweet, and with one bottle, you obtain a full week's worth of vitamin A. If pure carrot doesn't excite you, cut it with a splash of OJ.

Not That!

Ocean Spray Cranberry Juice Cocktail
(12 fl oz)

180 calories
0 g fat
45 g sugars

If this bottle contained 100 percent juice, it would still be an unusually high caloric load. As it stands, most of these calories come from added sugar.

Minute Maid Coolers Fruit Punch
(6.75 fl oz)

100 calories
0 g fat
25 g sugars

A full-size Hershey's chocolate bar contains 24 grams of sugar—1 fewer than this small pouch. Keep that in mind as you scan juice labels.

Nantucket Naturals makes some decent juices, but this just isn't one of them. Eighty percent of the calories in this bottle come from sugar.

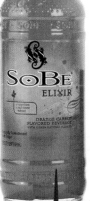

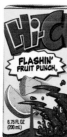

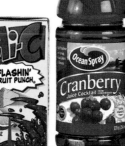

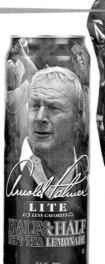

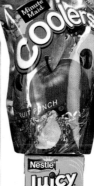

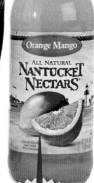

SoBe Elixir Orange Carrot
(20 fl oz)

220 calories
0 g fat
56 g sugars

Both oranges and carrots play minor supporting roles. The real star, as with all of SoBe's Elixirs, is sugar.

Hi-C Flashin' Fruit Punch
(6.75 fl oz)

90 calories
0 g fat
25 g sugars

See the "100% Vitamin C" claim on the package? That's Hi-C's attempt to align this punch with far-healthier 100 percent juices. Don't be fooled. Only 10 percent of this sugar comes from fruit.

AriZona Arnold Palmer Lite Half & Half Iced Tea Lemonade
(11.5 fl oz)

72 calories
0 g fat
19 g sugars

"Lite" it may be, but high-fructose corn syrup is still behind nearly every one of these calories.

Juicy Juice 100% Juice Apple
(4.23 fl oz)

60 calories
0 g fat
14 g sugars

Not a bad little box, but we'll take real fruit juice lightened with a bit of water over this any day.

Nantucket Nectars Orange Mango Juice Cocktail
(16 fl oz)

260 calories
0 g fat
65 g sugars

331

Smoothies & Shakes
Eat This

The 15 grams of protein in this box go a long way toward subduing hunger pangs. Keep one of these in your office fridge and you'll find it far easier to resist the doughnut tray in the break room.

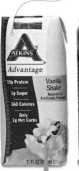

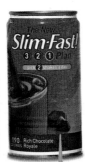

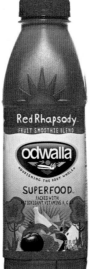

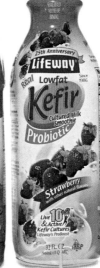

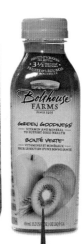

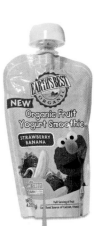

Atkins Advantage Vanilla Shake
(11 fl oz)

160 calories
9 g fat
(3 g saturated)
1 g sugars

Slim-Fast Rich Chocolate Royale Shake
(11 fl oz)

190 calories
5 g fat
(2 g saturated)
13 g sugars

Contains 15 grams of protein, 5 grams of fiber, and a multivitamin's worth of high-quality nutrients.

Odwalla Superfood Red Rhapsody
(12 fl oz)

160 calories
0 g fat
31 g sugars

This smoothie contains rooibos, a tea-like shrub that delivers a blend of antioxidants known to boost the immune system.

Lifeway Lowfat Kefir Strawberry-Banana
(8 fl oz)

140 calories
2 g fat
(1.5 g saturated)
20 g sugars

Kefir, a drinkable yogurt, has been linked to lower cholesterol.

Bolthouse Farms Green Goodness
(15.2 fl oz)

260 calories
0 g fat
51 g sugars

Each bottle contains more than 2 days' worth of immune-strengthening vitamin A.

Earth's Best Organic Fruit Yogurt Smoothie Strawberry Banana
(4.2 fl oz)

90 calories
0.5 g fat
15 g sugars

Packs a substantial load of bananas and strawberries.

Not That!

There are a lot of nutrients packed into this bottle, but that doesn't excuse the fact that water and sugar are the primary ingredients.

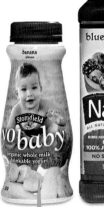

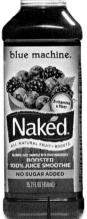

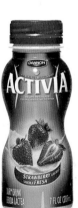

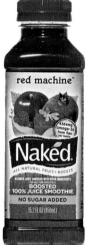

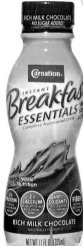

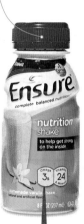

Stonyfield YoBaby Whole Milk Drinkable Banana Yogurt (6 fl oz)

180 calories
7 g fat
(0 g saturated)
22 g sugars

Not enough fruit to scare up even a single gram of fiber.

Naked Juice Blue Machine Smoothie (16 fl oz)

340 calories
0 g fat
58 g sugars

The ingredients list is impressive, but the calories are too high considering that stronger alternatives are readily available.

Dannon Activia Smoothie Strawberry Banana (7 fl oz)

160 calories
3 g fat
(2 g saturated)
25 g sugars

Activia's alleged digestive benefits have been disputed.

Naked Juice Red Machine Smoothie (16 fl oz)

340 calories
9 g fat
(1 g saturated)
50 g sugars

The first ingredient is apple juice. Look for smoothies made primarily with fruit purees instead.

Carnation Breakfast Essentials Rich Milk Chocolate Drink (11 fl oz)

260 calories
5 g fat
(1.5 g saturated)
39 g sugars

Packs more sugar than 2 scoops of ice cream.

Ensure Nutrition Shake Vanilla (8 fl oz)

250 calories
6 g fat
(1 g saturated)
23 g sugars

Teas & Fortified Drinks
Eat This

Honest Tea strikes the balance just right with this subtly sweetened tea, allowing the natural flavor of metabolism-elevating green tea to take the lead.

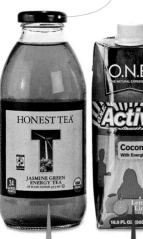

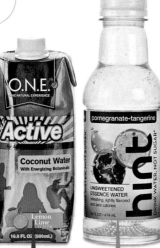

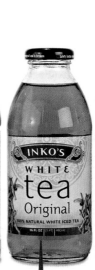

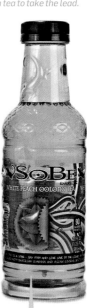

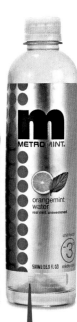

Honest Tea Jasmine Green Energy Tea
(16 fl oz)

34 calories
0 g fat
10 g sugars

O.N.E. Active Coconut Water Lemon Lime
(16 fl oz)

40 calories
0 g fat
8 g sugars

Coconut water is a natural source of electrolytes without a sports drink's sugar.

Hint Unsweetened Essence Water Pomegranate-Tangerine
(16 fl oz)

0 calories
0 g fat
0 g sugars

Purified water with natural flavorings and no funky stuff.

Inko's White Tea Original
(16 fl oz)

56 calories
0 g fat
14 g sugars

White tea contains high levels of catechins, polyphenols with a well-documented ability to reduce the risk of cancer.

SoBe Energize White Peach Oolong Tea
(20 fl oz)

90 calories
0 g fat
22 g sugars

Oolong boasts all the same health benefits as green tea.

Metromint Orangemint Water
(16.9 fl oz)

0 calories
0 g fat
0 g sugars

The mint in this bottle has been shown to improve digestion and help relieve stress.

Not That!

High-fructose corn syrup is the second ingredient, which makes this bottle more similar to soda than to tea.

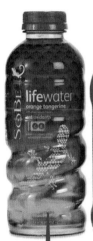
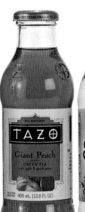
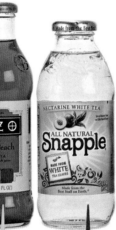
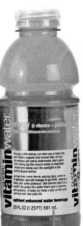
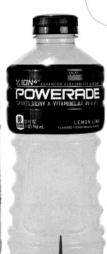
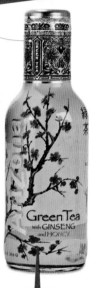

SoBe Lifewater Orange Tangerine (20 fl oz)
100 calories
0 g fat
24 g sugars
Drink 100 extra calories every day for a year and you'll pack on more than 10 pounds of flab.

Tazo Giant Peach Green Tea (16 fl oz)
180 calories
0 g fat
40 g sugars
Don't even think about it—this bottle contains more sugar than a small chocolate Frosty from Wendy's.

Snapple All Natural Nectarine White Tea (16 fl oz)
120 calories
0 g fat
30 g sugars
Contains as much sugar as three small nectarines—but with none of the fiber.

Glacéau Vitaminwater Energy Tropical Citrus (20 fl oz)
125 calories
0 g fat
32.5 g sugars
Know what's better than sugar-saturated water? Plain H₂O.

Powerade Lemon Lime (16 fl oz)
100 calories
0 g fat
25 g sugars
Powerade's electrolyte package comes polluted with more sugar than you'd find in three Krispy Kreme Original Glazed doughnuts.

AriZona Green Tea with Ginseng & Honey (16 fl oz)
140 calories
0 g fat
34 g sugars

Coffee & Energy Drinks
Eat This

Illy's drinks are made in the authentic Italian style: strong, bold, and without a torrent of sugar to bury the flavor.

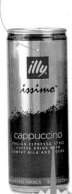
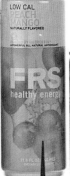
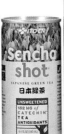
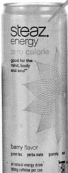
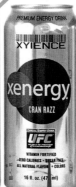
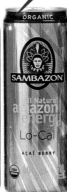
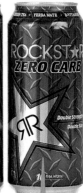

Illy Issimo Cappuccino
(8.45 fl oz)

100 calories
1.5 g fat
(1 g saturated)
18 g sugars

FRS Healthy Energy Low Cal Peach Mango
(12 fl oz)

20 calories
0 g fat
2 g sugars

A rare low-calorie energy drink, FRS also contains an antioxidant called quercetin, which may help alleviate allergies.

Ito En Sencha Shot
(6.4 fl oz)

0 calories
0 g fat
0 g sugars

One of our favorite sources of fuel. The blend of caffeine and green tea–derived antioxidants will keep you energized both short and long term.

Xenergy Xtreme Cran Razz Fuel
(16 fl oz)

0 calories
0 g fat
0 g sugars

Xenergy's drinks deliver an impressive load of B vitamins without the glut of sugar typically found in its competitors' cans.

Rockstar Zero Carb
(16 fl oz)

20 calories
0 g fat
0 g sugars

Rockstar's normal cans are among the worst energy drinks in the cooler, but this one is laced with yerba maté and green tea, two natural metabolism boosters that also provide plenty of energy.

Not That!

Rockstar Punched Energy + Punch
(16 fl oz)

260 calories
0 g fat
62 g sugars

Contains 13 percent of your day's energy, and virtually every calorie comes from sugar.

Inko's White Tea Energy
(16 fl oz)

160 calories
0 g fat
38 g sugars

Inko's tea line is commendable, but the energy drinks stray too far into cola territory.

Starbucks' bottled drinks are among the worst caffeinated beverages in the supermarket. Not even the chain's in-house espresso drinks are typically this bad.

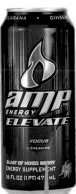
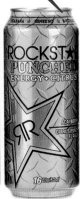
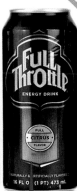
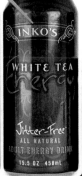
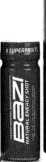
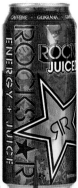
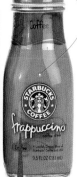

AMP Energy Elevate
(16 fl oz)

220 calories
0 g fat
58 g sugars

The sugar in this can provides short-lived energy followed by a steady decline to sluggishness. Stick to low-sugar beverages if you want your energy to last.

Full Throttle Citrus
(16 fl oz)

220 calories
0 g fat
58 g sugars

Most of the "throttle" comes from added sweetener. In fact, the sugar-to-caffeine ratio in this can is 295 to 1.

Bazi Natural Energy Shot
(2 fl oz)

64 calories
0 g fat
16 g sugars

This shot contains 2 teaspoons of sugar in every ounce.

Rockstar Juiced Mango Orange Passion Fruit
(16 fl oz)

280 calories
0 g fat
70 g sugars

This drink has more sugar than an entire box of Rice Krispies Treats.

Starbucks Frappuccino Coffee Drink Coffee
(9.5 fl oz)

200 calories
3 g fat
(2 g saturated)
32 g sugars

337

Flavored Milks & Milk
Eat This

Almonds are a calorie-dense food, but almond milk is anything but. In fact, it's the lightest nondairy alternative on the market.

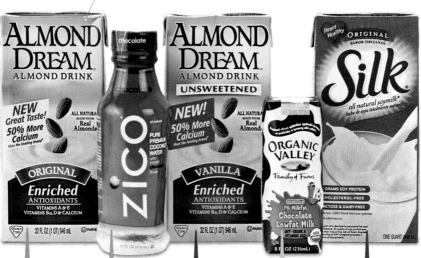

Almond Dream Almond Drink Original
(8 fl oz)

50 calories
2.5 g fat
(0 g saturated)
5 g sugars

Zico Coconut Water Chocolate
(14 fl oz)

110 calories
2 g fat
(0 g saturated)
18 g sugars

What coconut milk lacks in protein and calcium, it makes up for in magnesium and potassium.

Almond Dream Almond Drink Unsweetened Vanilla
(8 fl oz)

50 calories
3.5 g fat
(0 g saturated)
<1 g sugars

Fewer calories and sugar, more healthy fat.

Organic Valley 1% Milkfat Chocolate Lowfat Milk
(8 fl oz)

150 calories
2.5 g fat
(1.5 g saturated)
22 g sugars

Organic milk boasts higher amounts of healthy fat.

Silk Organic Original
(8 fl oz)

100 calories
4 g fat
(0.5 g saturated)
6 g sugars

One challenge vegetarians face is obtaining adequate amounts of B$_{12}$. Fortunately, Silk is fortified with plenty of it.

Horizon Lowfat Strawberry Milk Box
(8 fl oz)

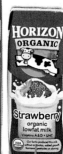

150 calories
2.5 g fat
(1.5 g saturated)
23 g sugars

Contains no artificial colors and a quarter of your day's calcium and vitamin D.

Substitutes

Not That!

Rice milk is one of the worst nondairy alternatives. Even when it's made with brown rice like Rice Dream's is, it contains zero fiber and a heavy load of quick-digesting starches.

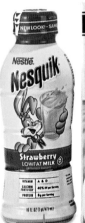
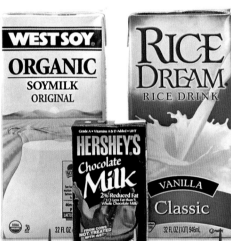
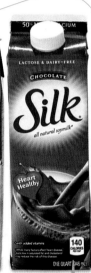
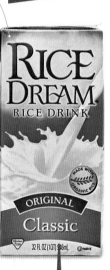

Nesquik Low Fat Milk Strawberry
(8 oz)

180 calories
2.5 g fat
(1.5 g saturated)
30 g sugars

Both of the dyes in this milk—Red 40 and Blue 1—have been linked to behavioral disorders.

WestSoy Organic Soymilk Original
(8 fl oz)

130 calories
3.5 g fat
(0.5 g saturated)
12 g sugars

WestSoy manages to pack in double the sugar of other leading brands.

Hershey's 2% Milk Chocolate
(8 oz)

200 calories
5 g fat
(3 g saturated)
29 g sugars

One box of this milk contains as much sugar as an entire Snickers bar.

Rice Dream Enriched Rice Drink Vanilla
(8 fl oz)

130 calories
2.5 g fat
(0 g saturated)
12 g sugars

Whether in liquid or solid form, almonds trump rice every time.

Silk Soymilk Chocolate
(8 fl oz)

150 calories
3 g fat
(0.5 g saturated)
21 g sugars

Don't make the mistake of thinking that soy milk is an infallible health food. This one is dangerously close to a milk shake.

Rice Dream Enriched Rice Drink Original
(8 fl oz)

120 calories
2.5 g fat
(0 g saturated)
10 g sugars

Beers

Eat This

Yuengling makes a complex American lager,
yet it keeps both calories and carbs within reasonable parameters.
It's a good beer to have if you're having more than one.

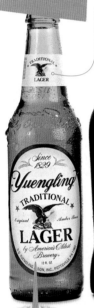

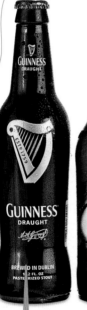

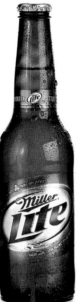

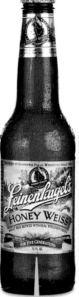

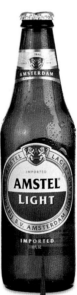

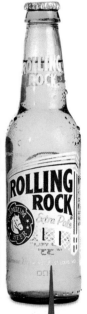

Yuengling Traditional Lager
(12 fl oz)

135 calories
12 g carbs
4.4% ABV

Guinness Draught
(12 fl oz)

125 calories
10 g carbs
4.2% ABV

This is the darkest beer you can find with fewer than 130 calories.

Miller Lite
(12 fl oz)

96 calories
3.2 g carbs
4.2% ABV

With only 96 calories, Miller Lite emerges as the light-beer champion of the classic domestics.

Leinenkugel's Honey Weiss
(12 fl oz)

149 calories
12 g carbs
4.8% ABV

One of the sweet beers with a reasonable calorie count.

Amstel Light
(12 fl oz)

95 calories
5 g carbs
3.5% ABV

This import is on par with the top low-calorie domestics like Michelob Ultra and Miller Lite, but it packs a richer and more robust flavor.

Rolling Rock Extra Pale
(12 fl oz)

132 calories
10 g carbs
4.5% ABV

Delivers a stronger flavor profile than the typical light beer in fewer calories than the typical heavy beer.

Not That!

Sam's most popular brew is one of the heaviest lagers you'll find. Shave 56 calories a bottle by switching to Sam Adams Light.

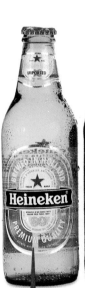

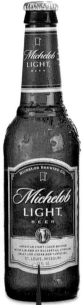

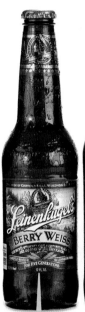

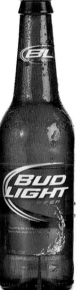

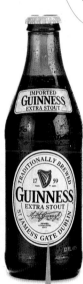

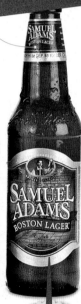

Heineken
(12 fl oz)

166 calories
9.8 g carbs
5.5% ABV

For this many calories, we expect a bit more flavor out of our beer.

Michelob Light
(12 fl oz)

123 calories
8.8 g carbs
4.3% ABV

Careful: In reality, Michelob's light beer is Michelob Ultra. This brew is as caloric as some of the full-flavor beers in the cooler.

Leinenkugel's Berry Weiss
(12 fl oz)

207 calories
28 g carbs
4.8% ABV

The name Berry Weiss implies a lighter ale, but this brew stands up to the heaviest of suds.

Bud Light
(12 fl oz)

110 calories
6.6 g carbs
4.2% ABV

The handful of extra calories in Bud Light will add up over the course of a long weekend.

Guinness Extra Stout
(12 fl oz)

153 calories
18 g carbs
4.3% ABV

Remember: Draught is for drinking, Extra Stout is for extra pounds.

Samuel Adams Boston Lager
(12 fl oz)

175 calories
18 g carbs
4.9% ABV

Mixers
Eat This

Schweppes Club Soda
(8 fl oz)

0 calories
0 g fat
0 g sugars

Club soda gives your cocktail sparkle and fizz without the waistline-expanding sugars.

Canada Dry Raspberry Sparkling Seltzer
(8 fl oz)

0 calories
0 g fat
0 g sugars

This fizzy mixer lends the perfect hint of raspberry without the added sugars.

V8's version not only contains less salt, but also provides 2 servings of vegetables per drink.

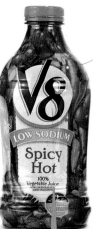
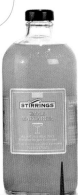
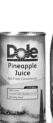
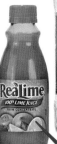
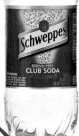
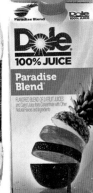
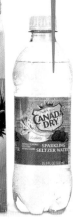

V8 Spicy Hot Low Sodium
(8 fl oz)

50 calories
0 g fat
140 mg sodium

Stirrings Simple Margarita Mix
(4 fl oz)

93 calories
0 g fat
24 g sugars

Lime juice is listed before sugar on the ingredients list. That's always a good sign.

Dole Pineapple Juice
(4 fl oz)

60 calories
0 g fat
0 g sugars

It's not marketed as a mixer, but it's got the right flavor and comes with a fraction of the calories.

ReaLime
(2 Tbsp)

0 calories
0 g fat
0 g sugars

Make a perfect low-cal margarita by combining this with a touch of agave syrup, a splash of triple sec, and a shot of tequila.

Dole Paradise Blend
(4 fl oz)

60 calories
0 g fat
12 g sugars

This blend is 100 percent juice—the gold standard for fruit-based cocktails.

Not That!

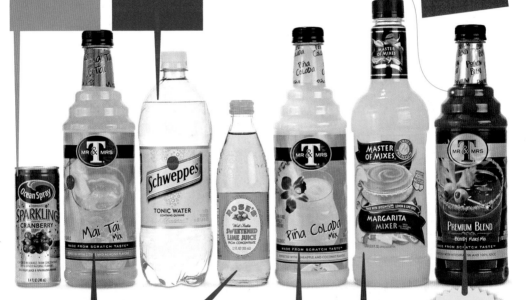

Ocean Spray Sparkling Cranberry
(8.4 fl oz)

90 calories
0 g fat
22 g sugars

Try mixing real cranberry juice with seltzer to cut the high sugar levels.

Schweppes Tonic Water
(8 fl oz)

90 calories
0 g fat
22 g sugars

Tonic's nutritional profile puts it nearer to soda than water.

One cup of this mix knocks out 92 percent of the recommended daily sodium limit for most people.

Mr. & Mrs. T Mai Tai
(4 fl oz)

140 calories
0 g fat
32 g sugars

An authentic Mai Tai gets its flavor from citrus liqueur and lime juice, but today's mixes are largely corn syrup and dyes.

Rose's Sweetened Lime Juice
(2 Tbsp)

60 calories
0 g fat
12 g sugars

This "lime juice" contains more high-fructose corn syrup than it does juice.

Mr. & Mrs. T Piña Colada Mix
(4 fl oz)

180 calories
0 g fat
42 g sugars

Prepared mixes are the fastest way to ratchet up your cocktail calorie counts.

Master of Mixes Margarita Mixer
(4 fl oz)

130 calories
0 g fat
30 g sugars

The primary flavoring agent is high-fructose corn syrup, and the fluorescent hue is the result of two artificial colors.

Mr. & Mrs. T Premium Blend Bloody Mary Mix
(8 fl oz)

80 calories
0 g fat
1,380 mg sodium

343

Index